PROCEDURES AND
TECHNIQUES IN
Emergency
Medicine

PROCEDURES AND TECHNIQUES IN
Emergency Medicine

Robert R. Simon, M.D.

Assistant Professor of Medicine
Division of Emergency Medicine
Assistant Director, Residency Training Program
Emergency Medicine Center
UCLA Center for the Health Sciences

Barry E. Brenner, M.D., Ph.D.

Assistant Professor of Medicine
Division of Emergency Medicine
Assistant Director, Emergency Medicine Center
Emergency Medicine Center
UCLA Center for the Health Sciences

Artwork by Leonard Morgan and Susan Gilbert

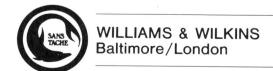

WILLIAMS & WILKINS
Baltimore/London

Copyright ©, 1982
Williams & Wilkins
428 East Preston Street
Baltimore, MD 21202, U.S.A.

Made in the United States of America

Library of Congress Cataloging in Publication Data

Simon, Robert Rutha.
    Procedures and techniques in emergency medicine.

    Includes index.
    1. Emergency medicine. I. Brenner, Barry E. II. Title. [DNLM: 1. Emer-
gencies.   2. Emergency   medicine—Methods.   WB   105   S596p]   RC86.7.S54
616'.025   81-19674   ISBN 0-683-07715-5   AACR2

Composed and printed at the
Waverly Press, Inc.
Mt. Royal and Guilford Aves.
Baltimore, MD 21202, U.S.A.

DEDICATIONS

Robert R. Simon, M.D., dedicates this book to an illiterate Lebanese villager who has contributed more than any other in both my personal development and the progression of my work, my mother.

Barry E. Brenner, M.D., Ph.D., dedicates this book to the patients in emergency medicine, the only justification for academic excellence; to my wife, Diane; and to my daughter, Rachel.

Preface

A number of manuals and texts relating to procedures and techniques have been published, especially in the past 5 years. All of these have a "cookbook" approach and subjectively relate the individual author's personal experience in performing a particular procedure. None are fully referenced complete works which review the literature and add objectivity to this vital area. Thus, the method for performing a procedure varies between authors and institutions. Currently, no academic and complete work exists on procedures and techniques performed in the emergency and outpatient setting. The purpose of this text is to fill this gap, to minimize personal opinion and subjectivity from this vital arena of medical practice and to supply the reader with an objective, researched work on procedures. The authors have reviewed the literature thoroughly, have compiled the data relating to each procedure, and have described this in as complete a form as possible.

In the majority of the text the format used to discuss a particular procedure is as follows: First the indications and contraindications for performing the procedure are listed. Following this the equipment necessary to perform the procedure is described. The steps necessary for performing the procedure are divided into three parts; the preparatory steps, followed by the procedural steps, and finally the aftercare. It is hoped that this format will enable a more organized approach to performing procedures in emergency centers. Finally, the complications of a procedure are listed. In the section on complications a detailed discussion usually follows, listing the measures which can be taken to prevent a complication and in some cases discussing how to deal with a complication once it occurs. Throughout the discussion, one will see *Caution!*, *Axiom,* and *Note.* Cautions are areas in which complications commonly occur, and these are placed in specific locations in the steps of performing a procedure in the hope that it will alert the reader and prevent the complication from occurring. The caution informs the reader how to avoid the complication. An Axiom is a major statement and should be regarded as a law in the performing of a procedure. Notes are detailed discussions which are of importance or of interest to the reader and are placed in various locations throughout the discussion of the procedures in the text.

Some chapters do not lend themselves readily to this type of format. The chapters on Plastic Surgery and Orthopedics are examples of chapters in which the format listed above is not used.

While the text is aimed at the emergency physician it is hoped that all physicians who deliver primary care including the clinical medical student, house officer, general surgeon, family practitioner, general internist, and critical care specialist will find it useful. It is the authors' hope that the text will add depth and understanding to each of the procedures and techniques which are discussed.

Acknowledgments

The authors would like to thank Karen Einstein for her excellent work in typing, editing, and preparing the manuscript.

We would like to express our deep appreciation to Leonard Morgan and Susan Gilbert for the fine diagrams which are featured in the text.

The authors would like to thank the publishers and authors who have permitted us to use diagrams which appear in the text.

We are deeply indebted to Doctors Constance Arnold and John Olsen for their detailed and critical review of the plastics chapter, Thomas Mudge for his review of the abdominal chapter, Fred Edelman for his comments and critique of the neurosurgical chapter, Mike Policar for his detailed and careful review of the obstetrical chapter, and George Boris for his review of the ENT chapter.

The authors would like to thank the UCLA Emergency Medicine Residents for their aid in reviewing and critiquing various sections of the text.

Contents

Abdominal Procedures

1

NASOGASTRIC INTUBATION

Nasogastric intubation is one of the most common procedures performed in the emergency center. Ideally, the patient should be in a semi-upright position. In the traumatized patient, however, this position may not be possible. The unconscious patient should have an endotracheal tube inserted before nasogastric intubation to decrease the chance of aspiration and prevent gastric dilatation secondary to ileus (19). A number of techniques have been described to aid in inserting the nasogastric tube where difficulties are encountered in its passage. These will be discussed in a separate section below.

Indications

There are numerous indications for nasogastric intubation, some of which are:
1. Emptying of gastric contents (overdose, poisoning)
2. In patients with an ileus or mechanical obstruction
3. To prevent gastric dilatation and aspiration in patients suffering from major trauma

Equipment

Nasogastric tube
K-Y jelly

Technique of Insertion

Preparatory Steps
1. Select the appropriate tube size: in the adult a 16 French nasogastric tube usually can be inserted. In children, a 12 French is the size usually selected.
2. Examine the nose and select the wider nares. Often patients have a deviation of the septum, making passage of the tube difficult on the narrower side.
3. Lubricate the tube well.

Procedural Steps
1. The nasogastric tube should be inserted along the floor of the nose directed posteriorly.

CAUTION!

The tube should not be pointed superiorly when it is inserted; otherwise it may impinge on the turbinates causing hemorrhage.

In patients with severe facial and skull trauma, passage superiorly may lead to entrance of the tube intracranially (20, 23, 24, 50, 59, 60).

NOTE

The cribriform plate is easily fractured and the dura in this area is quite thin and easily perforated by the nasogastric tube. Patients who have suffered significant facial and skull trauma may have nasal, orbital floor, zygomatic, maxillary, or palatal fractures. In addition, these patients may have suffered fractures of the cervical spine, frontal ethmoid, sphenoid sinuses, cribriform areas, or base of the skull. These fractures may be present with or without evidence of cerebrospinal fluid rhinorrhea (20, 23, 24, 50, 59, 60).

2. Pass the tube past the soft palate into the posterior pharynx. One can feel a "give" or decreased resistance once the tube has passed into the posterior pharynx in most patients. Most patients initially will feel like "gagging" once the tube is passed beyond this point.
3. The conscious patient who is not traumatized should be instructed to hold a sip of water in the mouth and to swallow while the tube is being passed down the esophagus.

CAUTION!

If the patient begins to cough during this passage, withdraw the tube back into the posterior pharynx and repeat the procedure as this indicates the tube has passed into the trachea.

NOTE

Passage of the nasogastric tube may be impeded by anterior and posterior choanal deviation, esophageal narrowing, or narrowing of the esophagus secondary to an inflated endotracheal tube (35). Inadequate relaxation of the cricopharyngeus muscle, a striated muscle of the upper pharynx, also has been implicated as a cause of difficult passage of the tube (35).

4. Aspirate the gastric contents to confirm proper placement of the tube within the stomach. Alternately, one may inject 20 to 30 ml of air, auscultating with a stethoscope over the left upper quadrant of the abdomen to ascertain proper placement.

NOTE

An alternate method to ensure proper positioning has been described by Fry (21). He injects 4 ml of water and 5 ml of air together down the tube while auscultating in the left upper quadrant. If the nasogastric tube is lying freely within the stomach, sounds can be heard on injection as well as aspiration. However, if the tube is lying within the cardiac sphincter or is kinked within the stomach, sounds will be heard only on injection. Water and air should be used together since either alone may enter and leave the stomach silently according to Fry. This test can be used to confirm both position and patency of the tube should gastric suctioning suddenly produce no aspirate.

Techniques to facilitate passage of a nasogastric tube

A. Chilling of the tube in either cold tap water or ice cubes has been advised to make the tube stiffer and easier to pass (12, 39, 54, 58). This is especially helpful when the problem is curling of the tube within the mouth.
B. The placement of two fingers into the mouth to hold the tube against the posterior pharyngeal wall while advancing the tube is another technique used to prevent or detect coiling in the oral cavity (12, 54, 58).

C. The nasogastric tube may be passed through an endotracheal tube previously positioned within the esophagus (12, 41, 54, 58). A technique introduced by Ogawa (41) is quite useful in the difficult patient. An endotracheal tube is lubricated and inserted orally into the esophagus (Fig. 1.1). The connector on the endotracheal tube is removed. A standard nasogastric tube is lubricated and inserted into the endotracheal tube (Fig. 1.1). Since the nasogastric tube follows the inside of the tracheal tube, no resistance is met and it can be easily inserted into the stomach. When resistance is encountered distal to the endotracheal tube, the tracheal tube should be passed further so that the nasogastric tube may be properly positioned. Passage of the nasogastric tube into the stomach should be ascertained either by the injection of air and auscultating over the epigastrium or the aspiration of gastric contents (Fig. 1.2). The endotracheal tube is then withdrawn and the gastric tube is left in position (Fig. 1.3). Following this, a small catheter with an outside diameter of approximately 3 to 5 mm or a suction tube is inserted nasally and the tip is pulled out through the oral cavity and is subsequently inserted into the

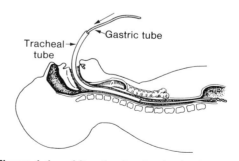

Figure 1.1. After the tracheal tube has been inserted perorally into the esophagus, the gastric tube is then inserted through the tracheal tube and into the stomach. (Reprinted with permission of Surgery, Gynecology Obstetrics, Ogawa, H., A reliable technique for insertion of a gastric tube during operation. 132:498, 1971.)

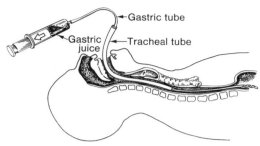

Figure 1.2. Verification that the inserted gastric tube is in the stomach is obtained by aspirating gastric juice through the nasogastric tube. (Reprinted with permission of Surgery, Gynecology Obstetrics, 132:498, 1971.)

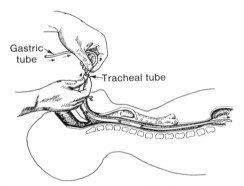

Figure 1.3. Remove the tracheal tube as shown. See text for details. (Reprinted with permission of Surgery, Gynecology Obstetrics, 132:498, 1971.)

gastric tube. This attachment is secured with a silk suture (Fig. 1.4). The catheter then is pulled out through the nostril, and the gastric tube is withdrawn from the oral cavity into the nose in a retrograde fashion.

NOTE

There are three sites where a nasogastric tube encounters narrowing in the esophagus and resistance in passage. The first is located behind the cricoid cartilage of the larynx, the second is located behind the bifurcation of the bronchus where it crosses the aorta, and the third is at the lower end of the esophagus where it passes into the stomach. The distance of these narrowed areas from the incisors of the

upper jaw in the average adult is 15, 25 and 40 cm, respectively (41). In most patients, difficulty in gastric tube insertion occurs when the tube becomes coiled in the oral cavity and fails to advance into the esophagus or when the tip is caught at the pharynx or larynx and does not advance further.

D. An alternate method has been described (39) for patients in whom the difficulty is at the narrowing in the esophagus posterior to the cricoid. In this situation the alae or wings of the thyroid cartilage should be grasped between the thumb and index fingers and lifted anteriorly. Normally in the supine patient the esophagus is collapsed due to gravity, and this maneuver opens the esophagus, and the tube passes readily into the stomach. Remember that vigorous palpation of the cricoid cartilage and adjacent structures may cause bradycardia reflexly, and this should be avoided (39).

E. In patients in whom there is a disorder of the esophageal motility or partial esophageal obstruction secondary to stricture, a technique has been described by Maher for passage of a nasogastric tube with the use of a bougie (38). The tube to be passed is fed either through the nares or perorally into the pharynx. A 20 to 25 French Maloney bougie (the bougie is a very firm catheter which, due to its stiffness, does not coil within the

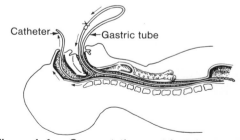

Figure 1.4. Connect the gastric tube to the catheter, which is inserted nasally, and pull the gastric tube in a retrograde fashion through the nose. (Reprinted with permission of Surgery, Gynecology Obstetrics, 132:498, 1971.)

esophagus) then is fed orally into the hypopharynx using the fingers as a guide, and the nasogastric tube is fed simultaneously into the esophagus. The bougie acts to keep the tube from curling in the esophagus. Occasionally this is not successful due to the extreme flexibility of the tube. This is especially true with the Sengstaken-Blakemore tube, which is extremely flexible (discussed in another section). In this situation, pass an O chromic catgut suture through the most distal portion of the nasogastric tube, being careful not to perforate any balloons. Form a loop with the suture material. The bougie then is placed through the loop and passed perorally into the stomach (Fig. 1.5). When the bougie is withdrawn, the loop releases the bougie without difficulty. When using this

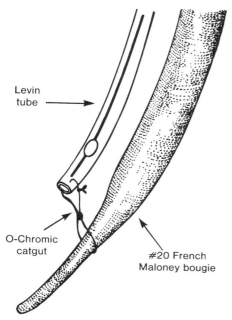

Levin tube

O-Chromic catgut

#20 French Maloney bougie

Figure 1.5. A chromic suture may be passed through the Levine tube and looped around the Maloney bougie as shown and discussed in the text. (Reprinted with permission of American Journal of Surgery, Maher, J., An aid in the passage of gastrointestinal tubes. 135:866, 1978.)

method it is best to do the procedure under fluoroscopic control.
F. In small children, passage of a tube may be quite difficult. A technique described by Robinson and Cox (47) has been used successfully. A 7 or 8 French pediatric feeding tube is used in conjunction with a straight, stainless steel spring guide which is 145 cm long and 0.6 mm in diameter. The pediatric feeding tube is first irrigated with normal saline which serves as a lubricant between the plastic and steel surfaces. The spring guidewire then is inserted into the feeding tube, and the flexible tip of the guidewire is advanced to within 1 cm of the tip of the catheter. The catheter then is introduced through the nose into the posterior pharynx, where the tip of the catheter can be manipulated into the esophagus and gently threaded into the stomach. When the tube is properly positioned as indicated by gastric aspiration or the injection of air accompanied by auscultation over the epigastrium, the spring guidewire is removed. In situations in which one is uncertain of proper placement, a radiograph may be obtained with the guidewire in place since the wire is radiopaque.

Aftercare

1. The tube should be secured with tape to the nose by placing one loop of tape around the tube and attaching the two distal ends of tape superiorly on the face or nose.

NOTE

A new method of stabilizing nasogastric tubes has been advocated to minimize the problem of decubitus ulcerations in the mucosa of the nose and pharynx in patients requiring prolonged nasogastric intubation (49). A heavy thread is tied around the tube and is held to the skin of the nose and forehead with adhesive tape. The free part of the thread must be 3 or 4 cm long to allow for short inward and outward movements of the tube during swallowing. In this way, pressure exerted on the tissues by the tube is alleviated periodically during swallowing, and erosions of the nasal mucosa are unlikely to occur.

Complications

1. Ulceration of the mucosa. The nasogastric tube can cause ulcerations at the site of the mucosa where the tube is positioned. This complication occurs with the double lumen (Salem sump) tube, contrary to what is commonly believed (22).
2. Sinusitis. Sinusitis has been described in patients following nasogastric intubation for prolonged periods (11, 16, 27, 59, 60).
3. Esophageal stricture (11, 26, 27, 59, 60).
4. Laryngeal obstruction (11, 26, 27, 59, 60).
5. Otitis media (11, 26, 27, 59, 60).
6. Rupture of esophageal varices (11, 26, 27, 59, 60). A nasogastric tube may induce pressure necrosis of the esophageal variceal wall, resulting in significant bleeding. It is unclear how long one may leave a nasogastric tube in place in the presence of esophageal varices.
7. Rupture of the esophagus or stomach (11, 26, 27, 59, 60).
8. Inability to remove the tube. The tube may coil or knot within the esophagus or stomach distal to a stricture, resulting in inability to remove the tube. When this occurs and is secondary to a stricture, dilatation may be necessary to facilitate removal of the tube.
9. Tracheoesophageal fistula. A nasogastric tube passed along with a rigid cuffed endotracheal tube has induced tracheoesophageal fistulas (52).
10. Nasogastric tube pushed hard during insertion has caused perforation of the esophagus and penetration into the pleural cavity and has actually drained a pleural effusion (30). This complication was contributed to by an enlarged heart which deviated the esophagus to the left (30).
11. Insertion of the nasogastric tube into the submucosa of the posterior pharynx (35).
12. Passage of the nasogastric tube intracranially. In normal patients as well as in patients with maxillofacial trauma, the nasogastric tubes have been placed intracranially, usually with fatal consequences. This complication has been described by numerous authors (20, 23, 24, 50, 59, 60). To prevent this complication, nasogastric intubation should be performed with a well-lubricated tube and should be done gently. In patients with maxillofacial trauma, it should be done only under direct visualization with the aid of a Magill forceps or passed orally (20, 23, 35, 59). The tube should be directed posteriorly and *not superiorly* (30, 35, 60). The initial aspiration through the tube followed by insufflation of air with concurrent auscultation over the epigastrium is recommended to ascertain proper positioning. Some authors suggest that a chest radiograph be obtained in all patients after nasogastric or orogastric intubation (30). When intracranial insertion does occur, the patient should be taken to the operating room where the nasogastric tube can be removed under direct vision allowing the neurosurgeon to deal immediately with the complications, particularly bleeding. The patient should be started on high doses of broad-spectrum antibiotics once this complication is recognized (23).
13. Nasal hemorrhage. In patients who are taking anticoagulants or who have coagulopathies, tumors, or infections of the nares, the tube should be passed through the oral route (35). In patients with a gastrointestinal bleed which is secondary to a coagulopathy, especially cirrhotics, cocaine should be instilled in the nostril before insertion of the nasogastric tube. This will shrink the nasal membrane and facilitate passage with less bleeding, which may be significant in such patients. In pa-

tients with a history of esophageal varices or coagulopathies, the tube should be inserted by spontaneous passage during swallowing rather than be forced down.

GASTRIC LAVAGE FOR HEMORRHAGE INTO THE UPPER GASTROINTESTINAL TRACT

Several types of double lumen tubes have been discussed in the literature (33, 37, 53). Each of these tubes, however, has a number of problems, including increased overall outside diameter causing discomfort and small outflow lumens on the sides of the tubes which limits the passage of larger blood clots. In contrast, a system devised by Atkenson (4) seems to be optimal in these patients. This system minimizes the discomfort to the patient and allows rapid evacuation of the large clots, because of its substantially larger outflow lumen size.

Technique

Two single lumen tubes are passed nasally. One is a size 18 French which functions as an inflow tube and is connected to an iced saline lavage solution. In Atkenson's method, an enema bucket functioned for this purpose (Fig. 1.6). Another nasogastric tube which is a 24 French functions as an outflow tube. This tube should have 3 side holes cut out and is inserted through the other nostril and is connected to an emptying bag with dependent drainage at the patient's bedside. A Toomey syringe is connected to the outflow tube through a wide connecter for aspiration should the outflow tube stop draining (Fig. 1.6). Irrigation begins when the inflow of iced saline solution occurs and breaks up the blood clots, enabling rapid movement of the clots out of the outflow tube. A grossly bloody and clot-laden return occurs through the outflow tube which rapidly clears as bleeding is brought under control. When this clearing occurs, the inflow tube is switched off and siphoning begins. In this phase, residual saline solution draining from the stomach may mix with hemorrhaging blood and the outflow changes from pink to red. This rate of color change

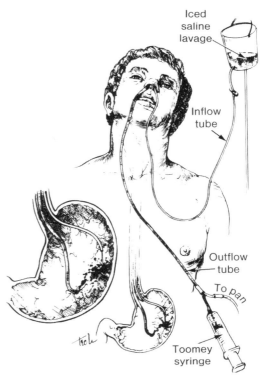

Figure 1.6. Flow of the iced saline solution occurs from the enema bucket, or iced saline lavage bag, through the inflow tube into the stomach. There, irrigation rates of up to 1 liter/minute break apart blood clots and prevent the collapse of the stomach around the outflow tube. See inset. The Toomey syringe is provided for the occasional clot which does not pass into and out of the outflow tube. (Reprinted with permission of Surgery, Gynecology Obstetrics, Atkenson, R. J., Nyhus, L. M., Gastric lavage for hemorrhage in the upper part of the gastrointestinal tract. 146:797, 1978.)

is proportional to the rate of bleeding. If the outflow tube becomes red, the irrigation is started once again. This system requires much less nursing care than does the single tube irrigation system that is commonly used. In the routine system, injections of 15 ml boluses and the frequently futile attempts to retrieve the injected fluid are avoided. In the system devised by Atkenson, nearly all the fluid is retrieved in the collecting system. Thus, overdistention of the stomach which may increase bleeding is avoided.

NOTE

The effectiveness of Atkenson's water sump irrigator is based on irrigation and simultaneous gravity drainage. Irrigation rates of up to 1 liter/minute can occur, breaking up clots and allowing gastric emptying. Outflow of clots and saline solution occurs at comparable rates. These rates never can be achieved by simple syringe irrigation or other techniques involving a single lumen tube. With this technique there is continuous irrigation of the stomach, avoiding the interruption of outflow by irrigating fluids and the conventional methods. With this system there is no need for wall suction as the technique relies on the siphon principle and avoids adherence of the gastric mucosa to the portals of the nasogastric tube which is a common problem when wall suction is used obstructing outflow.

It has been found that during lavage of the gastric contents, gentle palpation over the left upper quadrant to "massage" the stomach will achieve better mixing of the gastric contents with the lavage fluid and removal of these contents. This is particularly helpful when using lavage for gastric emptying in an overdose patient (38b).

SENGSTAKEN-BLAKEMORE BALLOON TAMPONADE

The Sengstaken-Blakemore tube is a triple lumen tube which is used to control massive bleeding from esophageal varices. The three lumens are conduits for a gastric balloon, an esophageal balloon, and an accessory tube, essentially a simple nasogastric tube for drainage of gastric fluid. Since the introduction of this method for control of esophageal variceal bleeding, many articles have reported on the high incidence of complications, including death (14, 19). The complication rates reported range as high as 35 to 38% of cases, with death being reported in 22 and 18%, respectively (14). These complications are directly related to the tube itself. Other authors have reported a complication rate of 9.2% and have advocated the use of the balloon for control of variceal hemorrhage.

One concludes that its use should be palliative and only for brief periods pending definitive surgical intervention (14) when possible, although few are acceptable candidates for surgery.

By far the most common method of inserting the tube is through the nose, similar to that used for insertion of a nasogastric tube. The size of the tube and the attached balloons makes this difficult, even for those experienced in its use. Interestingly, those authors who use the nasal route also have the highest reported complication rates and fatalities (14, 19). The method advocated below is that of Pitcher (13, 46), whereby he reports the highest incidence of successful control of bleeding as well as the lowest incidence of complications by using the oral route.

Indication

Due to the high complication rate, the procedure should be reserved for those patients with proven unequivocal bleeding from esophageal varices in whom massive bleeding continues despite conservative therapy and/or in whom surgical intervention is impossible (14). Many physicians reserve use of the Sengstaken-Blakemore tube to patients with esophageal varices hemorrhage who have been unresponsive to intravenous vasopression.

Equipment

20 French Sengstaken-Blakemore tubes (Davol, Inc., Providence, RI)
18 French plastic nasogastric tube and syringe
2 rubber-shod heavy surgical clamps
High intermittent suction (Gomco) iced saline for irrigation—4 x ⅛ inch keyhole plywood retainer
1 inch adhesive tape
Mouthpiece
Manometer

Technique

Preparatory Steps

1. Check the balloons for leaks.
2. Lubricate the tube well with viscous xylocaine.
3. Anesthetize the pharynx with 10% cocaine solution in a spray.

4. Empty the stomach of blood clots and/or food before insertion of the tube (13, 46).

NOTE

Nasogastric intubation is optimally performed after emergency endoscopy to verify if bleeding is from esophageal varices. In this situation the stomach is usually empty. If delay occurs between intubation and endoscopy and bleeding is brisk, lavage should be performed before intubation (46).

Procedural Steps

1. Place the patient in the left lateral decubitus position (46).
2. Insert the lubricated 20 French Sengstaken-Blakemore tube (Davol, Inc.) through the mouth until the gastric balloon is well within the stomach, usually by the 50 cm mark. When the stomach has been reached, blood can be aspirated. Instill 20 ml of air and auscult over the left upper quadrant to confirm that the tube is properly positioned (Fig. 1.7).
3. After the gastric tube is flushed with air, the gastric balloon is slowly inflated with 250 to 275 ml of air while the clinician simultaneously ausculs over the epigastrium to insure inflation of the gastric balloon and positioning of the gastric tube within the stomach and not the esophagus (46). One can usually auscult the air being instilled into the balloon over the epigastrium.
4. Once the gastric balloon is inflated, it is double clamped with a rubber-shod heavy surgical clamp; firm traction is applied manually at the mouth and the gastric lumen inlet is connected to high-intermittent suction (Gomco).
5. The stomach is lavaged with copious amounts of iced saline until the return is clear. If bleeding continues, the esophageal balloon is inflated.
6. The esophageal balloon is inflated to a pressure of 25 to 45 mm mercury

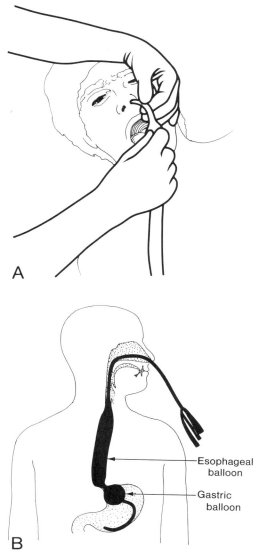

Esophageal balloon

Gastric balloon

Figure 1.7. *A.* The placement of a Sengstaken-Blakemore tube is shown. In passing the tube, the empty balloon should be folded around itself and the patient given appropriate analgesia. *B.* The gastric and esophageal balloons are shown inflated in proper position. See text for details.

(this can be ascertained using a simple manometer), using the lowest pressure which appears to control variceal bleeding as determined by gastric lumen and accessory tube lavage (46). Double-clamp the esophageal lumen with a rubber-shod heavy surgical clamp, at the balloon pressure which stops the bleeding.

7. While maintaining firm traction on the Sengstaken-Blakemore tube, a padded 4 × ⅓" keyholed plywood retainer is positioned around the tube at the angle of the mouth and is held in place by strips of adhesive tape fixed to the retainer and tube. This maintains the traction on the gastric varices. Alternately, a catcher's mask or football helmet may be used to secure the Sengstaken-Blakemore tube. The tube may easily be bitten through by an uncooperative, agitated patient (34). A rubber mouthpiece should be inserted and taped into position with the retainer.

8. Suction on the accessory tube should be switched to low-intermittent (Gomco).

9. After the esophageal balloon is inflated, a small nasogastric tube should be inserted through the nose to check for bleeding proximal to the esophageal balloon and to remove secretions. The nasogastric tube usually extends from the top of the Sengstaken-Blakemore esophageal balloon to the mid-hypopharynx (46).

10. Continue inflation for 24 to 48 hours. The head of the bed can be kept up to prevent hiccups and aspiration of vomitus.

NOTE

Using this technique, up to 92% of patients with variceal bleeding can be safely controlled (46). Overdistention of the gastric balloon can be avoided by checking balloon pressure every 2 hours. If air is continually needed to maintain pressure, then suspect complications with the balloon. One can check the balloon size with an anterior-posterior x-ray of the abdomen and add air only when there is a decrease in the balloon size by radiograph (40). Air is usually used for inflation of the balloon even though some authors have used wa-

ter. Water makes the tube heavy and increases the risk of pressure necrosis of the mucosa (34).

Complications

1. Difficulty in insertion.
2. Unintentional deflation or rupture of one or both balloons.
3. Inability to maintain constant traction on the gastric or esophageal balloon due to improperly securing the catheter to the helmet or wood.
4. Failure of the gastric balloon to deflate. When this occurs, the tube may have to be cut to deflate the balloon.
5. Persistent hiccups.
6. Cardiac arrhythmias.
7. Pulmonary edema may occur due to pressure of the inflated esophageal and gastric balloons on mediastinal structures.
8. Regurgitation and aspiration of gastric contents during insertion and when the tube is in place. This can be prevented partially by placement of the nasogastric tube as indicated above.
9. Dislodgement or herniation of the esophageal balloon causing airway obstruction (7, 14, 46). One must always keep a scissors at the bedside of a patient with a Sengstaken-Blakemore tube. If the esophageal balloon obstructs the airway, it can be immediately deflated by cutting the air inlet of the balloon.
10. Pressure necrosis at several levels along the tube: alae nasi (this is with nasal insertion of the tube), pharynx, esophagus, and stomach.
11. Damage to the esophagus, including laceration or rupture (7, 61).

ABDOMINAL STAB WOUNDS— SINOGRAM

Abdominal stab wound sinograms, once commonly used to detect peritoneal penetration in stab wounds of the abdomen, are not commonly performed today. Stab wounds of the abdomen are treated by close observation and peritoneal lavage when indicated to ascertain significant intraperitoneal injury. In one large study involving 172 patients with stab wounds of the abdomen, 65 underwent sinography and 62% demonstrated penetration of the peritoneal cavity (3). Of those patients with penetration, 30% had no visceral injury and another 10% had only a minor intraperitoneal injury which did not require laparotomy. The authors concluded that the cost/benefit ratio for sinograph was not worthwhile and indicated that if doubt existed as to significant intraperitoneal pathology the patient should be followed with close observation without a sinogram (3, 57). Most centers today advise elective observation of abdominal stab wounds with or without penetration of the abdominal cavity and do not use sinography (25).

One situation in which abdominal stab wound sinograms may be helpful is in the patient with an abdominal stab wound of the epigastrium in which one would like to ascertain whether the pericardium has been penetrated (9, 25, 29).

Technique

The technique advocated here is the introduction of a 16 French catheter threaded in through the wound as far as possible. A continuous locked silk suture is placed around the catheter to make the wound watertight. Sixty to 100 ml of 50% sodium diatrizoate (Hypaque) mixed with 1 ml of ethylene blue should be injected into the stab wound. This is done with enough pressure to force the solution into the abdominal cavity (and pericardium) if a penetration exists. Following this, anterior, posterior, and lateral x-rays are taken. An abdominal radiograph should be obtained 10 minutes after the initial radiograph to determine if a nephroureterogram effect occurs. If this effect is noted, then the dye has reached the peritoneum and has been rapidly absorbed and excreted by the kidneys (10). This indicates peritoneal penetration of the puncture. An alternate technique has been described with the use of a Foley catheter; however, inflation of a Foley catheter balloon placed in

the stab wound is difficult, and this technique is not recommended here.

ABDOMINAL STAB WOUND EXPLORATION

Abdominal stab wound exploration has been advocated by a number of authors (6, 55). Abdominal stab wound exploration combined with peritoneal lavage increases the diagnostic accuracy of peritoneal lavage. The incidence of negative laparotomies following peritoneal lavage when combined with local exploration to determine peritoneal penetration was 4% in one study involving 135 patients (55). Currently, a number of centers advocate observation in patients with abdominal stab wound with or without penetration. In view of this, one may wonder why exploration of a stab wound to the abdomen is necessary at all. If the stab wound is explored and penetration into the abdominal cavity is *definitely* ruled out, then the patient may be discharged from the emergency center with no further studies or observation necessary. When the stab wound penetrates the abdominal cavity, the patient must be admitted to the hospital for observation and should have peritoneal lavage. In a number of cases, local exploration does not permit differentiation between penetration and nonpenetration of the abdominal cavity; in this situation, the patient must be observed for signs of abdominal injury and should undergo peritoneal lavage.

Technique

The technique of abdominal stab wound exploration is simple. Using a #10 blade the stab wound is extended for 1 to 2 cm on each end (Fig. 1.8). The stab wound is carefully dissected through the fascia and the abdominal musculature and followed to the abdominal fascia. If the fascia has been entered, then penetration into the abdominal cavity is diagnosed and the wound margins should be closed. To make exploration easier, an angiocath can be inserted into the stab wound before exploration and a solution of methylene blue injected through the catheter. This may

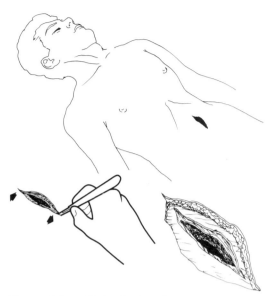

Figure 1.8. Abdominal stab wound exploration. See text for details.

aid in visualizing the tract of the stab wound and is preferred by the authors. The stab wound then is closed primarily. In patients with grazing gunshot wounds to the abdomen in which peritoneal penetration is in question, wound exploration should be used in a similar fashion to ascertain penetration.

PERITONEAL LAVAGE

To detect hemoperitoneum, peritoneal lavage is one of the most common procedures performed in the emergency center on the traumatized patient. Three techniques have been described in the literature, each of which has advantages and disadvantages and all three will be described and discussed here: insertion of the catheter through a midline incision, percutaneous insertion of a catheter, and insertion of the catheter through an infraumbilical incision. The accuracy of peritoneal lavage in detecting hemoperitoneum and the presence of significant abdominal injury has been reported variably by different authors. Some authors (2) have reported an accuracy rate of 97%, indicating significant intraabdominal injury, while others have reported a false positive rate of 30% (51).

The problem which arises is in deciding how much blood indicates a positive lavage. Olsen divided the patients with peritoneal lavage into three groups (5). In Group I, a strongly positive lavage indicating greater than 25 ml of blood/liter of fluid was found to be associated with a 90% incidence of significant intraabdominal injury at laparotomy. In Group 2, a negative lavage with no blood and no positive findings was associated with a very low incidence of significant intraabdominal injury. In Group 3, lavage fluid which was weakly positive (8 drops to 15 ml of blood/liter) was associated with an incidence of significant intraabdominal injury of 32%. In interpreting the peritoneal lavage aspirate, one should place the intravenous tubing containing the returned lavage fluid over newspaper. If the newspaper cannot be read through the tubing, this indicates a positive peritoneal lavage and correlates with a blood count of approximately 100,000 erythrocytes/ml of fluid. In addition, some authors report that the presence of greater than 500 leukocytes/ml of lavage fluid or the presence of greater than 100 Somogyi units of amylase also is indicative of significant intraabdominal injury (45, 56). The significance of the WBC count has been questioned by some. In one study, only 1 of 18 patients with greater than 500 WBCs in the lavage fluid had significant intraabdominal injury (45).

Indications

A number of authors have verified the unreliability of physical examination in patients with blunt abdominal trauma in detecting significant intraabdominal injury. In one study, 40% of the patients who were felt to have surgically significant intraabdominal injury based on the initial physical examination were found to have no significant intraabdominal injury on laparotomy (44). In this same study there was a 6% incidence of false negative examinations felt to be due to the lack of release of intestinal contents into the peritoneal cavity and only blood was present. Many patients with only blood in the peritoneal cavity have no findings on physical examination. It has been recommended that those patients who have a questionable peritoneal lavage should undergo abdominal ultrasound and arteriography (44). Any patient with significant abdominal injury who has abdominal pain, tenderness, rigidity or abdominal distention should have peritoneal lavage (45). In a large series of over 400 patients in which peritoneal lavage was performed in patients without evidence of abdominal injury but who had sustained significant trauma elsewhere, the following findings were reported: in patients with head injury with unconsciousness, 26% of the patients had positive peritoneal lavage (45); in those with unexplained hypotension, 42% had a positive lavage; in patients who had multiple-system injuries, 13% had a positive lavage (45). In this study, it was found that pelvic fractures and a falling hematocrit were not valid indications for peritoneal lavage (45). In children who sustained blunt abdominal injuries, physical examination has been documented to be very inexact. The indications for lavage in children are any evidence of abdominal signs or symptoms, altered sensorium, unexplained shock, major thoracic injuries, multiple-system injury, and major orthopedic injuries (such as a fractured pelvis, femur, or hip) (17).

Physical examination does not allow prompt and reliable assessment of intraabdominal injury from blunt trauma and was misleading in 45% of patients in one study (42). The role of peritoneal lavage for penetrating wounds of the abdomen has received little emphasis until recently, reflecting the former policy of exploring all patients with penetrating abdominal wounds (36). The incidence of organ injury in patients at Cook County Hospital having sustained peritoneal penetration by a missile was 98.6% (36). At Detroit General Hospital, peritoneal lavage is performed in patients having sustained gunshot wounds of the abdomen in whom peritoneal penetration is questionable and in patients with hemothorax from stab or gunshot wounds to the lower thorax, especially the left side. In a recent study at Detroit General Hospital involving 135 patients with stab wounds to the lower chest and abdo-

men, it was concluded that chest wounds located between the two anterior axillary lines and below the fifth rib and all abdominal wounds are indications for peritoneal lavage even when an abdominal examination is negative (55). With abdominal wounds, if the physical examination was negative and the stab wound was located between the two anterior axillary lines, local exploration of the stab wound was performed and was followed by peritoneal lavage if the exploration indicated peritoneal penetration. If the exploration revealed no penetration to the peritoneal cavity, the patient was observed. If the lavage was positive in those with penetration, the patient underwent surgery. In this study, 70% of patients were spared an unnecessary operation (55). The incidence of negative laparotomy was reduced to 4.0%, and it was concluded that the combination of local exploration and peritoneal lavage increased the diagnostic accuracy and decreased the incidence of negative laparotomies in patients with abdominal stab wounds (55). Remember that a negative physical examination is associated with a 23% incidence of positive laparotomy in abdominal stab wounds (6). A negative lavage can occur with significant abdominal injuries which do not produce hemoperitoneum, including retroperitoneal injuries to the pancreas, great vessels, duodenum, rectosigmoid and subcapsular injuries to the liver and spleen; even transsection may not produce sufficient hemoperitoneum to cause a positive lavage (42).

Peritoneal lavage also has been used to diagnose acute pancreatitis in patients with a normal amylase since an elevated amylase will persist within the peritoneal fluid for 3 to 5 days following pancreatitis (42). Primary peritonitis also may be diagnosed by finding pneumococci or staphylococci. Intestinal flora and debris found on a Gram stain of the sediment of the lavage may signify perforation of the gastrointestinal tract (42).

Contraindications

The following are contraindications to the use of peritoneal lavage:

1. Multiple previous abdominal operations (32).

NOTE

In the patient who has a midline scar in the infraumbilical region, a midline incision can be made above the umbilicus to introduce the catheter for a lavage. Alternately, an incision can be made lateral to the rectus abdominus muscles, and the catheter can be introduced into the peritoneal cavity under direct vision to avoid adhesions. The supraumbilical incision is made approximately 3 to 4 cm above the umbilicus in the midline, using the same technique as is described in the cutdown approach with direct visualization of the peritoneum. When using an incision lateral to the rectus abdominus muscles, the incision is placed at the lateral border of the rectus abdominus muscle on the side selected (opposite the scar of the previous surgery, i.e., appendectomy). Here also, a direct cutdown approach is utilized, using the same technique and length of incision as is described below.

2. Peritoneal lavage is contraindicated in the pregnant patient (44). It is unclear whether peritoneal lavage is contraindicated in the first trimester.
3. In the unstable patient requiring immediate surgical intervention, peritoneal lavage is not indicated (44).
4. Inability to catheterize bladder (here the cutdown approach is not contraindicated).

Equipment

The equipment necessary will depend on whether the incisional technique is used or the percutaneous puncture technique is selected.

Standard peritoneal dialysis catheter and trochar
20 ml syringe
4 mosquito hemostats
#11 blade
Suture material 4-0 silk, 4-0 vicryl, 5-0 nylon
Scissors
Adhesive tape
Local anesthetic 1% Xylocaine^R with epinephrine
Betadine solution for prep
Shaver
5 ml syringe

18 ga and 25 ga 1½ inch needle
Standard intravenous tubing with an extension tube
Needle-holder
4 x 4 gauze pads

Technique

Before this procedure is performed, when possible the patient should have an upright or left lateral decubitus abdominal film to exclude free air. During peritoneal lavage, air may be introduced and may produce a false positive finding of free air under the diaphragm. In this section, three techniques will be described and discussed with regard to their advantages and disadvantages.

Peritoneal lavage using the midline incision technique (2, 8, 17, 18, 44, 48)

Preparatory Steps

1 Place the patient in the supine position.
2. Catheterize and empty the urinary bladder even if patient has voided.
3. Shave the area between the symphysis pubis and the umbilicus in the midline.
4. Prepare the shaved area with Betadine^R solution and drape.
5. In the average adult, anesthetize an area 6 cm long, below the umbilicus in the midline. In the smaller patient, the area which should be anesthetized is one third the distance between the umbilicus and the symphysis pubis. The area of anesthesia should extend approximately 3 cm.

Procedural Steps

1. Make a 3 cm vertical midline incision approximately 3 cm below the umbilicus. The incision must remain in the midline and should be carried down to the linea alba. Ligate any bleeders encountered in the subcutaneous tissue. A self-retaining retractor should be placed as one carries the dissection down to the linea alba.

NOTE

This method offers the advantage of being able to directly visualize the peritoneum and avoid perforation into a viscus by the trochar or catheter (2). In the patient who has had previous surgery in the lower abdomen, one can safely do the lavage through an upper midline incision 2 to 3 cm above the umbilicus (44).

2. After visualization of the peritoneum, pick up the fascia of the abdomen along the linea alba with 2 small hemostats (Fig. 1.9).
3. An assistant should lift up the hemostats and a small 2 mm incision should be made between the hemostats with a #11 blade. The peritoneum thus is visualized and opened.
4. Insert a standard peritoneal dialysis catheter through the incision, directing the catheter toward the pelvis until all the side holes are within the abdominal cavity (Fig. 1.10). The trochar which comes with the catheter should be removed before insertion. Some authors prefer to direct the peritoneal dialysis catheter away from the midline so as to avoid the shallowest area of the abdomen (8).
5. Aspirate the catheter with a 20 ml syringe to ascertain whether there is any free blood in the abdominal cavity. If 20 ml of blood are withdrawn, the test is considered positive and the procedure is concluded. If less than 20 ml of blood are withdrawn, one liter of Ringer's lactate solution is in-

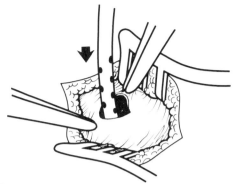

Figure 1.10.   A catheter is passed through a 2 mm incision and directed toward the pelvis. See text for details.

fused through the catheter in the average adult. This infusion should be done rapidly.
6. The patient is shifted briefly from one side to the other as the clinical condition permits (17, 42, 44, 48).
7. The infusion bottle now is placed on the floor to permit the fluid to return to the bottle. A positive lavage is defined as an inability to read a newspaper through the lavage fluid, which correlates with significant intraabdominal injury and allows for early operative intervention (36). Usually, approximately 90% of the lavage fluid is recoverable (48).

NOTE

If the lavage is equivocal and signs and symptoms of abdominal injury are present, a catheter can be left in place and the wound sutured and the lavage repeated again in 2 to 3 hours to determine if the lavage changes to a positive test (18). An aliquot of the lavage fluid can be sent for leukocyte count and amylase as well as Gram stain of the sediment if so desired (45).

Aftercare

1. The catheter should be removed and a single suture of silk should be placed in the fascia of the abdominal wall.
2. The subcutaneous tissue and skin are closed and the wound is dressed.

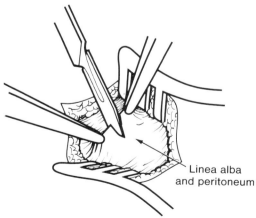

Linea alba and peritoneum

Figure 1.9.   An incision is made between two hemostats which pick up the peritoneum and fascia as shown. See text for details.

Peritoneal lavage in children

In children the preferred technique is the incisional method, using a small vertical infraumbilical midline incision which is made approximately one third of the way between the umbilicus and the symphysis pubis. The child should be sedated, and the catheter should be placed in the peritoneal cavity under direct vision after dissection down to the peritoneum. After emptying the bladder and following essentially the same procedures as above, the catheter should be directed toward the pelvis. In a child, the test is considered positive if more than 10 ml of blood are returned before lavaging. If not, administer 15 to 20 ml of Ringer's lactate per kilogram of body weight into the peritoneal cavity (17, 18, 44). The child should gently be turned from side to side if the condition permits, and the remainder of the examination should be performed similarly to the adult.

NOTE

The criticism raised for the incisional method of peritoneal lavage is that this technique is essentially a mini-laparotomy (31, 32). In addition, in the obese patient the cutdown technique may be quite difficult and significant bleeding may be encountered and may lead to a false positive lavage.

Percutaneous technique of peritoneal lavage (31, 32, 42, 52)

1. Select a point in the lower midline approximately 2 to 3 cm below the umbilicus.
2. Decompress the urinary bladder in the routine fashion.
3. Cleanse the skin and prep with iodinated antiseptic solution after shaving a small area at the puncture site.
4. Raise a wheal with 1% lidocaine at the puncture site.
5. A stab wound is made in the skin with a #11 blade, and hemostasis is obtained with local pressure.
6. A standard peritoneal dialysis cath-

eter attached to a trochar is inserted through the puncture site. The optimal method of inserting the catheter to avoid puncturing a viscus with the trochar is as follows:

a. Rotate the trochar and advance it to the linea alba. A firm resistance will be felt at this point.
b. Place the index finger and thumb of the left hand around the trochar and catheter at the puncture site holding it firmly (Fig. 1.11). The trochar should be angulated at approximately 60 degrees inferiorly toward the pelvis.
c. If the patient is able to do so, he should be instructed to raise his head, tensing the abdominal musculature and thus permitting easier introduction of the trochar.
d. With a back and forth rotary motion with the left hand and firm pressure on the trochar applied with the right hand, the trochar

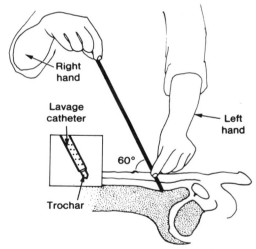

Figure 1.11. Using the percutaneous approach the index finger and thumb of the left hand hold the trochar (see inset) and resist the pressure applied by the right hand, thus preventing penetration too deeply into the peritoneal cavity. A rotary motion is applied by the right hand to pass the trochar. The angle of penetration is 60 degrees. After the trochar is inserted, the lavage catheter is passed over it into the peritoneal cavity (see inset).

is advanced through the fascia. While this is done the index finger and thumb of the left hand guard against passage of the trochar beyond the fascia and hold the trochar firmly, preventing further advancement once a "give" is felt and the trochar has entered into the peritoneal cavity.

NOTE

Using this technique of introducing the trochar the authors have not had a single instance of viscus injury from the trochar. Most of the complications listed below are secondary to inadvertent advancement of the trochar too deeply into the peritoneal cavity due to "uncontrolled introduction."

7. Once the trochar has been introduced the catheter is advanced into the peritoneal cavity over the trochar, and the trochar is removed (Fig. 1.11, inset).
8. Aspirate for blood and if none is present, introduce one liter of saline over a 5 to 10 minute period as indicated above (Fig. 1.12).
9. Turn the patient from side to side to disperse the fluid in the peritoneal cavity (42, 43, 56). This should not be done, however, in the presence of a pelvic fracture (56).

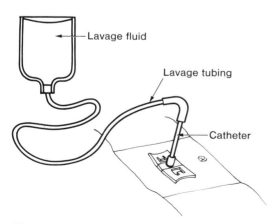

Figure 1.12. The lavage catheter then is attached to the tubing and the bag of lavage fluid as shown.

10. Place the bottle on the floor and allow the abdominal cavity to drain into it. The criteria for a positive lavage are similar to those discussed above.

Umbilical approach for peritoneal lavage

NOTE

Most authors use either the percutaneous insertion technique in the midline or the incision methods already described. There are a number of complications which have been reported with each of these two procedures. A technique has been described using an umbilical incision over the inferior portion of the umbilical ring. Fibrous changes within the vessels of the umbilical cord and urachus form a scar which draws against the superior circumference of the umbilical ring and retraction occurs around the umbilical vein. A similar scar forms inferiorly by fibrosis of the two arteries and urachus, which are likewise obliterated. The inferior adhesion is more dense and adherent than the superior one. There is a central papilla surrounded by a circular bulge created by subcutaneous fat. Between these two areas lies a circular or elliptical depression which is free of subcutaneous fat; here the skin is quite thin and fused directly to the ring margins and is adherent to the underlying peritoneum (51).

Technique. Decompress the urinary bladder and prepare and drape as in the routine fashion. Raise a skin wheal in the inferior portion of the umbilical ring. The area of incision is not infraumbilical but rather is in the inferior portion of the umbilical ring itself, formed by the umbilical papilla centrally in the umbilicus and a circular bulge made by the presence of subcutaneous fat (Fig. 1.13). Between these two areas is a depression free of fat, and this is the ring over which the incision is made. Incise the ring with a #11 blade, and introduce a standard dialysis catheter, advancing the trochar grasped as indicated above to provide good control of the catheter and trochar. Once inserted, the trochar is removed immediately, and the

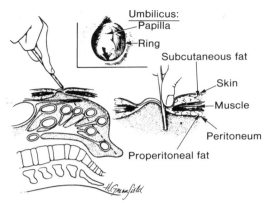

Figure 1.13. Technique of diagnostic peritoneal lavage performed by percutaneous insertion through the inferior portion of the umbilical ring. See text for details. Inset shows the anatomy of the umbilicus with the arrow demonstrating the precise location of the puncture. (Reprinted with permission of Surgery, Gynecology Obstetrics, Slavin, S., A new technique for diagnostic peritoneal lavage. 146:447, 1978.)

catheter is advanced toward the pelvis. After aspirating for blood, instill a liter of saline and follow the same procedures as for the percutaneous method. The authors state that in a small number of cases reported there were no false positive or false negatives in the peritoneal lavage and no complications using this technique (51).

Alternate Technique

A method has been described using a sharp needle and a guidewire to introduce the catheter; this technique has been associated with a lower incidence of complications than with the standard percutaneous technique. A 3 mm vertical skin incision is made with a #11 blade inferior to the umbilicus in the midline following adequate preparation and anesthesia. A 3 mm vertical skin incision is made with a #11 blade over the puncture site. An 18 ga needle is introduced through the incision and is carefully introduced into the peritoneal cavity. Once the linea alba is penetrated, the needle is advanced an additional 2 to 3 mm and the floppy end of a guidewire is introduced through the needle. Once the guidewire moves freely within the abdominal cavity, a 9 French

catheter is introduced over the guidewire using a twisting and pushing motion so that it will penetrate the fascia. Following this, the guidewire is removed and the catheter is aspirated; if the aspiration is negative, 1000 ml of fluid are introduced. The remainder of this procedure is similar to that described above (31, 32).

COMPLICATIONS

The complication rate of peritoneal lavage varies from 1 to 6% (31). A number of complications have been reported in the literature.

1. Bleeding within the rectus sheath with a false positive result (31, 51).
2. Bleeding at the puncture site with a false positive result (51).
3. Infusion of the lavage fluid into the abdominal wall (38a).
4. Lack of fluid return. This is not an uncommon problem. When only a portion of the fluid returns, one must analyze that portion which is obtained. The remainder will be absorbed by the peritoneum. When there is no fluid return, the catheter may be withdrawn slightly or the patient may be turned, once again from side to side. This may result in return of lavage fluid into the drainage bag. Alternately, the patient may be placed in 10 to 15 degrees of reverse Trendelenburg position which may result in drainage through the catheter if the catheter has been placed in the pelvis. Finally, if none of the above has worked, an additional 500 cc of fluid may be instilled which may promote drainage through the catheter.
5. Laceration of the mesenteric vessels, iliac artery or vein (31, 45, 51).
6. Perforation of the small intestine or colon (31, 45, 51). As the catheter and trochar pass through the abdominal wall, the trochar should be removed as soon as the peritoneum is pierced, otherwise visceral or vessel perforation occurs.
7. Inadvertent entry into the mesentery or retroperitoneal space (5). This occurs more commonly with the per-

cutaneous technique, as do any of the visceral or vessel injuries indicated above. This can be prevented by using the technique indicated earlier for introducing the trochar.

8. Penetration of the bladder (31, 51). Always empty the bladder before insertion of the catheter to prevent this complication. Inability to drain the bladder is a contraindication to this procedure.
9. Incisional hernia (31).
10. Wound infection (31).
11. Wound separation (31).

SIGMOIDOSCOPY

Sigmoidoscopic examination of the rectum and sigmoid colon is a very useful procedure which unfortunately is not utilized as often as it should be within the emergency center.

Indications

1. Sigmoid volvulus. In a patient with large bowel obstruction in whom one suspects sigmoid volvulus, sigmoidoscopy can be performed for both diagnostic and therapeutic purposes.
2. Gastrointestinal hemorrhage. When the nasogastric lavage does not demonstrate a cause proximally.
3. Bleeding from the anal canal in which a diagnosis cannot be demonstrated.
4. Purulent or mucoid discharge from the anal canal.
5. Recurrent diarrhea lasting for several days.
6. Undifferentiated pain in the anoperineal region or lower abdomen.

Contraindications

1. An uncooperative, agitated patient.
2. Patients with obstruction in the rectum prohibiting advancement of the sigmoidoscope.

Equipment

Sigmoidoscope and obturator. Sigmoidoscopes come in various sizes, usually the length is 25 cm.
A long metal suction device
Cotton swabs on a long applicator

An insufflation bag and tubing to dilate the rectum
A good suction source such as a Venturi-type adapter that can be connected to a water faucet or other dependable, powerful suction apparatus
An electrical light source

Technique

Preparatory Steps

1. Prep the bowel. To empty the lower rectum, a nonirritating enema such as tap water should be administered 30 minutes to 1 hour before sigmoidoscopy is performed. Caution should be exercised in patients with colitis. In patients with sigmoid volvulus, severe gastrointestinal hemorrhage, or perianal abscess, preparation of the bowel is not necessary.
2. Position the patient. When the procedure is performed at the bedside, the left lateral Sims position is preferred with left knee flexed and right knee extended. The pelvis should be at or beyond the edge of the table. Optimally the patient should be in Trendelenburg in the knee-chest position (Fig. 1.14A). A special table is

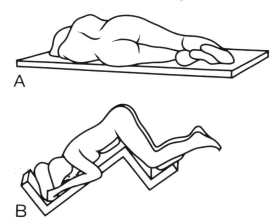

Figure 1.14. Two positions are shown for performing sigmoidoscopy in the adult. *A.* The knee-chest position with the left knee and hip flexed and the right knee and hip slightly extended. This position is used on the examining table in the emergency center. When a sigmoidoscopy table is available as shown in *B*, this is preferred.

available for this procedure and the jackknife position is preferred when such a table is available within the emergency center (Fig. 1.14B). Sedation is usually not necessary.

3. Examine the perianal and buttocks area for any lesions. Ask the patient to strain to see if there is any prolapse of the mucosa or internal hemorrhoids. Following this, a rectal examination must be performed to ascertain any lesions before introducing the sigmoidoscope, to relax the sphincter before the procedure, and to ensure patency of the anal canal.

4. Insert the obturator into the sigmoidoscope and lubricate the tip.

Procedural Steps

1. Insert the sigmoidoscope into the rectum, aiming it anteriorly in the direction of the umbilicus (Fig. 1.15-1). The sigmoidoscope should be directed in the midline and inserted into the anus with gentle and firm pressure.

2. Remove the obturator when the scope has been passed 4 cm into the canal. After removal of the obturator the anal mucosa should be visualized and fluid and fecal material suctioned (Fig. 1.16A and B).

3. A glass covering should be secured over the end of the sigmoidoscope and the insufflator and electric light

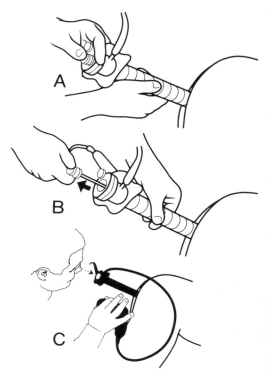

Figure 1.16. *A.* The obturator should be removed so that direct visualization can be performed when passing the sigmoidoscope. *B.* A suction catheter can be used to suction out secretions and fecal material during passage of the tube. *C.* Periodic insufflation of the rectum and sigmoid will permit direct visualization of the canal and aid in passage of the tube. See text for full discussion.

source should be attached (Fig. 1.16C).

4. *Advance the sigmoidoscope into the bowel lumen only under direct vision* (Fig. 1.16C). The insufflation of air dilates the rectal lumen and facilitates identification of the mucosal structures and aids in passing the scope. However, it also increases the risk of perforation.

5. After passing through the anal canal the sigmoidoscope should be directed posteriorly (Fig. 1.15-2), keeping the sigmoidoscope in the midline toward the hollow of the sacrum. If resistance is met withdraw slightly and visualize the lumen then pass the sig-

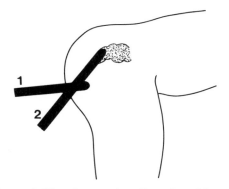

Figure 1.15. In passing the sigmoidoscope into the anus and anal canal, it is first aimed toward the umbilicus (*1*). After passing the anal canal, the sigmoidoscope is directed posteriorly (*2*). See text for details.

moidoscope, instilling only small amounts of air to aid in visualizing the lumen. If the patient notes that the rectum has become uncomfortable, remove the glass shield, permitting air under pressure to be released.

6. At approximately 10 to 12 cm the rectosigmoid junction is encountered and the bowel angulates. At this point the sigmoidoscope should be directed anteriorly and to the left side. One may encounter difficulty in passage of the instrument should acute angulation be present.

NOTE

In patients with diverticulitis it is often impossible to advance the scope beyond 15 cm because of pain. In some patients the angulation of the rectosigmoid juncture is so acute that one is unable to advance the scope beyond this point. The sigmoid colon can be identified by its transverse folds in contrast to the smooth mucosa of the rectum.

In patients with a sigmoid volvulus, the mucosa at the site of the obstruction may be sloughed or have ulcerations with dark blood noted. If this is not seen in a patient with a sigmoid volvulus and if obstruction is met at the site of the volvulus, then a soft rubber tube which is well-lubricated may be advanced through the obstructed segment, thus permitting decompression and rapid and often explosive passage of air and liquid. Caution must be exercised in doing so as the examiner may be sprayed with this material. The rectal tube should be left in place for several days until bowel function returns to normal. After so doing, the sigmoidoscope is removed and the rectal tube is taped to the buttocks.

7. When the sigmoidoscope has been inserted to its maximal extent, the sigmoidoscope should be withdrawn and careful inspection should be performed. This is best done with frequent insufflations of small amounts of air to separate the bowel walls and

with aspiration of any fluid and feces or wiping the area with cotton swabs.

Complications

1. Perforation. Perforation may occur at the antimesenteric border. This occurs most frequently at the rectosigmoid junction at approximately 15 cm due to overzealous advancement of the sigmoidoscope. Perforation may be noted by a sudden "give" during sigmoidoscopy or by visualizing bowel serosa. Look for any evidence of peritonitis. An upright abdominal radiograph should be taken in all patients with suspected perforation after sigmoidoscopic examination to exclude this complication. One must exercise extreme caution in performing sigmoidoscopic examination in the patient with colitis or inflammatory bowel disease, as perforation is most likely to occur in inflamed bowel.
2. Trauma to the mucosa following instrumentation.
3. Bacteremia. Bacteremia has been found to occur in 8 to 10% of all patients undergoing sigmoidoscopic examination.
4. Bursting of a thin-walled sigmoid colon or rectum due to excessive insufflation of air.

ANOSCOPY

The rectum is approximately 15 cm long and extends approximately from the pectinate line to the sigmoid. The anal canal extends from the pectinate line distally and is approximately 3.5 cm long. An anoscope is a short instrument with an obturator which is used to examine the anal canal and distal aspect of the rectum. This procedure can be done without any bowel preparation or enema. The procedure is quite useful in examining the patient with suspected hemorrhoids, fistulas, and other lesions involving the anus.

Technique

Always perform a digital rectal examination before anoscopy (see "Sigmoidoscopy"). Place the patient in the lateral decubitus position. Insert a well-lubricated anoscope gently into the anus. Direct the anoscope gently toward the midline anteriorly, following the direction of the anal canal. While the anoscope is being advanced, the obturator should be held in place with the thumb until the instrument is fully inserted. After the anoscope is fully inserted, the obturator should be removed. Rotate the anoscope through a 360 degree arc to inspect all the areas of the anus circumferentially as the instrument is withdrawn. Illumination is provided by an ordinary flashlight or a gooseneck lamp. Cotton swabs on a forceps may be necessary to clean the area. As the instrument is withdrawn the examiner should check for hemorrhoids, polyps, fistulas, or other lesions of the anal canal causing the patient's symptomatology.

PROCTOSCOPY IN THE INFANT (28)

Proctoscopic examination is a procedure which is not commonly performed in the infant but which can be quite useful in ascertaining the cause of symptoms referred to this area.

Indications

1. Prolonged or unexplained diarrhea
2. Passage of bloody stools, pus or mucus
3. Abdominal pain of unknown etiology
4. Perineal fistulas or abscesses
5. Imperforate anus

Equipment

The anoscope comes in various sizes and one should have an anoscope with an outer diameter of approximately 1 cm and a length of 8 to 10 cm for the newborn and one with a diameter of 1.5 cm and a length of 12 to 25 cm for the older infant and child (28).

Technique

1. Position the infant on his back (Fig. 1.17). A nurse puts her forearms alongside the child's body and grasps the thighs of the infant with her

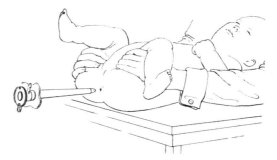

Figure 1.17. Position for proctoscopy for small infants. (Reprinted with permission of American Journal Diseases of Children. Hijmans, J., Proctoscopy of the infant. 105:298, 1963.)

hands. She then abducts the thighs and flexes them so they touch the child's abdomen but do not compress the abdominal wall. The buttocks are placed at the edge of the table so the instrument can be depressed easily during the procedure. Examine the child for fissures, hemorrhoids, or inflammatory changes before insertion of the instrument. Digitally examine the rectum to ascertain the size of the sphincter and the patency of the canal. No sedation is necessary for this procedure and, in fact, it is contraindicated. Sedation may prevent a pain response which warns against an accident and, in addition, the sphincter relaxes during the inspiratory gasp following a prolonged cry permitting the scope to slide more easily into the anal canal. Laxatives, suppositories, and enemas are not used as these may cause changes in the anal mucosa, leading to an erroneous diagnosis.

2. Grasp the instrument with the thumb held firmly over the obturator. Lubricate the tip and then press the instrument gently and evenly against the anal sphincter. Do not attempt to pass the instrument forcefully through; it will pass with gentle, even pressure when the sphincter relaxes. The examiner must wait patiently for this to happen. Once the tube is in the canal then the obturator should be removed

and advanced; the instrument is advanced only under direct vision. The mucosa should be cleansed with a cotton swab or suction until the lumen is visualized and the mucosa examined. Do not use air to inflate in the infant and small child as this may cause tears or pneumatic perforations (15). One should examine for pitting edema, friability, inflammation, submucosal hemorrhagic ulcers, masses, or polyps. Cultures can be taken when necessary. The instrument should not be passed beyond the angulation of the rectosigmoid junction. Instrumentation beyond this level should be performed only by an expert. One can easily tell when this junction is reached as the rectum passes backward and has longitudinal folds whereas the sigmoid has transverse folds.

EXTERNAL THROMBOSED HEMORRHOIDS

The arterial and venous supply of the rectum consists of, from top to bottom, the superior, middle, and inferior hemorrhoidal arteries and the superior, middle, and inferior hemorrhoidal veins. The middle hemorrhoidal vein anastomoses with the superior hemorrhoidal vein and also with the portal system. Therefore, in patients with portal hypertension, such as cirrhosis of the liver, high portal pressure is communicated to the middle hemorrhoidal vein and results in venous dilatation under a considerable amount of pressure.

Hemorrhoids represent a mass of dilated venules. If the hemorrhoid originates above the dentate line, they are called internal hemorrhoids. If they originate below the dentate line, they are termed external hemorrhoids. A prolapsed internal hemorrhoid is an internal hemorrhoid which extends lower than the dentate line. This type of hemorrhoid can prolapse outside the rectum.

Acute external thrombosed hemorrhoids present as a sudden, painful lump in the anus. On physical examination a dark-blue tender nodule is noted at the anal verge. This nodule is covered with normal skin. The lesion is extremely painful and treatment is directed to relieve this pain. If the patient has no pain, then only conservative treatment is necessary.

Technique of Incision

The patient should be given intravenous analgesics (Demerol®). The authors recommend intravenous analgesics in any operative procedure performed in the emergency center involving the anal region. After the patient is relaxed and in less pain, the lesion is anesthetized by infiltrating 1% lidocaine with epinephrine in the area under and around the thrombosed mass. An elliptical incision with a #11 blade is made over the thrombosed mass and the point of the ellipse is picked up with a hemostat or Allis forceps (Fig. 1.18A and B). The scalpel then is carried downward to "scoop out" and remove the thrombosed area. Almost always there is more than one clot, and it is important to express a series of clots within the thrombosed area. If all the clots are not expressed from the hemorrhoid, recurrence of thrombosis is likely. After removal of the clots, the tip of a gauze compress is inserted into the wound (Fig. 1.18C). No further dressing is necessary, and the buttocks are taped together to create a pressure dressing. This pad and pressure are left in place for approximately 8 hours, following which the patient removes the pack while in a sitz bath.

SEVERE HEMORRHOIDAL BLEEDING

The usual therapy of intravenous fluids for the hypotensive patient or a massively bleeding patient should be employed. Hemorrhoidal bleeding usually presents with a "squirting of blood" with defecation. To treat this entity with moderate or severe bleeding, the patient should be asked to bear down. If the bleeding site is visible, apply a hemostat to the bleeding site and tie a ligature around the hemostat. If the lesion is not visible, try to visualize the bleeding spot through the anoscope.

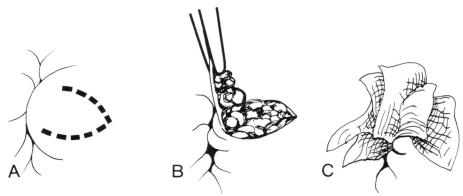

Figure 1.18. *A.* An elliptical incision is made around a thrombosed external hemorrhoid. *B.* The skin wedge containing the thrombus is then uplifted and excised. *C.* A gauze pack is inserted and the buttocks taped together. See text for details.

When the bleeding point is visualized, apply a hemostat to the bleeding site and leave the hemostat in place for 5 minutes. After this period of time, cauterize the bleeding site with silver nitrate. If the hemorrhoidal bleeding is mild, the usual symptomatic therapy for hemorrhoids is recommended.

POST-HEMORRHOIDECTOMY BLEEDING

Ten to 14 days following a hemorrhoidectomy, the patient absorbs the sutures and in 1.3% of cases bleeding may ensue. Bleeding may be severe and require the insertion of a pack. Post-hemorrhoidectomy bleeding packs are commercially available for this purpose. The packs should be inserted through the anoscope, and the strings pulled down to engage the pack against the bleeding site, causing tamponade (Fig. 1.19). The patient should be admitted for hospitalization. When such a pack is not available, the emergency physician may insert a Foley catheter and inflate the balloon for temporary control of the bleeding. With either of these procedures, proper sedation should be administered as pressure from the pack or balloon causes significant discomfort to the patient.

ANORECTAL ABSCESSES

The dentate or pectinate line represents a transverse series of openings or crypts in the anal mucosa. These crypts are the openings of the anal glands which are in the connective tissue of the anus. The anal glands are mucus-secreting glands that drain via ducts into the anal crypts at the dentate line (Fig. 1.20). When a blockage occurs in the duct of the anal gland, inflammation and abscess formations are likely to occur. When an abscess occurs in an anal gland, one has a perianal abscess. The anal abscess may extend into several potential spaces (Fig. 1.20A). When the abscess extends to the skin surface, it is considered a perianal abscess. When extension occurs into the space between the sphincters in the posterior midline, it is called an intersphincteric abscess. Extension into the submucosal space of the ischiorectal fossa leads to an ischiorectal abscess. Two other rectal abscesses which present to the emergency center are submucosal and supralevator abscesses. Each of these abscesses will be discussed separately below.

Perianal Abscesses

The patient should lie in the prone position. The buttocks are separated and taped with 3 inch adhesive tape to the lateral aspect of the hip, thus exposing the anus. The area around the abscess is infiltrated with 1% Xylocaine® with epinephrine, and the roof of the abscess is likewise infiltrated. If adequate analgesia cannot be achieved, the patient needs general anesthesia. One of two techniques can be used

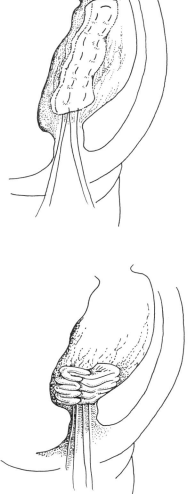

day and each day thereafter until healing is complete. Due to pain and complications, some institutions do not permit drainage of these in the emergency center.

Submucosal Abscess

Most submucosal abscesses may be drained within the emergency center. These patients present with a deep, dull pain in the area of the rectum and usually have a history of diarrheal episodes or a mucous or purulent discharge from the rectum. These abscesses can be visualized with a proctoscopic or sigmoidoscopic examination and incision and drainage performed in the normal fashion.

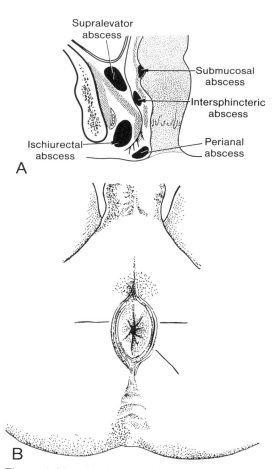

Figure 1.19. A post-hemorrhoidectomy pack is inserted. This accordion-like pack contains two strings which are then pulled down to secure the pack in place in the anal canal; the pack tamponades bleeding.

to drain these abscesses. Either an elliptical wedge is excised, using a radial incision from the roof of the abscess thus permitting wide drainage, or a cruciate incision is made with the edges excised to expose the abscessed cavity adequately (Fig. 1.21). Either method will permit adequate drainage of the abscess. A gauze pad is applied to the anal region and the buttocks released around it. The patient should be advised to take a sitz bath the following

Figure 1.20. Various locations of rectal abscesses. A radial incision should be used in draining a perianal abscess. The incision should be lateral to the sphincter muscle.

Ischiorectal and Supralevator Abscesses

Because of their size and extension, ischiorectal and supralevator abscesses should be drained in the operating room.

Pilonidal Abscesses

A pilonidal abscess results from an infection in a pilonidal cyst. A pilonidal cyst results from the posterior neuropore failing to close, resulting in a structure that becomes fluid-filled. The cyst may develop

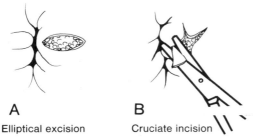

A Elliptical excision   B Cruciate incision

Figure 1.21. The most common type of rectal abscess drained in the emergency center is the perianal or perirectal abscess. In draining this abscess, an elliptical excision should be used to provide adequate opening for proper drainage to occur, as shown in *A*. Alternately, a cruciate incision can be used when deeper abscesses are being drained, as shown in *B*.

tracts called pilonidal sinuses. When a cyst fails to drain, infection and abscess formation are likely to occur. The pilonidal sinus may become plugged with keratin, desquamated epithelial cells, or debris. Pilonidal cysts derive their name from the fact that many of the cysts have hair within the cavity. The abscesses which form may be treated in the usual manner; however, they almost always recur and the patient should be referred following incision and drainage for definitive excision of the underlying lesion.

The pilonidal abscess should be drained, using a midline vertical incision following adequate anesthesia by local infiltration. Loculations should be opened and the abscess cavity irrigated with half-strength hydrogen peroxide. The cavity then is packed with iodoform gauze. The gauze packing should be removed in 48 hours while the patient is in a sitz bath. The patient is instructed to continue sitz baths daily until healing is complete.

Foreign Bodies in the Anus

Foreign bodies in the anus and rectum may present a formidable problem. The patient may or may not complain of pain in the rectal area. Occasionally, foreign

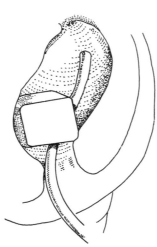
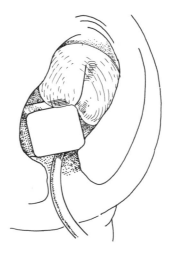

Figure 1.22. A size 24 French Foley catheter with a 50 cc balloon at its tip is used to stabilize a foreign body in the rectum while manipulating it for extraction.

bodies may be removed in the emergency center; however, some patients may require a general anesthetic to remove the object. The foreign body must be stabilized before removal, as attempts to remove the object without stabilization may result in displacing it further and further away from one's grasp. A 24 French Foley catheter with a 50 ml balloon can be inserted into the rectum through an anoscope and inserted past the foreign body. The balloon then is inflated proximal to the foreign body. Traction is applied on the Foley catheter, thus stabilizing the foreign body in position (Fig. 1.22). If the object is small and round, the inflated balloon may actually be used to remove the object. In situations in which the object is either irregular or has sharp edges, the inflated balloon of the Foley catheter is used to stabilize the object and a long forceps is introduced through the anoscope to grasp the foreign body and remove it.

References

1. Abcarian, H., Acute suppurations of the anorectum. Surg. Annual 8:305, 1976.
2. Ahmad, W., Polk, H.C., Blunt abdominal trauma. Arch. Surg. 111:489, 1976.
3. Aragon, G.E., Eiseman, B., Abdominal stab wounds: Evaluation of sinography. J. Trauma 16:792, 1976.
4. Atkenson, R.J., Nyhus, L.M., Gastric lavage for hemorrhage in the upper part of the gastrointestinal tract. Surg. Gynecol. Obstet. 147:797, 1978.
5. Breen, P.C., Rudolf, L.E., Potential sources of error in the use of peritoneal lavage as a diagnostic tool. J. Am. Coll. Emerg. Phys. 3:401, 1974.
6. Bull, J. C., Jr., Mathewson, C., Jr., Exploratory laparotomy in patients with penetrating wounds of the abdomen. Am. J. Surg. 116:223, 1961.
7. Byrne, W.D., Samson, P.C., Dugan, D.J., Complications associated with the use of esophageal compression balloons. Am. J. Surg. 104:250, 1962.
8. Caffee, H.H., Benfield, J.R., Is peritoneal lavage for the diagnosis of hemoperitoneum safe? Arch. Surg. 103:4, 1971.
9. Caralps-Riera, J.M., Diagnostic value of hypaque injection in the conservative management of upper abdominal stab wounds. Am. J. Surg. 123:612, 1972.
10. Carter, J.W., Sawyers, J.L., Pitfalls in diagnosis of abdominal stab wounds by contrast media injection. Am. Surg. 35:107, 1969.
11. Complications of gastro-intestinal intubation. Ann. Surg. 130:113, 1949.
12. Cohen, D.D., Nasogastric intubation in the anesthetized patient. Anesth. Analg. 42:578, 1963.
13. Conn, H.O., Sengstaken-Blakemore tube revisited (editorial). Gastroenterology 61:398, 1971.
14. Conn, H.O., Simpson, J.A., Excessive mortality associated with balloon tamponade of bleeding varices: A critical reappraisal. JAMA 202:135, 1967.
15. Crohn, B.B., Trauma from sigmoid manipulation. Am. J. Dis. Child. 2:678, 1936.
16. Daly, W.M., Unusual complication of nasal intubation. Anesthesiology 14:96, 1953.
17. Drew, R., Perry, J.F., Fischer, R.P., The expediency of peritoneal lavage for blunt trauma in children. Surg. Gynecol. Obstet. 145:885, 1977.
18. Engrav, L.H., Benjamin, C.I., Strate, R.G., et al., Diagnostic peritoneal lavage in blunt abdominal trauma. J. Trauma 15:854, 1975.
19. Fenig, J., Richter, R.M., Levowitz, B.S., Gastric ulceration caused by Sengstaken-Blakemore balloon tamponade. N.Y. State J. Med. 76:404, 1976.
20. Fremstad, J.D., Martin, S.H., Lethal complication from insertion of nasogastric tube after severe basilar skull fracture. J. Trauma 18:820, 1978.
21. Fry, E.N.S., Positioning of nasogastric tubes (letter). Brit. Med. J. 1:110, 1978.
22. Greene, J.F., Jr., Sawicki, J.E., Doyle, W.F., Gastric ulceration: A complication of double-lumen nasogastric tubes. JAMA 224:338, 1973.
23. Gregory, J.A., Turner, P.T., Reynolds, A.F., A complication of nasogastric intubation: Intracranial penetration. J. Trauma 18:823, 1978.
24. Gustavsson, S., Albert, J., Forsberg, H., et al., The accidental introduction of a nasogastric tube into the brain. Acta Chir. Scand. 144:55, 1978.
25. Haddad, G.H., Pizzi, W.F., Fleischmann, E.P., et al., Abdominal signs and sinograms as dependable criteria for the selective management of stab wounds of the abdomen. Ann. Surg. 172:61, 1970.
26. Hafner, C.D., Wylie, J.H., Jr., Brush, B.E., Complications of gastrointestinal intubation. Arch. Surg. 83:147, 1961.
27. Hanselman, R.C., Meyer, R.H., Complications of gastrointestinal intubation. Surg. Gynecol. Obstet. Internat. Abstr. Surg. 114:207, 1962.
28. Hijams, J., Proctoscopy of the infant. Am. J. Dis. Child. 105:297, 1963.
29. Hyatt, D.F., Gordon, L.A., Abdominal stab wound sinogram. Arch. Surg. 104:340, 1972.
30. James, R.H., An unusual complication of passing a narrow bore nasogastric tube. Anaesthesia 33:716, 1978.
31. Lazarus, H.M., Nelson, J.A., A technique for peritoneal lavage without risk or complication. Surg. Gynecol. Obstet. 149:889, 1979.
32. Lazarus, H.M., Nelson, J.A., Peritoneal lavage with low morbidity. JACEP 8:316, 1979.
33. Liebman, R., New tube for the diagnosis and treatment of upper gastrointestinal hemorrhage. Am. J. Surg. 127:171, 1974.
34. Liedberg, G., Esophageal tamponage in the treatment of massive bleeding from esophageal varices, with special reference to volume and pressure in the balloons. Acta Chir. Scand. 134:249, 1968.
35. Lind, L.J., Wallace, D.H., Submucosal passage of a nasogastric tube complicating attempted intu-

bation during anesthesia. Anesthesiology 49:145, 1978.

36. Lucas, C.E., The role of peritoneal lavage for penetrating abdominal wounds (editorial). J. Trauma 17:649, 1977.
37. Madureri, V., Sonda de doble circulacion para lavado, gastrico. GEN 26:411, 1972.
38. Mahar, J., An aid in the passage of gastrointestinal tubes. Am. J. Surg. 135:866, 1978.
38a.Markovchick, V.J., Elerding, S.C., Moore, E.E., et al., Diagnostic peritoneal lavage. JACEP 8:326, 1979.
38b.McDougal, K., Modifications in the technique of gastric lavage. Ann. Emerg. Med. 10:514, 1981.
39. Mundy, D.A., Another technique for insertion of nasogastric tubes. Anesthesiology 50:374, 1979.
40. Nickell, M.D., Schwitzer, G.A., Gremillion, D.E., Jr., Overdistension of the gastric balloon: Complication with the Sengstaken-Blakemore tube. JAMA 240:1172, 1978.
41. Ogawa, H., A reliable technique for the insertion of a gastric tube during operation. Surg. Gynecol. Obstet. 132:497, 1971.
42. Olsen, W.R., Hildreth, D.H., Abdominal paracentesis and peritoneal lavage in blunt abdominal trauma. J. Trauma 11:824, 1971.
43. Olsen, W.R., Redman, H.C., Hildreth, D.H., et al., Quantitative peritoneal lavage in blunt abdominal trauma. Arch. Surg. 104:536, 1972.
44. Parvin, S., Smith, D.E., Asher, W.M., et al., Effectiveness of peritoneal lavage in blunt abdominal trauma. Ann. Surg. 181:255, 1975.
45. Perry, J.F., Jr., Strate, R.G., Diagnostic peritoneal lavage in blunt abdominal trauma: Indications and results. Surgery 71:898, 1972.
46. Pitcher, J.L., Safety and effectiveness of the modified Sengstaken-Blakemore tube: A prospective study. Gastroenterology 61:291, 1971.
47. Robinson, E.P., Cox, P.M., Jr., Feeding tube introduction—an easier way. Crit. Care Med. 7:349, 1979.
48. Root, H.D., Hauser, C.W., McKinley, C.R., et al., Diagnostic peritoneal lavage. Surgery 57:633, 1965.
49. Sader, A.A., New way to stabilize nasogastric tubes. Am. J. Surg. 130:102, 1975.
50. Seebacher, J., Nozik, D., Mathieu, A., Inadvertent intracranial introduction of a nasogastric tube: A complication of severe maxillofacial trauma. Anesthesiology 42:100, 1975.
51. Slavin, S., A new technique for diagnostic peritoneal lavage. Surg. Gynecol. Obstet. 146:446, 1978.
52. Spencer, G.T., Tracheostomy and endotracheal intubation in the intensive care unit. In Gray, T.C., Nunn, J.F. (eds) General Anaesthesia, 3rd ed. Butterworths, London, 1973, vol. 2, p. 566.
53. Stenapien, S.J., Dagradi, A.E., A double lumen tube for gastro-esophageal lavage. Gastrointest. Endosc. 12:26, 1966.
54. Tahis, A.H., A method of inserting a gastric tube during operation. Surg. Gynecol. Obstet. 132:497, 1971.
55. Thal, E.R., Evaluation of peritoneal lavage and local exploration in lower chest and abdominal stab wounds. J. Trauma 17:642, 1977.
56. Thal, E.R., Shires, G.T., Peritoneal lavage in blunt abdominal trauma. Am. J. Surg. 125:64, 1973.
57. Trimble, C., Stab wound sinography. Surg. Clin. North Am. 49:1217, 1969.
58. Virtue, R.W., Simple and reliable method for inserting nasogastric tube during anesthesia. Br. J. Anaesthes. 45:234, 1973.
59. Wyler, A.R., Reynolds, A.F. An intracranial complication of nasogastric intubation. J. Neurosurg. 47:297, 1977.
60. Young, R.F., Cerebrospinal fluid rhinorrhea following nasogastric intubation. J. Trauma 19:789, 1979.
61. Zeid, S.S., Young, P.C., Reeves, J.T., Rupture of the esophagus after introduction of the Sengstaken-Blakemore tube. Gastroenterology 36:128, 1959.

Bibliography

1. Altemeier, W.A., Culbertson, W.R., Fullen, W.D., et al., Intra-abdominal abscesses. Am. J. Surg. 125:70, 1973.
2. Bizzarri, D., Giuffrida, J., Latteri, F., et al., Esophageal intubation for prevention of aspiration of gastric contents. Acta Anesth. Scand. Supp. 24:19, 1966.
3. Bizzarri, D., Gremillion, M.D.E., Jr., Simple method for passage of small-bore nasogastric feeding catheter. Ann. Intern. Med. 91:655, 1979.
4. Blades, B., Ruptured diaphragm. Am. J. Surg. 105:501, 1963.
5. Borja, A.R., Lansing, A.M., Immediate control of intermediate vascular bleeding. Surg. Gynecol. Obstet. 132:494, 1971.
6. Bray, P.F., Herbst, J.J., Johnson, D.G., et al., Childhood gastroesophageal reflux. JAMA 237:1342, 1977.
7. Burcharth, F., Malmstrom, J., Experiences with the Linton-Nachlas and the Sengstaken-Blakemore tubes for bleeding esophageal varices. Surg. Gynecol. Obstet. 142:529, 1976.
8. Child, C.G., Braunstein, P.W., Gastroduodenal intussusception with massive hemorrhage. Surgery 34:754, 1953.
9. Clarke, J.M., Culdocentesis in the evaluation of blunt abdominal trauma. Surg. Gynecol. Obstet. 129:809, 1969.
10. Conway, K., Letter to the Editor. Anesth. Analg. 50:1010, 1971.
11. Dennis, C., The gastrointestinal sump tube. Surgery 66:309, 1969.
12. Durham, M.W., Holm, J.C., Simple perforated ulcer of the colon. Surgery 34:750, 1953.
13. Elerding, S.C., Aragon, G.E., Moore, E.E., Fatal hepatic hemorrhage after trauma. Am. J. Surg. 138:883, 1979.
14. Galloway, D.C., Grudis, J., Inadvertent intracranial placement of a nasogastric tube through a basal skull fracture. So. Med. J. 72:240, 1979.
15. Grant, G.N., Elliott, D.W., Frederick, P.L., Post-

operative decompression by temporary gastrostomy or nasogastric tube. Arch. Surg. 85:844, 1962.

16. Jahadi, M.R., Diagnostic peritoneal lavage. J. Trauma 12:936, 1972.

17. James, R.H., An unusual complication of passing a narrow bore nasogastric tube. Anaesthesia 33:716, 1978.

18. Lawler, N.A., McCreath, N.D., Gastro-oesophageal regurgitation. Lancet. 2:369, 1951.

19. Ledgerwood, A.M., Kazmers, M., Lucas, C.E., The role of thoracic aortic occlusion for massive hemoperitoneum. J. Trauma 16:601, 1976.

20. McCoy, J., Wolma, F.J., Abdominal tap: Indication, technic, and results. Am. J. Surg. 122:693, 1971.

21. Markovchick, V.J., Elerding, S.C., Moore, E.E., et al., Diagnostic peritoneal lavage. JACEP 8:326, 1979.

22. Moss, C.M., Levine, R., Messenger, N., et al., Sliding colonic Maydl's hernia: Report of a case. Dis. Col. and Rect. 19:636, 1976.

23. Nance, F.C., The early management of abdominal trauma. Curr. Concepts in Trauma Care 9–16 Summer, 1979.

24. Notaras, M.J., A simple technique for continuous gastric aspiration. Lancet 2:476, 1966.

25. Orloff, M.J., Snyder, G.B., Experimental ascites. I. Production of ascites by gradual occlusion of the hepatic veins with an internal vena caval cannula. Surgery 50:789, 1961.

26. Palmer, E.D., The vigorous diagnostic approach to upper-gastrointestinal tract hemorrhage. JAMA 207:1477, 1969.

27. Palmer, E.D., Soderstrom, C.A., DuPriest, R.W., et al., Pitfalls of peritoneal lavage in blunt abdominal trauma. Surg. Gynecol. Obstet. 151:513, 1980.

28. Palmer, E.D., Tucker, A., Lewis, J., Passing a nasogastric tube. Brit. Med. J. 281:1128, 1980.

29. Requarth, W., Theis, F.V., Incarcerated and strangulated inguinal hernia. Arch. Surg. 57:267, 1948.

30. Richards, J.H., Bacteremia following irritation of foci of infection. JAMA 99:1496, 1932.

31. Sealy, W.C., Rupture of the esophagus. Am. J. Surg. 105:505, 1963.

32. Tobias, S., DeClement, F.A., Cleveland, J.C., Management of abdominal stab wounds. Arch. Surg. 95:27, 1967.

33. Wavak, P., Zook, E.G., A simple method of exsanguinating the finger prior to surgery. JACEP 7:125, 1978.

34. Wright, R.N., Arensman, R.M., Coughlin, T.R., et al., Hernia reduction en masse. The Am. Surg. 43:627, 1977.

35. Yurko, A.A., Williams, R.D., Needle paracentesis in blunt abdominal trauma: A critical analysis. J. Trauma 6:194, 1966.

Airway Procedures

2

I. Essential Anatomy of the Airway and Basic Airway Maneuvers
  A. Stages of Obstruction
    1. Common Traumatic Conditions
  B. Breathing Adequately without Obstruction
    1. Nasal Cannula   3. Venturi Mask
    2. Plastic Face Mask   4. Oxygen Reservoir Mask
  C. Breathing Spontaneously with Obstruction
    1. Search for Foreign Body   4. Jaw Thrust Maneuver
      Obstruction of the Airway   5. Oropharyngeal Airway
    2. Head Tilt Maneuver   6. Nasopharyngeal Airway
    3. Chin Lift Maneuver
  D. Apnea with Complete Airway Obstruction
    1. Heimlich Maneuver
  E. Apnea without Airway Obstruction
    1. Mouth-to-Mouth Breathing   4. Oxygen Powered Manually
    2. Pocket Mask   Triggered Breathing Device
    3. Bag Valve Mask

II. Neonatal Resuscitation
  A. Congenital Causes of an Obstructed Airway in the Newborn
    1. Choanal Atresia   3. Micrognathia
    2. Macroglossia   4. Other Causes
  B. Asphyxia and the Airway
  C. Cardiac Compression and Defibrillation in the Neonate
  D. Guidelines for Neonatal Resuscitation

III. Intubation of the Trachea
  A. Endotracheal Intubation per Orotracheal Route
    1. Advantages of   4. Equipment
      Endotracheal Intubation   5. Technique
    2. Indications   6. Special Considerations
    3. Contraindications   and Helpful Hints
  B. Nasotracheal Intubation
    1. Indications   4. Technique
    2. Contraindications   5. Complications
    3. Equipment
  C. Esophageal Obturator Airway
    1. Advantages   5. Equipment
    2. Disadvantages   6. Technique
    3. Indications   7. Aftercare
    4. Contraindications   8. Complications
  D. Esophageal Gastric Tube Airway

IV. Tracheotomy
  A. Cricothyroidotomy
    1. Indications   4. Technique
    2. Contraindications   5. Complications
    3. Equipment
  B. Tracheostomy
    1. Indications   4. Technique
    2. Contraindications   5. Aftercare
    3. Equipment   6. Complications
  C. Tracheotomy in the Patient with Massive Neck Swelling

V. Ancillary Procedures
  A. Percutaneous Transtracheal Catheter Ventilation
    1. Indications   3. Technique
    2. Equipment   4. Complications
  B. Bronchoscopy
    1. Indications   3. Technique
    2. Equipment
  C. Transtracheal Aspiration
    1. Technique   2. Complications
  D. Pulmonary Aspiration and Nasotracheal Suctioning

ESSENTIAL ANATOMY OF THE AIRWAY AND BASIC AIRWAY MANEUVERS

A thorough understanding of both the surface and structural anatomy of the airway, particularly that of the upper respiratory tract, is fundamental to the emergency physician. A detailed description and discussion of the upper respiratory tract anatomy is beyond the scope of this text.

The upper airway is best thought of as a "Y," with one arm of the "Y" being the oral passage and the other the nasal and the two joining in the hypopharynx. The problems in either arm of the "Y" which the emergency physician deals with are primarily obstructive in nature. If either "arm of the Y" is obstructed, the patient will still be able to breath adequately; therefore, respiratory obstruction must have either both arms obstructed or an obstruction at the area where they join, the hypopharynx, or else an obstruction proximal to this site.

In the oral passage, obstruction is usually due to the tongue which tends to fall posteriorly and cause obstruction when in the supine position. In the nasal passage, obstruction is usually due to swelling from nasal fractures and/or maxillofacial injuries and is less consequential than obstruction of the oral passage.

There are four causes of respiratory inadequacy that present to the emergency center:

1. Obstruction
2. Respiratory failure
   a. Parenchymal (emphysema, tension pneumothorax, tracheal tear)
   b. Neurogenic (drug induced, depression of the respiratory center due to metabolic causes)
3. Musculoskeletal disorders
   a. Chest wall trauma
   b. Diseases of muscles (myasthenia gravis)
4. Cardiorespiratory arrest

CRITICAL QUESTION

The physician must first ask himself—Is the patient breathing normally, ventilating and moving air adequately or is there evidence of obstruction?

Stages of Obstruction

The symptoms and signs of respiratory obstruction have been graded by Forbes (27) according to severity and this system has been modified by Verrill (89).

Stage I   This stage is a mild form of upper airway obstruction characterized by hoarseness, cough, and stridorous respirations on moderate exertion. Generally, these patients have either oral or nasal obstruction alone and not both.

Stage II   These patients present with stridor on slight exertion and have associated signs of increased work of breathing, rib retraction on inspiration, use of accessory muscles of respiration, alae nasi dilating on inspiration, and suprasternal retraction.

Stage III   Stridor occurs at rest, the patient is apprehensive and restless with sweating, pallor, increased pulse rate and blood pressure. These patients have severe obstruction.

Stage IV   This stage represents very severe obstruction with slowing of respirations, hypotension, cyanosis, and impaired consciousness. If these patients are not treated immediately, death ensues shortly.

It is those patients who are in stages III and IV who are of most immediate concern to the emergency physician and in whom accurate assessment of the cause and relief of symptoms are urgently needed. Verrill (89) has divided the common causes of airway obstruction into five groups: oral obstruction, nasal obstruction, pharyngeal obstruction, laryngeal obstruction, and finally tracheal obstruction. A modification of this system into those disorders which should be considered in the patient presenting to the emergency center are grouped in Tables 2.1 through 2.4.

Table 2.1.   Causes of Oral Obstruction Seen in the Emergency Center

Neoplastic
Tumors of the palate and floor of the mouth, jaws, or tongue
Inflammatory
Oral Infections
Osteomyelitis of the mandible
Dental Infections with association trismus
Ludwig's angina
Temporomandibular joint (TMJ) syndrome and TMJ arthritis
Caustic agents ingested
Traumatic
Fractures of the facial bones or mandible with swelling
Swelling associated with severe facial injuries
Neurological
Tetanus
Allergies
Angioneurotic edema or severe allergic reactions

Table 2.3.   Causes of Pharyngeal Obstruction Presenting to the Emergency Center

Neoplastic
Carcinoma
Inflammatory
Hypertrophy of uvula
Hypertrophied tonsils
Peritonsillar abscess
Retropharyngeal abscess
Severe pharyngitis
Traumatic
Caustic burns with acids or alkali
Posteriorly displaced tongue in facial trauma
Blood and vomitus following facial and oral injuries
Neurologic
Bulbar palsy
Foreign bodies
Fish and chicken bones
Allergies
Angioneurotic edema
Stings

Table 2.2.   Causes of Nasal Obstruction Presenting to the Emergency Center

Congenital
Deviated septum
Postchoanal atresia in the neonate
Neoplastic
Polyps
Cysts
Carcinoma
Inflammatory
Coryza
Abscesses
Adenoids
Traumatic
Septal hematoma
Nasal fracture
Allergic
Allergic rhinitis
Foreign body
For example, buttons and beads (especially in children)

Table 2.4.   Causes of Laryngeal and Tracheal Obstruction Presenting to the Emergency Center

Congenital	Traumatic
Stenosis	Fracture of the larynx
Cysts	Tracheal rupture
Neoplastic	Allergic
Carcinoma	Glottic edema
Polyps	Angioneurotic edema
Inflammatory	Neurologic
Laryngitis	Laryngeal spasm
Diphtheria	Laryngeal tetany
Epiglottitis	Foreign body
Tracheitis	Laryngeal obstruction
Croup	most common; tracheal obstruction is rare.

COMMON TRAUMATIC CONDITIONS

Maximal edema is reached in 24 to 48 hours following facial trauma (58). In patients with fractures of the mandibular arch, collapse may allow the base of the tongue to obstruct the entrance to the larynx and lead to signs of airway obstruction. When it is not possible to easily pass an oral or nasal airway in these patients, a large towel clip or suture passed through the anterior tongue will permit traction to be used to bring both the tongue and the mandibular arch forward (29).

In obtunded patients with or without trauma, a common misconception is that "swallowing of the tongue" is prevented by placing the patient in a prone position. Studies have shown no difference in the incidence of or the degree of pharyngeal obstruction with patients in either the prone or supine position (69). Flexion of the neck was found to worsen obstruction significantly in both positions (69).

Some controversy is found in the literature regarding the management of patients with laryngotracheal trauma. Some authors prefer emergency tracheostomy (2, 14), while others feel that careful endotracheal intubation yields excellent results (46, 77). In our opinion, it would seem that careful endotracheal intubation via the orotracheal route yields good results and is advocated whenever possible.

Foreign Bodies

The sixth most common cause of accidental death in the United States is foreign body obstruction of the airway (83). Most foreign bodies in the trachea that cause severe obstruction are located in the subglottic area (83). If the particle is distal to the cricoid cartilage, a bronchoscope is needed to remove it. In patients with airway obstruction so severe that the patient cannot speak, the Heimlich maneuver should be used. Otherwise, the patient should be manipulated as little as possible and emergency bronchoscopy used. The removal of foreign bodies in children is best done under general anesthesia.

The procedures listed and described in this chapter are divided into those useful when there is an adequate airway with no obstruction and those used when there is not an adequate airway with or without obstructive symptoms.

Breathing Adequately without Obstruction

If the patient is breathing adequately with no evidence of obstruction but needs supplemental oxygen, four modalities or modifications thereof are available for delivering oxygen.

NASAL CANNULA

NOTE

This delivers an unpredictable amount of oxygen varying between 25 and 40% with a flow rate of 6 liters/minute, de-

pending on the ratio of mouth to nose breathing in a given patient.

Procedure

1. Place the cannula into the patient's nostrils.
2. Lead the tubing around the patient's ears and tighten.

PLASTIC FACE MASK (SIMPLE MASK)

NOTE

This supplies 50 to 60% oxygen at a flow rate of 10 liters/minute.

VENTURI MASK

NOTE

The Venturi mask is used in the patient whose respiratory failure is secondary to chronic lung disease or who has hypercarbia, in whom it would be dangerous to administer an unpredictable volume of oxygen which may induce respiratory arrest by suppressing the respiratory center "drive to breath." These masks are available to deliver 24, 28, 35, and 40% FiO_2 and require a flow rate of 4, 4, 8, and 8 liters of oxygen per minute respectively.

OXYGEN RESERVOIR MASK

NOTE

This mask stores oxygen in a reservoir during expiration; when the patient inspires, this oxygen is inhaled from the reservoir. If a very tight seal is maintained, one can delivery an oxygen concentration of 90%. Fifty to 60% of the stored oxygen is the maximum delivered with the usual fit of a mask.

Breathing Spontaneously with Obstruction

With incomplete obstruction, the patient has labored breathing, excessive use of the accessory muscles, intercostal retraction, supraclavicular retraction, and a "crowing" sound on inspiration. The patient may be ashen gray or cyanotic, and there may be posterior displacement of the tongue. In the patient with signs of respiratory distress and signs of incomplete obstruction, consider the causes listed in Tables 2.1 through 2.4. Perform the following maneuvers, as indicated.

SEARCH FOR FOREIGN BODY OBSTRUCTION OF THE AIRWAY

The search for a foreign body obstructing the airway should be a very quick and superficial examination. One has no time to do a meticulous examination of the patient. Search for a bolus of food or foreign particle lodged in the posterior pharynx, dentures occluding the airway, or a large posteriorly displaced tongue. When one must provide an airway immediately, if the superficial search including jaw thrust or chin lift maneuvers discloses no obvious foreign body obstruction which can be relieved immediately, then a cricothyroidotomy should be performed next.

Ruben (68) evaluated three airway maneuvers and found the chin lift, jaw thrust, and head tilt useful techniques in the flaccid subject. For the chance rescuer, the head tilt method is perhaps the easiest to master. When mouth to nose ventilation is used, the head tilt is the procedure of choice. With the exception of its use in the cardiac arrest victim, the traditional head tilt maneuver is no longer advocated, however. Recent studies demonstrate the ineffectiveness of this procedure in relieving upper airway obstruction when compared with the chin lift or jaw thrust.

HEAD TILT MANEUVER (Fig. 2.1)

1. In the supine patient, place one hand behind the neck under the patient's occiput.
2. Place the heel of the other hand on the patient's forehead.
3. Displace the forehead back and lift the occiput up, thereby extending the head.

Contraindications

1. Suspected cervical spine injury (52).

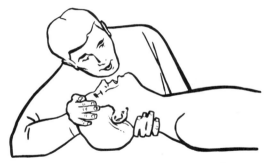

Figure 2.1. The head tilt maneuver. See text for details. (Reprinted with permission of Aspen Systems. Guildner, G.W., Resuscitation—Opening the airway. J.A.C.E.P. 5:589, 1976.)

CHIN LIFT MANEUVER (29, 52) (Fig. 2.2)

1. Place the heel of the hand on the forehead.
2. The first two fingers of the other hand are placed on the underside of the patient's chin.
3. Traction on the chin and tilting motion on the forehead extends the neck and opens the airway. This method is the most adequate and consistent means of relieving airway obstruction (5).

Contraindications

1. Cervical spine injury (52).

JAW THRUST MANEUVER (TRIPLE AIRWAY MANEUVER) (29, 52) (Fig. 2.3)

1. While standing above the patient's head, place the fingers of each hand behind the angle of the mandible, lifting and displacing the jaw forward. While doing this, the patient's lower lip may be retracted to insert an oral airway.
2. Tilt the head backwards, while the thumbs retract the lower lip and jaw.

In many instances the airway is improved by the above maneuvers. One should attempt these before resorting to any adjuncts. If they work, then place an oropharyngeal or nasopharyngeal airway as described below.

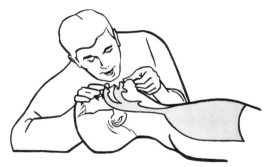

Figure 2.2. The chin lift maneuver. See text for details. (Reprinted with permission of Aspen Systems. Guildner, G.W., Resuscitation—Opening the airway. J.A.C.E.P. 5:589, 1976.)

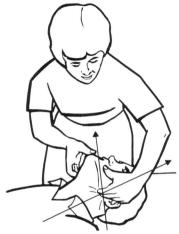

Figure 2.3. The jaw thrust maneuver or triple airway maneuver. See text for details. (Reprinted with permission of Aspen Systems. Guildner, G.W., Resuscitation—Opening the airway. J.A.C.E.P. 5:589, 1976.)

OROPHARYNGEAL AIRWAY (52)

The airway comes in various sizes from 000 for neonates to 4 for large adults. It is semicircular in shape and curved to fit behind the tongue in the lower portion of the posterior pharynx. The airway is usually made of plastic but may be made of metal or rubber. The hard plastic form is the most commonly used. When in place it extends from the lips to the posterior pharynx. The distal 2 cm includes a hard plastic guard to prevent the patient from biting and occluding the airway.

Contraindication

1. It is contraindicated in a patient with an intact gag reflex.

Technique (Fig. 2.4)

1. Insert the airway between the patient's teeth with the convexity pointing toward the patient's feet (Fig. 2.4*A*).
2. As the airway passes the back of the tongue, it is rotated around to its resting position with the concavity point-

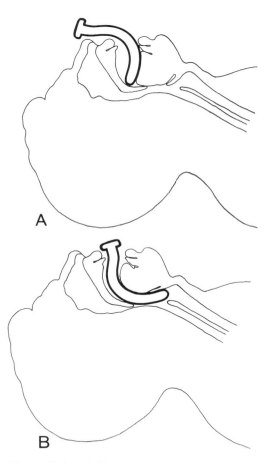

Figure 2.4. *A.* The oropharyngeal airway. The airway is inserted between the patient's teeth, with the convexity pointing toward the patient's feet. *B.* As the airway passes the back of the tongue, it is rotated around into its resting position so the concavity points toward the feet.

ing toward the feet. The airway is then inserted to the hub (Fig. 2.4B).

Alternate Method

One can also insert the airway into its proper position by using a tongue depressor to depress the tongue inferiorly while passing the airway into the pharynx.

CAUTION!

If the airway is not properly placed, it can increase the obstruction by pushing the tongue back into the pharynx.

Complications

1. Retching and vomiting
   a. Prevention and treatment
      1) Do not use the airway in the conscious patient
      2) Remove the airway and suction the oropharynx

NASOPHARYNGEAL AIRWAY (Fig. 2.5)

NOTE

The nasopharyngeal airway is made of soft rubber and is approximately 6 inches in length.

Indications

1. This airway is better tolerated in the conscious patient.

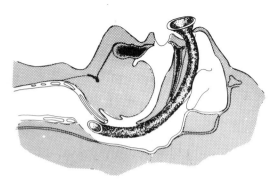

Figure 2.5.   The position of the nasopharyngeal airway. (Reprinted with permission of Annals of Internal Medicine. Warner, A., Nasopharyngeal airway: A facilitated access to the trachea. 75:594, 1971.)

Contraindications

1. Severe nasal fractures which occlude the nasal passage.

Technique

1. Select the size of airway desired, judged by the largest size which will fit into the patient's nostril.
2. Look into both nostrils for septal deviation, polyps, etc. and select the nostril which appears more open.
3. Lubricate the airway with an anesthetic lubricating solution (Xylocaine® ointment).
4. Pass the airway, with the bevel facing the nasal septum along the floor of the nose.

CAUTION!

The floor of the nose lies parallel to the oral cavity. If one recalls this anatomical point in passing the tube, then the most common complication with this procedure can be avoided, i.e., nasal bleeding.

5. Rotate the tube as it reaches the hypopharynx so that the tube sits as shown.

Complications

1. Nasal bleeding
   a. Prevention and treatment
      1) See step 4 under Technique above.
      2) No treatment is usually indicated, as the bleeding will subside spontaneously. If bleeding is significant, a nasal pack may have to be inserted.

Apnea with Complete Airway Obstruction

HEIMLICH MANEUVER

Indications

1. Upper airway obstruction due to a bolus of food or any aspirated foreign material unrelieved by coughing and traditional means which now is causing complete airway obstruction and threatening asphyxiation.

Contraindications

1. The patient who has any chest injury such as fractured ribs or flail, cardiac contusion, sternal fracture, etc.

Technique

NOTE

Recent studies have shown that the traditional Heimlich maneuver causes more complications and is not as effective as the modified technique shown in this text.

1. Sit the patient upright or have the patient stand. In patients who are lying on the ground, place them in the supine position.
2. In the patient who is sitting or standing, wrap both arms around the patient's chest with the right hand closed in a fist and placed over the midsternal region (between the nipples) while the left hand grasps the right "fist" (Fig. 2.6). In the supine patient, place the hands over the lower sternum with the right hand over the left and compress. Alternately, one may place the right hand over the lower sternum just above the xyphoid process as shown in Figure 2.7. The technique remains the same except for positioning of the hand over the sternum. Both methods are equally acceptable.
3. With a rapid forceful thrust compress the chest and the bolus will dislodge.

NOTE

In that situation in which repeated thrusts fail to dislodge the bolus and the patient is asphyxiating, one should immediately resort to a cricothyroidotomy or cricothyroid membrane puncture.

NOTE

A technique for dislodging a foreign body in a small child is shown in Figure 2.8. The child can be placed upside down,

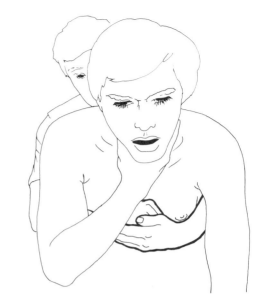

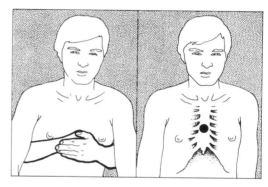

Figure 2.6. Heimlich maneuver. Wrap both arms around the patient's chest with the right hand closed in a fist and placed over the midsternal region, while the left hand grasps the right hand as shown in the inset in the lower left-hand corner. The hand should be placed between the nipples as shown in the lower left inset. Compression should be forceful and directed posteriorly.

held in the examiner's hand as shown in the figure. Forceful compression is applied with the right hand while the left hand is over the lower sternum. The authors have found this method to be quite successful in dislodging foreign bodies in smaller children. Its value compared to the Heimlich maneuver remains to be determined.

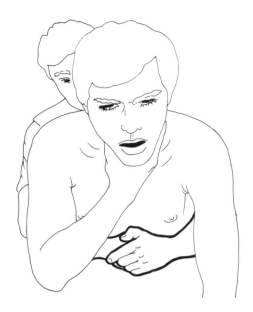

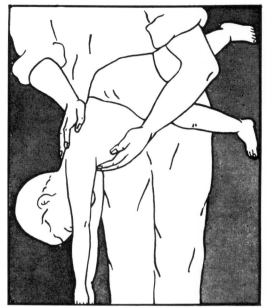

Figure 2.8. The technique for dislodging a foreign body in a small child. The child should be inverted and a sharp blow applied between the shoulder blades. (Reprinted with permission of J.A.M.A. 172:815. Copyright © 1960, American Medical Association.)

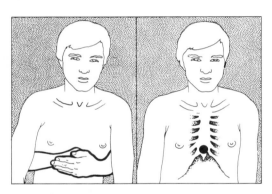

Figure 2.7. Heimlich maneuver—alternate technique. One may place the right hand over the lower sternum, just above the xyphoid process. The technique remains the same except for positioning of the hand over the sternum, as shown in the inset. See text for details.

Complications

1. Fractured ribs
   a. Prevention and treatment
      1) Unavoidable, particularly in the elderly patient with brittle rib cage.
      2) Treat as with any rib fracture.
2. Rupture of the liver or spleen.
   a. Prevention and treatment
      1) Not associated with the proce-

dure described above. A common complication of the traditional Heimlech maneuver.

Apnea without Airway Obstruction

If there is no spontaneous breathing and the possibility of complete airway obstruction is unlikely or has been eliminated by examination, proceed with the following:

MOUTH-TO-MOUTH BREATHING

NOTE

Exhaled air delivers 16 to 17% FiO_2 to the patient. Ideally this would provide a PO_2 of 80 torr; however, due to the decreased cardiac output, ventilation-perfusion abnormalities, and physiologic shunting, the actual PO_2 is much less.

Technique

1. Stand at the patient's right side and extend the head by placing the right

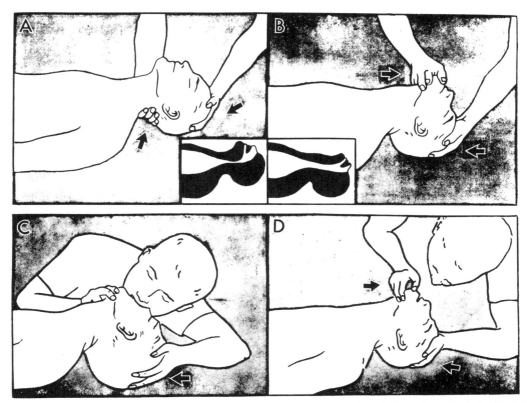

Figure 2.9.   Technique for mouth-to-mouth breathing using the head-tilt oral method. *A.* Neck is lifted. *B.* The head is fully tilted back. *C.* The lungs are inflated via the nose or mouth. *D.* Victim exhales by himself, as necessary, through his mouth. (Reprinted with permission of J.A.M.A. 172:814. Copyright © 1960, American Medical Association.)

hand under the neck. Apply upward pressure on the neck as a downward pressure is applied concomitantly over the head with the palm of the left hand (Fig. 2.9A).

2. With the thumb and index fingers of the left hand pinch the nostrils shut so as not to permit the egress of air while using upward traction on the jaw or the patient's neck to open the mouth.

3. Take a deep breath, cover the patient's mouth with yours, and forcibly exhale air into the patient's oral cavity.

Alternate Technique—Mouth to Nose Breathing

An alternate technique which can be used effectively is that of providing mouth-to-nose artificial ventilation. In this procedure, one stands at the patient's right side and extends the head as indicated above and as shown in Figure 2.9A. The left hand is used to hyperextend the neck by placing it over the patient's forehead and applying downward and backward pressure while the right hand is used to hyperextend the jaw and close the mouth (Figure 2.9B). With the patient's mouth closed, the physician can then effectively give mouth-to-nose ventilation (Fig. 2.9C). In order for this technique to be effective, there must be a patent nasal passage. *It is particularly useful in those patients in whom one cannot give mouth-to-mouth ventilation because of either vomitus, profuse bleeding from the mouth, or severe mandibular fractures. The mouth is then permitted to open slightly in order to per-*

mit exhaling of air, as shown in Figure 2.9D.

NOTE

In an infant or small child, one can exhale into both the oral and nasal passages by covering the infant's nose and mouth

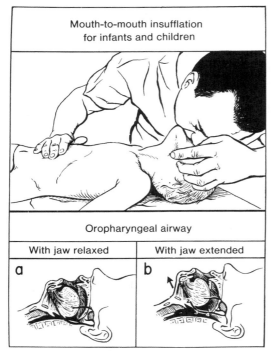

Figure 2.10 inset labels:

Mouth-to-mouth insufflation
for infants and children

Oropharyngeal airway

With jaw relaxed	With jaw extended
a	b

Figure 2.10. Technique for mouth-to-mouth resuscitation in an infant or small child. The infant is placed in the supine position with the head extended. The rescuer positions himself at the side of the head. He places the fingers of both hands beneath and behind the angles of the lower jaw and lifts vertically upward, so that it juts out into a position shown above. This is the most important step in the entire procedure since it effectively clears the oropharynx of obstruction by the tongue. In the unconscious patient, the jaw relaxes and the tongue gravitates against the posterior pharyngeal wall to occlude the oropharynx as shown in *A* above. When the mandible is extended by lifting it upward, the airway is opened as shown in *B* above. (Reprinted with permission of J.A.M.A. 167:322, Copyright © 1958, American Medical Association.)

with that of the rescuer (Fig. 2.10). An alternate method of providing mouth-to-mouth ventilation in an infant is shown and discussed in Figure 2.11.

For those patients who have vomited, it is extremely important that aspiration be prevented and that an airway be maintained. The technique of providing this is shown and discussed in Figure 2.12.

POCKET MASK

NOTE

The pocket mask has an inlet nipple for providing supplemental oxygen. With a 10 liter flow rate the mask will deliver an oxygen concentration of 50%. If the flow rate is increased to 30 liters the mask will supply oxygen at a concentration of 100% and the rescuer can occlude the portal intermittently and provide adequate ventilation to the patient without any mouth-to-mask breathing!

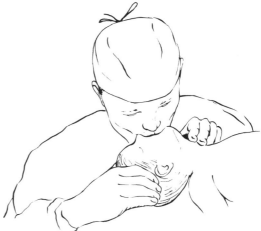

Figure 2.11. The application of gentle cricoid pressure during mouth-to-mouth resuscitation of a small infant. The use of cricoid pressure controls regurgitation of gastric contents. This also prevents inflation of the stomach during ventilation by a face mask or mouth-to-mouth. (Reprinted with permission of Anesthesiology 40:97, Copyright © 1974, Lippincott/Harper Co.)

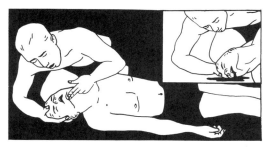

Figure 2.12.   The semilateral position for gravity drainage of fluid from the victim's oropharynx is shown. The victim's shoulders should be pulled up and stabilized with the rescuer's knee. Gentle pressure should be applied over the epigastrium to facilitate emptying fluid from the stomach. (Reprinted with permission of J.A.M.A. 172:815, Copyright © 1960, American Medical Association.)

Technique

1. The mask is applied to the patient's oral and nasal passages and held firmly by placing the thumbs on either side of the mask while index, middle and ring fingers grasp the mandible pulling it upwards, which opens the airway for ventilation.

Advantages of Pocket Mask

1. Eliminates contact with the patient.
2. Provides good ventilation.
3. Easier to use than the bag valve mask devices.
4. Contains an inlet for the provision of supplemental oxygen.

BAG VALVE MASK (LAERDAL BAG[R])

NOTE

This device is very familiar to all emergency personnel. It is found in every emergency center and ambulance. While it is perhaps the most popular modality for providing artificial ventilation, it has numerous disadvantages when compared with the pocket mask and other adjuncts to ventilation which have up to now not been adequately appreciated.

Features this device should contain

1. The bag should be self-refilling and contain no sponge-rubber on the inside lining. The sponge rubber can become friable and also is difficult to sterilize in cleaning the bag.
2. The bag must feature a non-jam valve system. The purpose of this is that some valves may become jammed with vomitus and may function poorly or not at all. The newer bags contain a non-jam valve system which does not permit this to happen.
3. The mask should be transparent and made of plastic. A clear transparent plastic will permit the examiner to see if there are any foreign particles or vomitus contained in the bag, which the black bags previously used do not allow.
4. Provisions for delivering supplemental oxygen.
5. A non pop-off valve. The pop-off valve contained on some pediatric bags will pop off once a predetermined pressure is reached during the delivery of the air contained within the bag. Thus, the patient does not receive the full volume of air contained within the bag when high pressures are necessary to deliver that volume.
6. The capability to be used with an oropharyngeal airway.

NOTE

The Ambu[R] bag does not meet all of the requirements listed above, and the authors recommend the Laerdal[R] bag which is available in several sizes for both pediatric and adult age-groups.

NOTE

When attached to supplemental oxygen at 12 liters/min, the bag valve mask will deliver only a 40% FiO_2 providing there is a tight seal. If one attaches an oxygen reservoir and adapter, an oxygen concentration of 90% can be achieved.

Technique

1. Remove foreign material. Leave dentures in place unless obstructing the airway. Dentures may render a good mouth-bag seal which is almost impossible to achieve in the edentulous patient.
2. Insert an oral airway.
3. Extend the neck and elevate the mandible to open the hypopharynx.
4. Apply the mask over the nose and mouth.

NOTE

Various size masks are available for children and adults. Select the mask which provides the tightest seal and conforms best to the patient's nose and mouth.

5. Squeeze the mask with the right hand and produce a tight seal, using the last 2 or 3 fingers to support the mandible while the thumb and first one or two fingers are placed over the mask on either side of the valve connection. The left hand is then used to squeeze the bag. When enough personnel are available, a better seal is provided with two operators—one to hold the mask in place and mandible extended while the other squeezes the bag.
6. Tilt the head and inflate the lungs.
7. Observe for chest movement.
8. For prolonged ventilation using this device, one should place a nasogastric tube to prevent gastric distension.

Advantages of the Bag Valve Mask

1. Provides an immediate means of ventilating the patient.
2. Enriched oxygen can be supplied.
3. Permits the operator to assess the compliance of the lungs. This clinical determination is lost when oxygen-powered devices are used.

Disadvantages of Bag Valve Mask

1. A lower tidal volume is delivered than with the mouth-to-mouth technique or the pocket mask.

2. Difficult for even the skilled practitioner to provide a perfect seal.
3. Gastric distension is a very common sequela.

Contraindications

1. Oral bleeding or vomiting.
2. Upper airway obstruction or injury.
3. Severe maxillofacial fractures.

OXYGEN-POWERED MANUALLY TRIGGERED BREATHING DEVICE

In an arrest situation, one cannot use pressure-cycled respirators. When chest compression is performed, this triggers the device to shut off prematurely due to the increase in intrathoracic pressure associated with chest compressions. This abbreviated respiration causes the patient to receive an inadequate volume. Volume-cycled respirators cannot be used either since one cannot properly synchronize compressions with ventilations.

With the oxygen-powered breathing devices, both these problems are overcome due to the manual triggering of the device (timing) and the delivery of high-flow oxygen at 100 liters/min. Do not use these devices for long periods, as they are associated with a high incidence of gastric distension.

Two additional modalities should be mentioned although not used. The *S-tube* is a device similar to the oral-pharyngeal airway in that it does assist in keeping the mouth open; however, it does not provide an adequate seal in the oropharynx and may induce emesis by irritating the oropharynx.

The *Accordian bag mask* is totally unacceptable and should never be used. This device is no longer available in most facilities as it does not meet any of the requirements of a good bag valve mask device.

CAUTION!

Remember to suction the patient's mouth and pharynx periodically while using any of the adjuncts described above in the patient who is not *spontaneously breathing*.

NEONATAL RESUSCITATION

Neonatal resuscitation is perhaps the most mentally taxing situation which confronts the emergency physician. An approach must be devised which will permit the rapid assessment and judicious care of the neonate. The approach advocated below can be modified according to the individual needs of the neonate. The emphasis here is on the newborn as this is the most common situation for neonatal resuscitation by an emergency physician.

Congenital Causes of an Obstructed Airway in the Newborn

Intrinsic obstructing lesions of the larynx and trachea are rare. When they occur they cause almost immediate asphyxiation after birth. They are manifested by stridor or crowing and usually require endoscopy to confirm the diagnosis (66).

CHOANAL ATRESIA

All infants are obligate nasal breathers until 9 months of age. Infants with choanal atresia will develop respiratory distress, especially during feeding. Catheter probing of the nose demonstrates a block bilaterally. If this patient presents in the first month of life to the emergency center with a compatible history, the treatment consists of an oral airway, tube feeding and admission for operative perforation of the posterior membrane (66).

MACROGLOSSIA

These infants usually have a lymphangioma. The treatment consists of positioning the neonate in the prone position for mild obstruction, and tracheostomy or percutaneous transtracheal ventilation in the emergency center may be necessary in severe cases.

MICROGNATHIA

This condition often presents in association with cleft palate. In severe cases, sternal retraction, cyanosis, and sudden asphyxia may be noted. For mild cases, the treatment consists of placing the infant in the prone position and a temporary anterior glossopexy by a suture placed through the mid or posterior tongue and tied in the anterior sublingual region to displace the tongue forward.

OTHER CAUSES

Other causes include tumors, e.g., cystic hygroma, of the mouth, pharynx, or neck which may require emergency treatment when the patient presents with airway obstruction. A congenital goiter may obstruct the airway of the child of a mother who is on goitrogenic drugs, especially iodides. Usually respiratory difficulty subsides with appropriate treatment after delivery.

Asphyxia and the Airway

In studies on puppies and monkeys (20) who were asphyxiated at birth, the first stage observed was very rapid dyspneic breathing. After 1.5 to 2.5 minutes of asphyxia, apnea ensued. This stage is called *primary apnea* and lasts for approximately 2 minutes. If the asphyxia continues, then the animal begins gasping which continues for 3 minutes. After 8 minutes of total asphyxia the last gasp occurs and *secondary apnea* ensues. This period of apnea continues until death. If asphyxia is relieved after primary apnea, the animal will recover and begin gasping. If secondary apnea has occurred, recovery will not be spontaneous. The duration of secondary apnea will determine the time needed for assisted ventilation before breathing occurs on its own. As a rough rule, for every minute of secondary apnea before the onset of ventilation 2 minutes of ventilation will be required before breathing begins on its own and 4 minutes before spontaneous regular ventilation occurs. Thus, for 5 minutes of secondary apnea a total of 20 minutes of ventilation will be needed before breathing occurs on its own.

The newborn is sensitive to hypoxia. Eight to 10 minutes of total anoxia will result in permanent brain damage (20). Bradycardia in the newborn usually means hypoxia (66). To clear the airway, the nares and anterior oral cavity should be aspirated with a bulb syringe. Suction should precede bagging. If the newborn is meconium-stained, bag-mask ventilation is contraindicated before the cords are exposed by a laryngoscope and direct suctioning is performed, otherwise meconium aspiration and severe pneumonitis are likely (1). Any child can be adequately ventilated by bag-mask ventilation without endotracheal intubation unless unusual circumstances exist. If bag-mask ventilation does not suffice and an airway is needed, orotracheal intubation should be performed in the infant with agonal or no spontaneous breathing. If the child has spontaneous respirations, some authors prefer nasotracheal intubation with a small Magill forceps (1) due to the more stable fixation of the tube. A nasotracheal tube of similar size to the orotracheal tube may be used. No cuff is needed because the subglottic tracheal diameter is narrow, which ensures a good tracheal seal. With orotracheal intubation, do not hyperextend the head but rather slightly elevate the head with the neck flexed in a sniffing position. If time permits, insert a gastric tube before endotracheal intubation and suction the stomach. Remove this tube (suctioning while removing it), when the infant is to be endotracheally intubated.

Cardiac Compression and Defibrillation in the Neonate

There are two acceptable methods advocated for cardiac compression in the neonate (1, 8, 20, 23). The physician wraps both hands around the infant's chest, encircling the chest, and with both thumbs at the midpoint of the sternum compresses the sternum approximately 1.5 to 2 cm at a rate of 100 to 120/min. Alternatively, one hand can be placed beneath the infant and the other over the sternum with the index and middle fingers touching the midsternum and compressing in a similar fashion. When these two methods were compared and the pressures generated were quantitated via a femoral catheter, the two-handed method encircling the infant's chest was found to be superior (85).

The energy dose needed for defibrillat-

ing a neonate is 2 w-sec/kg or about 1 w-sec/lb. This energy is adequate for defibrillating children under 50 kg. If the first attempt does not work, then one can double the energy dose and repeat (34).

Guidelines for Neonatal Resuscitation

On the basis of the foregoing considerations, the following guidelines are suggested for treating infants who have depressed respirations after delivery (8, 20, 23).

1. The mouth and nares of the newborn should be gently aspirated with a bulb syringe as soon as the head is delivered. The newborn should be held in the head-down position to permit gravity to aid in the drainage of secretions. After delivery, continue this position and further suctioning should be performed with the bulb syringe or a DeLee suction trap. The DeLee suction trap has a catheter connected to a small container, which permits suctioning of copious secretions and analysis of the secretions retained within the trap.

CAUTION!

Overvigorous suctioning of the posterior pharynx will result in vagally induced bradycardia and laryngospasm.

The newborn is unable to shiver to produce heat and generates heat through the oxidation of its brown fat which consumes oxygen. This oxidation induces further hypoxia and acidosis so the infant must be placed on a warm resuscitation table with a radiant heater over it.

2. Place neonate on warm resuscitation table in head-down position with heat source overhead.
3. Quickly check for congenital causes of airway obstruction. This check includes probing the nose with a small catheter to demonstrate a block bilaterally (choanal atresia).

An examination of the mouth to check for macroglossia, micrognathia, cleft palate, a goiter in the neck or "tumors" in the mouth, the pharynx, or the neck should also be made. A detailed discussion of these is in the section "Congenital Causes of Airway Obstruction in the Newborn" above.

4. If the infant does not respond to these measures, moderate depression exists. The airway must be cleared before ventilating with a bag and mask.

NOTE

Neonates born through particulate meconium are prone to develop aspiration pneumonitis. When this occurs the infant should be delivered and passed to the resuscitation table with minimal stimulation. Stimulation of the infant who has meconium staining may cause aspiration of the meconium as the infant takes a breath. The trachea should then be cleared by passing an endotracheal tube under direct vision with a laryngoscope and suction on this tube as it is withdrawn from the infant's trachea. This will remove the large plugs or meconium which are too large to be aspirated by a suction catheter. This procedure should be repeated until the aspirate is clear. Remember that oxygenation of the infant is necessary after each endotracheal intubation and suction. This oxygenation is provided by gently bagging the patient, using supplemental O_2, after suctioning through the endotracheal tube. Meconium may not be present in the pharynx in these infants and may still be present in the trachea, so this procedure should be followed in all meconium-bathed infants.

5. The infant should be ventilated by mouth-to-mouth resuscitation if a bag and mask are not available. Remember that in the newborn, it is necessary to cover the baby's nose and mouth for effective ventilation. In those infants who have sponta-neous respirations in whom mouth-to-mouth or bag mask ventilation is not necessary, supplemental O_2 can be supplied by a small O_2 mask held over the patient's mouth and nose. In this early stage, retrolental fibroplasia, while being a concern, should not prevent the physician from giving high concentrations of oxygen in the *immediate* efforts to resuscitate the infant.

If these initial resuscitative measures have produced no response by 1½ minutes after delivery, the progressing asphyxia may lead to diminished muscular tone and a fall in heart rate.

6. A small plastic oropharyngeal airway should be inserted into the mouth, and the infant should be ventilated with a bag mask with supplemental oxygen applied (ideally under a pressure of 16 to 20 cm of water) for 1 to 2 seconds. It is difficult to estimate this pressure unless previous experience shows what this amount of pressure feels like.

NOTE

The newborn generates negative intrathoracic pressures of 80 cm of water spontaneously on its first breath. The bag and mask oxygen will not produce these kinds of pressure; however, oxygen will be forced down to the level of the terminal bronchioles where some gas exchange does take place. The increase in intrabronchial pressure stimulates the pulmonary stretch receptors and will initiate a gasp in about 85% of infants (23).

7. If there is no respiratory effort and the heart rate continues to fall, the larynx should be visualized with a laryngoscope; if foreign material obstructs the larynx quick brief suction is indicated. When the glottis is visualized, a curved endotracheal tube is inserted. Brief puffs of air blown through the tube with enough force to cause the lower chest to rise will

usually initiate spontaneous respiration. With the first or second application of positive pressure, the infant usually makes an effort to breath and the endotracheal tube may be withdrawn after the infant has taken 5 or 6 breaths (23). A severely depressed infant may need 6 to 8 minutes of artificial ventilation before spontaneous gasping ensues (23).

NOTE

In infants born to heroin-addicted mothers, naloxone should be administered. The dose is 10 $\mu g/kg$ over 1 to 3 times. Since the narcotically depressed infant has normal circulation, the drug is effective intramuscularly (20).

8. If, despite adequate ventilation and external massage for 2 or 3 minutes, there is no improvement in the color, muscle tone, or heart rate, then an umbilical catheter should be inserted (see "Vascular Procedures") and sodium bicarbonate administered.
    a. Dilute 5 ml of bicarbonate with 5 cc of 5% dextrose and water. This 10 ml solution then contains 5 mEq of sodium bicarbonate and can be administered to the neonate who weighs 3 kg at a dose of 1.5 mEq/kg. If no response is elicited then an additional 0.75 mEq/kg can be administered.
    b. Obtain blood for pH, PO_2, PCO_2 and bicarbonate as soon as possible.
9. Administer 1 to 2 ml/kg of 50% glucose if there is no response to the above steps.
10. If no marked improvement is elicited after the preceding steps, dilute 1 ml (1 mg) of a 1:1000 epinephrine solution in 10 ml of isotonic saline and give 0.5 to 2.0 ml of this solution until the heart rate is increased to above 70 beats per minute.
11. Continue ventilation and cardiac massage throughout this period, as indicated by the infant's status. Remember to minimize heat loss and oxygen consumption.
12. Place the infant in a bassinette after resuscitation and transfer to the nursery.

INTUBATION OF THE TRACHEA

Endotracheal Intubation per Orotracheal Route

Advantages of Endotracheal Intubation

1. Protects against aspiration and achieves complete control of airway.
2. Eliminates gastric distension associated with mouth-to-mouth, mouth-to-mask, bag valve mask, and O_2 powered devices used for ventilation.
3. Suctioning of the trachea is possible.
4. Permits better elimination of CO_2.

Indications

1. Respiratory arrest or cardiorespiratory arrest.
2. Hypoventilation or hypoxia. Patients who have neuromuscular disturbances which impair respiratory function may require endotracheal intubation because of hypoventilation and hypoxia (13).
3. Inability to ventilate a patient who is unconscious by other conventional means.
4. Prolonged artificial ventilation.
5. Moderate to severe flail chest.
6. To isolate the trachea and prevent aspiration.
7. Some feel that endotracheal intubation can be performed with little difficulty in acute epiglotitis (45).
8. To prevent airway obstruction and aspiration of vomitus in CNS depressed patient (65).

NOTE

Endotracheal intubation is indicated if the lash reflex is absent, response to stimulation is not purposeful, or airway obstruction develops when the patient's neck is flexed (65).

A misconception exists about an empty stomach. The stomach is never completely empty no matter how long the depressed patient may have been without food. In the absence of recent food ingestion, the normal stomach will secrete at least 50 ml of gastric juice per hour (40). Patients are often thought of as having an empty stomach if intake has not occurred in the preceding 8 hours; however, in some situations food ingested before this time may remain in the stomach, i.e., ulcers and obstructing lesions may delay gastric emptying. In addition, any acute abdominal process will delay gastric emptying. Sepsis, systemic diseases, and medications also may delay emptying.

Aspiration of blood, mucus, and saliva does not lead to serious complications in such patients (40). The acidic fluid is a severe respiratory irritant, causing large secretions and respiratory compromise.

Contraindications

1. Severe injury to the larynx. Controversy exists on laryngotracheal trauma. Some authors (2) prefer emergency tracheotomy in these patients, while others (77) recommend careful endotracheal intubation. Careful endotracheal intubation has many advocates (46).
2. Severe maxillofacial trauma.
3. Fracture or possible fracture of the cervical spine.

Equipment

Laryngoscope with assorted sized blades.

NOTE

Two types of blades are available, the MacIntosh and the straight blade (Fig. 2.13). Each is available in a variety of sizes for children and adults. The practitioner usually finds one or the other type more comfortable to him. While the choice between the MacIntosh and the straight blade is primarily that of personal preference, there are some distinct situations in which one is preferred over the other.

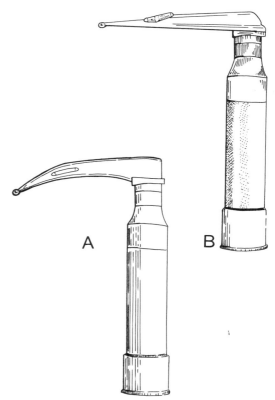

Figure 2.13. The MacIntosh (A) and straight (B) blades are shown.

These are discussed in the appropriate area in the section on procedure.

Endotracheal tubes in sizes 3 through 9.5.

NOTE

All of these tubes have a standard 15 mm adapter to fit bag or ventilator. Tubes less than 7 mm do not have a cuff. Generally, patients under 8 years of age do not need a cuffed tube, as the cartilaginous trachea is "soft" and a well-fitting endotracheal tube will sufficiently "seal" the airway.

Lubricating jelly
Stylet
Topical spray anesthetic
10 cc syringe
Suction catheters

NOTE

One should have both tracheal suction catheters to suction secretions from the tube and rigid (tonsil) suction for oral secretions and vomitus.

Technique

Preparatory Steps

1. Select the proper tube. In urgent situations remember that in the average adult an 8 mm tube works well.

NOTE

The adult male patient generally takes an 8.5 to 9.5 mm tube. The average adult female takes a 7.5 to 8.5 mm tube. In the child, the tube size should approximately equal the diameter of the patient's small finger.

> In the patient with a narrow pharynx, a smaller tube than one would otherwise judge appropriate is indicated to facilitate visualization and placement (72). In determining whether a patient has a narrow pharynx, clinical judgment must be used. Those patients with a narrow, long neck and a small mouth and those with long faces can be assumed to have a narrow pharynx and a smaller tube size would be used, such as a 7 mm tube in the average adult male.

2. Attach a syringe with 10 ml of air to the portal of the tube. A child between 8 and 12 years of age needs only 5 cc of air in the syringe. One must use clinical judgment here, as some 12-year-olds are large enough to be considered adults.
3. If time permits, check the cuff for air leaks.
4. If one is going to use a stylet, insert it into the tube at this time. The stylet must be recessed one-half inch from the end of the tube.

CAUTION!

A stylet which sticks out of the end of the tube may cause tracheal perforation or injury to the vocal cords! This potential danger is the prime reason that many anesthesiologists do not permit stylets into their operating suites.

5. Select a blade, either the MacIntosh or straight blade of appropriate size to negotiate the oropharynx.

NOTE

In patients with a short thick neck, the MacIntosh blade may be somewhat easier to use in visualizing the glottic opening. These patients tend to have a more posteriorly placed tongue and epiglottis. In infants and small children the straight blade is preferred, due to the large size of these patients' heads as compared with the rest of the torso. While the curved blade can be used in these patients, due to the proximity and small size of the epiglottis in relation to the glottic opening, the curved blade may not provide sufficient visualization of the opening as it does not displace the epiglottis as does the straight blade. Some individuals who have been well-trained in the use of the curved blade, however, have not found this to be a problem.

6. Lubricate the tube.

Procedural Steps

Ideally, intubation should take no more than 20 to 30 seconds. If particular attention is paid to those steps which are in italics, the requisite skill will be attained. In a survey of difficult or unsuccessful intubations involving anesthetists, medical students, and physicians, one of these steps was either omitted or performed improperly and this led to the difficulties encountered in the majority of cases (72).

CAUTION!

Ventilate the patient well before attempting intubation, including between unsuccessful attempts! If this is not done, one may cause arrhythmias or sudden death (78). No attempt at endotracheal intubation should persist for more than 50 to 60 seconds without artificial ventilation.

1. *Align the axis of the mouth, pharynx, and larynx in a straight line (53, 72). This is accomplished by extending the head at the atlanto-occipital joint and flexing the neck (Fig. 2.14) (note flexion of neck by small towel placed beneath the head). This maneuver of aligning the mouth with the posterior pharynx and the larynx converts their normal relationship to each other from that of a semicircular curve to more of a gentle curve approximating that of a straight line. One can facilitate this maneuver by locating the tracheal axis first and then proceed to align the mouth and posterior pharynx with this axis. This places the patient in what is commonly referred to as the "sniffing" position.*

NOTE

In the endotracheal intubation in which visualization of the glottis is difficult, two maneuvers may be of use. Place a *folded towel* under the occiput which will flex the neck, aiding in aligning the axes of the larynx and the mouth (Fig. 2.14). Compression of the larynx often facilitates visualization of the glottis.

CAUTION!

Do not permit the head to hang over the bed (extension of neck rather than flexion) during endotracheal intubation as this displaces the desired axes. At the very least the head should be horizontal with the shoulders. Extension of the neck will cause anterior displacement of the larynx and make it difficult to visualize the glottis.

2. *Use two fingers to open the mouth widely (thumb and index finger of left hand) and a third (middle finger) to displace the tongue to the left (72).*

NOTE

A common error is in not opening the patient's mouth wide enough for adequate visualization.

3. Remove dentures and foreign material with the right hand and suction any secretions, blood, or vomitus from the oral cavity, using the tonsil suction. Keep dentures nearby. If the

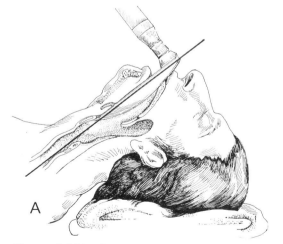
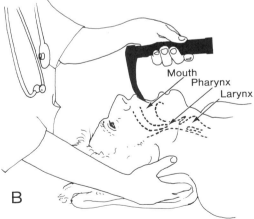

Figure 2.14. *A.* Aligning of the axis of the mouth, pharynx, and larynx. *B.* This is accomplished by extending the head at the atlanto-occipital joint and flexing the neck. Note flexion of the neck by a small towel placed beneath the head for difficult cases.

initial attempts at endotracheal intubation is unsuccessful, dentures may be needed for good seal with bag mask ventilation.

4. *With the laryngoscope held in the left hand, insert the blade from the right aiming toward the posterior midline of the tongue, while displacing the tongue to the left with the blade (34).*

5. Applying forceful leverage to the blade in an upward direction and *not traction* (the *arrow* in Figure 2.15 shows the direction in which the traction is applied with the laryngoscope blade), advance the blade until the epiglottis is visualized. The eyes of the intubationist need to be in line with the epiglottis for visualization of the glottis, which often requires the physician to crouch down.

CAUTION!

One must be careful not to use the laryngoscope as a lever against the upper incisors, as this process may fracture a tooth which can later be aspirated!

6. *MacIntosh*—If the MacIntosh is used, position the tip of the blade into the vallecula (Fig. 2.16).
Straight blade—If the straight blade is used, uplift the epiglottis with the blade (Fig. 2.15).

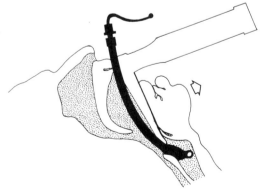

Figure 2.15. Applying forceful leverage to the blade in an upward direction as shown by the *arrow*. Advance the blade until the epiglottis is visualized.

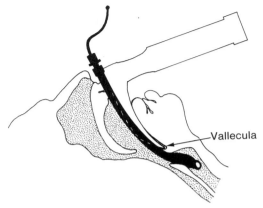

Figure 2.16. If the MacIntosh blade is used, position the tip of the blade into the vallecula.

7. *MacIntosh*—While applying upward leverage to the epiglottis with the blade positioned anterior to the epiglottis and in the vallecula, visualize the arytenoid cartilages or the glottic opening and advance the endotracheal tube into the trachea. Figure 2.17 shows the vocal cords and glottic opening as visualized through the laryngoscope. When using the curved blade (MacIntosh) one may see only the epiglottis and the arytenoid cartilages through the laryngoscope; however, the glottis lies between these two structures. All that is necessary in order to insert the endotracheal tube accurately into the trachea is visualization of the epiglottis and arytenoid cartilages through the curved blade. With the straight blade the vocal cords are usually visualized, making accurate placement more definitively assessed by the physician.
Straight blade—Lift the epiglottis upward and visualize the vocal cords as you apply leverage, displacing the epiglottis. Pass the endotracheal tube into the trachea once the glottis is seen.

NOTE

The tube should be passed only during inspiration in the patient who is sponta-

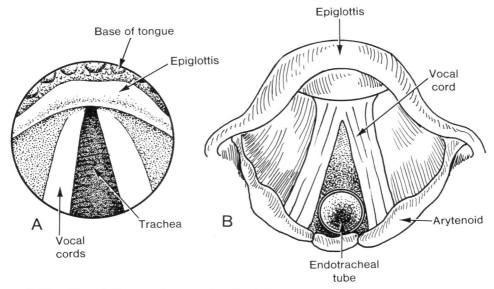

Figure 2.17. The glottic opening, as visualized through the laryngoscope. With the straight blade, the epiglottis will be uplifted and all that one will see are the vocal cords and trachea through the channel of the laryngoscope. With the MacIntosh blade, one may see only the epiglottis (*above*) and the arytenoid cartilages posterior to the vocal cord.

neously breathing. This technique will avoid damage to the vocal cords.

External pressure on the larynx may bring an anteriorly placed larynx into view.

8. *In passing the tube, always insert it from the right side with the upper end of the tube pointing toward the patient's right side. Do not pass the tube down the channel of the blade as this obscures adequate visualization.*
9. Inflate the cuff and auscult both sides of the chest. If the right thorax is the only side on which breath sounds are heard, retract the tube 1 or 2 cm and recheck the breath sounds.

NOTE

The left main stem bronchus comes off at a 45 degree angle to the trachea, while the right main stem bronchus is essentially continuous with the trachea. This anatomical difference causes one to pass the tube into the right main stem bronchus more commonly than into the left.

CAUTION!

A tube in the esophagus may cause laryngospasm (50).

NOTE

Malposition of the tube is a hazard. If doubt exists about the location of the tip of the tube, advance the tube until breath sounds are lost then withdraw the tube 1 or 2 cm until bilaterally *equal* sounds are heard (90). In one study of 49 patients the tube remained in the right main bronchus in 25 of the cases despite distinct breath sounds ausculted on both sides of the chest. (37). Therefore, radiographs should be obtained to confirm the position of the tube (33, 90). Ideally the tube tip is 5 ± 2 cm from the carina of the trachea with the head in the neutral position (33). To determine if the head was in the neutral position, on the anteroposterior film of the neck the mandible should lie over C_5 or C_6.

With the neck flexed, the mandible is at T1. The tube moves significantly with movement of the head. In one large study the tube moved an average of 1.9 cm toward the carina with flexion from the neutral position and 1.9 cm away from the carina with extension. With lateral head rotation the endotracheal tube moved 0.7 cm away from its neutral position (17) (Fig. 2.18). Thus, it is best to place the tip of the tube in the middle third of the trachea with the neck in neutral or 5 ± 2 cm above the carina rather than at the carina in the average adult.

10. Insert an oral airway to prevent bit-

ing on the tube and secure the tube in place. Always restrain the patient; it is part of securing the airway. There are a number of devices on the market for securing the endotracheal tube in place. The devices are made of synthetic plastics which encompass the endotracheal tube and serve as a bite block as well as safeguarding the tube while in position. If one of these is not available, adhesive tape may be used to secure the tube in its proper position; however, this requires frequent rechecking of the patient as perspiration and motion often loosens the tape.

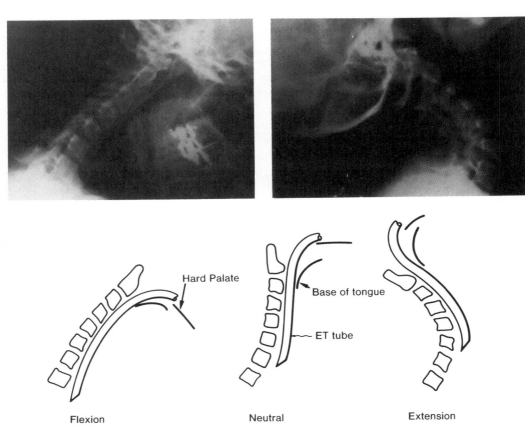

Figure 2.18. The occurrence of endotracheal tube movement is shown. The endotracheal tube is diagrammed so that the length is constant from the base of the hard palate to the tube tip. See text for details. (Reprinted with permission of Critical Care Medicine 4:10. Copyright © 1976, Williams & Wilkins Co., Baltimore.)

SPECIAL CONSIDERATIONS AND HELPFUL HINTS

Endotracheal intubation in the patient who has vomitus and secretions in the oral cavity can be a very challenging problem. Adequate suctioning is critical for visualization of the glottis to insert the endotracheal tube. However, suctioning is often followed by refilling of the oral cavity with secretions from the esophagus or stomach. In this situation it is not always easy to visualize the vocal cords. An important landmark is the esophageal surface of the larynx. The mucosal surface on the posterior (esophageal) surface of the larynx is unique and can usually be visualized with the laryngoscope which has been passed too far, as is often the case in such patients. The larynx is convex and the mucosa is loosely attached, giving the appearance of transverse folds. This mucosal pattern is distinctive and is not present in the mucosal lining of the pharynx or the esophagus in which the mucosa is smooth. If in passing the blade this distinctive surface is seen, then the blade is in the midline and is in too far. Withdraw the blade slightly and the glottis will fall into place, making endotracheal intubation possible. An esophageal obturator airway can be used effectively in these patients when endotracheal intubation remains difficult.

Retrograde Intubation

In difficult endotracheal intubations, one may pass a 14 gauge, 12 inch intercath, as shown in Figure 2.19, through the cricothyroid membrane and into the oral cavity. The endotracheal tube then is threaded over this catheter (72, 90). Retrograde intubation is indicated when the patient requires endotracheal intubation and an esophageal obturator airway cannot be used (e.g., awake patient) and in whom several attempts at endotracheal intubation have been unsuccessful due to either

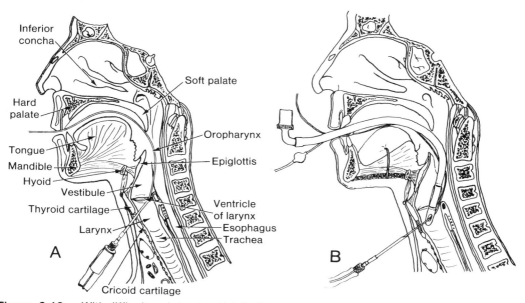

Figure 2.19. With difficult endotracheal intubations, one may pass a 14 gauge, 12 inch intracath as shown above. *A.* Position of intracath after percutaneous insertion through the cricothyroid membrane for oral intubation. The endotracheal tube is then threaded over the catheter as shown in *B.* The position of the Intracath before cutting and withdrawing the catheter is shown in *B.* (Reprinted with permission of Anesthesia and Analgesia 46:232–233, Copyright © 1967, International Anesthesia Research Society.)

abnormal anatomy or the patient's condition (e.g., multiple facial injuries resulting from an auto accident). Retrograde intubation can also be used in medical situations such as patients suffering acute respiratory distress from asthma, emphysema, or a neck tumor in whom nasotracheal intubation is either unsuccessful or cannot be performed. When performing endotracheal intubation over the catheter it must be held tightly at both ends to provide a "rigid" channel over which the endotracheal tube may pass.

Fiberoptic Endoscopes

Fiberoptic endoscopes were thought to be the answer to difficult endotracheal intubations but they have significant shortcomings, making their usefulness in the emergency center limited. Secretions accumulate over the scope and make visualization difficult, and it is often harder to identify structures with the endoscope than with conventional laryngoscopy (72). They are very useful in the patient who does not have a problem with secretions, vomitus, or blood.

Exchanging a Damaged Endotracheal Tube (Cuff Ruptured)

A flexible stylet 4 mm in diameter and twice the length of the endotracheal tube may be passed through the damaged endotracheal tube; the old tube is removed over the stylet and a new tube is placed over the stylet (24).

Guidelines to the Obstructed Endotracheal Tube (40)

CAUTION!

Be prepared to bag-ventilate the patient.

1. First turn and hyperextend the head.
2. If obstruction persists, deflate the cuff as the cuff may herniate around endotracheal tube orifice.
3. If obstruction persists, insert catheter into endotracheal tube and if it can be passed only part way, place a finger in the mouth to see if the endotracheal tube is kinked.

NOTE

Using a large endotracheal tube diminishes the risk of kinking.

4. If this obstruction persists, withdraw the tube a short distance and if it is still obstructed withdraw the tube entirely.

Suctioning an Endotracheal Tube

Suction catheters should be handled as sterilely as possible, and suction should be applied only upon withdrawal of the catheter after it has been inserted through the endotracheal tube into the trachea and bronchi. Suction for 15 seconds and avoid high intratracheal pressures greater than 50 cm of H_2O (25). Turning the patient's head to the right does not promote catheter insertion into the left main stem bronchus as has been the popular belief (25, 35). By bending the tip of the plastic catheter or using a catheter with an angled tip, catheterization into the left main stem bronchus may be achieved (25, 35, 45). One must always use an aseptic technique. Sterile gloves and a sterile catheter should be used during suctioning of the endotracheal tube. Forty seconds of suctioning resulted in a decrease in PO_2 more than twice as large as the decrease in PO_2 from only 20 seconds of suctioning (10). Therefore, bag-mask ventilate with oxygen three times before suctioning to prevent arrhythmias (78).

Guidelines to the Difficult Endotracheal Intubation

If, after following standard technique, one either does not see the glottis or cannot pass the tube, what then do the authors suggest? Five common situations, in addition to the ones already indicated above, are discussed separately and some helpful hints are given to aid with the difficult intubation.

1. *Normal anatomy.* In the patient with normal anatomy in whom the physician cannot pass the tube, one should check the following as these are the common causes for inability to pass a tube:

a. The patient's neck should be flexed rather than extended. One may have to place a folded towel or a small pillow under the patient's head to facilitate this position (sniffing position) so that the larynx is aligned with the posterior pharynx and the mouth to facilitate visualization of the glottis (Fig. 2.14).

b. An assistant can apply pressure over the laryngeal notch or cricoid cartilage to displace the glottis posteriorly and facilitate visualization.

c. Check the size of the laryngoscope blade and be certain that it is not too narrow (the tongue will "fold" around the blade, obstructing visualization) or too short. The laryngoscope blade should be approximately one half the width of the tongue to properly displace it.

d. A smaller tube may have to be placed if the size routinely used causes obstruction of visualization of the glottis due to a narrow oral cavity or pharynx.

2. *Large tongue.* When a large tongue causes difficulty with visualization of the glottis or epiglottis, a wider blade than routinely used is suggested. In the authors' experience a MacIntosh blade facilitates endotracheal intubation of these patients more readily than does a straight blade.

3. *A patient with a short, squat neck.* These patients are perhaps the most difficult to intubate endotracheally. One must check to be certain that the axes of the larynx, pharynx and mouth are accurately aligned. One of the authors (RS) routinely places a folded towel beneath the head of such patients before endotracheal intubation, as accurate alignment of the structure seems most difficult in these patients. A MacIntosh blade permits more adequate visualization of the glottic opening than does the straight blade, which requires more displacement anteriorly of the epiglottis and tongue. A smaller size endotracheal tube is suggested in these patients to facilitate visualization and accurate placement. When all else fails and endotracheal intubation is mandatory, the authors suggest either nasotracheal intubation, retrograde intubation, or cricothyroidotomy as a last resort.

4. *Glottic edema.* When glottic edema following an allergic reaction is a problem, either a small endotracheal tube is used or a nasotracheal intubation with a small nasotracheal tube is suggested.

5. *Abnormal anatomy*

a. *Epiglottitis.* As is indicated in the section on "Nasotracheal Intubation," a number of studies have shown that patients with epiglottitis can be intubated using the nasotracheal route without difficulty. The authors recommend that when dealing with a patient with epiglottitis, one uses the same philosophical approach as when examining a third trimester bleed, that is, have a cricothyroidotomy set ready and open, resuscitative drugs (including succinylcholine) nearby, an intravenous route established, and have a catheter for retrograde intubation should this become necessary. The decision whether to perform nasotracheal intubation or cricothyroidotomy in these patients must be individualized, based on the physician's experience, skill, and preference. Retrograde intubation as described above is not suggested in these patients, as the swollen epiglottis may be displaced over the glottis by the passing endotracheal tube and may obstruct passage of that tube.

b. *Congenital anomaly.* In the patient with a congenital anomaly, endotracheal intubation may be difficult depending on what the anomaly involves. Obviously one must individualize each situation. In the patient in whom the anomaly causes a narrow pharynx and oral cavity, a smaller tube could be used. When the anomaly makes it difficult to visualize adequately the structures necessary to intubate a patient and intubation is necessary, a cricothyroidotomy may have to be performed.

c. *Cancer.* A number of patients who have received radiotherapy to the head and neck have stiffening of those structures, and one is unable to extend the head or flex the neck in these patients to perform endotracheal intubation. In such patients, nasotracheal intubation is the preferred route; when this is not possible, one should go directly to a cricothyroidotomy.

d. *Maxillofacial trauma.* In patients with maxillofacial trauma causing an abnormal anatomy, the authors recommend either a cricothyroidotomy or nasotracheal intubation when possible.

When a patient comes into the emergency department and is difficult to intubate endotracheally for any of the reasons listed above and he either has an esophageal obturator airway in place or is unconscious and an esophageal obturator airway can be inserted, this should be done. Following insertion of the esophageal obturator airway and ventilation through it, endotracheal intubation should then be performed over the esophageal obturator airway. The technique is the same as for endotracheal intubation except that a smaller endotracheal tube is usually used, particularly in the patient with a small mouth and oropharynx. The esophageal obturator airway should be left in place during endotracheal intubation and should be removed only after the patient has been successfully intubated and the cuff inflated. Removal of the esophageal obturator airway often is accompanied by vomiting and, if an endotracheal tube is not in place to protect the trachea, aspiration may result. Following endotracheal intubation, the esophageal obturator airway cuff is deflated and the tube is removed.

The roles of nasotracheal intubation, cricothyroidotomy, and retrograde intubation have either been discussed in this section or will be discussed in their respective sections.

Infant and Child Endotracheal Intubation

Prominence of the maxilla is usual until the fifth postnatal month and mandibular retrusion also may exist. Either anatomic variation (posterior displacement or mandibular retrusion) may lead to poor support of the tongue of the infant by the muscles attached; obstruction of the airway occurs more easily in the child than in the adult (19). The cranium dominates the small body of the infant, and excess adenoidal tissue also may be present. The larynx is more anterior and cephalad and so the angle between the laryngeal opening and the pharynx is even more acute; thus, even though large heads of infants give some degree of flexion, usually there must be additional flexion which is aided by a pillow placed under the head. The laryngoscope blade with a curve (MacIntosh) will increase the anterior displacement of the glottis; therefore, a straight blade should be used in the manner recommended with the tip of the blade lifting the epiglottis. In the child it is difficult to lift the epiglottis, and slight posterior pressure exerted by hand placed on the skin anterior to the larynx will give full view of the glottic opening. Due to the softness of the neck structures and cartilage, the larynx is easily displaced.

During endotracheal intubation it is important to be extremely gentle in the infant. When the vocal cords are tightly apposed, a 1.5 cm depression of the sternum for 1 second duration by an assistant using the tips of the fingers will open the glottis during a forced expiration at which time a tube can be safely passed (57).

A formula which may be used for calculating tube sizes in infants and children is the following (64):

below 6.5 years, tube size (mm) = (age years/3)+3.5
above 6.5 years, tube size (mm) = (age years/4)+4.5

Complications

1. Perforation of the trachea with the stylet.

a. Prevention and treatment: See step 4 in Preparatory Steps.
2. Esophageal intubation.
   a. Prevention and treatment.
      1) Adequate visualization of either the glottis or the vocal cords will prevent passage into the esophagus.
      2) One must auscult both sides of the chest after endotracheal intubation. If no breath sounds are heard remove the tube and reintubate or check tube for proper placement. When vomiting occurs leave the tube in place as this acts as a conduit for the vomitus and endotracheally intubate around the endotracheal tube in the esophagus.
3. Injury to the vocal cords.
   a. Prevention and treatment.
      1) Use a lubricated tube and if the patient is breathing, pass the tube only during inspiration, when the vocal cords are retracted and the glottic opening is widest.
4. Injury to the teeth.
   a. Prevention and treatment: See step 5 in Procedural Steps.
5. Intubation of the right main stem bronchus (29). In a recent series, this complication occurred 11% of the time and, interestingly enough, often was not detected by chest radiography. If the left bronchus is not totally occluded, the air that comes from the right main stem bronchus may successfully partially ventilate the left lung. On all occasions, one should listen and make sure that both lungs are being equally ventilated and should confirm the position of the tube by careful inspection of the chest radiograph.
6. Dislodged tube. This complication occurs in up to 2.5 to 3.0% of the reported cases. One must secure the tube properly with either tape or, preferably, with one of the commercially available devices for holding the endotracheal tube in place and restrain the patient.

7. Obstruction of the tube. Thick secretions or particulate foreign matter (78) aspirated into the lungs may obstruct the endotracheal tube. Should ventilation become ineffective, one should expect this obvious complication and either suction to relieve the obstruction or replace the tube (see "Guidelines to Obstructed Endotracheal Tube") (29).
8. Aspiration of stomach contents. In a recently published series, this complication occurred in 14% of endotracheal intubations involving drug overdoses (32). The incidence of aspiration during endotracheal intubation is increased when the patient is hypotensive or difficult to intubate. Aspiration is associated with a definite increase in pneumonia and mortality rates.
9. Pneumothorax (29). Pneumothorax occurs in patients with decreased pulmonary compliance who, therefore, require high ventilatory pressures or those with endotracheal intubation of the right main stem bronchus. Frequent chest auscultation and appropriate chest radiographs would alert the physician to the development of a pneumothorax.
10. Atelectasis. This may occur with intubation into the right main stem bronchus in which the left side of the lung is not ventilated and atelectasis will result (93).
11. Cuff damage. Cuff damage may occur with repeated attempts at endotracheal intubation or with a defective cuff. Gastric distension may result from an air leak. After three or four attempts at intubation, one should switch the endotracheal tube or check the cuff again for air leak (78).
12. Arrhythmias. Hypoxia may result from poor ventilation between attempts at endotracheal intubation or from prolonged attempts at intubating a patient. Hypoxia may result in the development of arrhythmias. One should not prolong an attempt at intubation beyond 40 seconds. If

unsuccessful, immediately ventilate the patient with a bag-mask device. Arrhythmias may also result secondary to vagal stimulation during intubation. Bradycardia is the most common arrhythmia noted in patients who have increased sensitivity of the vagus during attempts at endotracheal intubation (85).

13. Laryngospasm - Laryngospasm has been reported after attempts at endotracheal intubation, particularly in the patient with inflammation around the glottis which would predispose him to laryngospasm or polyps in this region (78).

Nasotracheal Intubation

There are many advantages to nasotracheal intubation, especially in patients with oral injury or in preoperative patients. Some feel it is better than tracheostomy when oral intubation is not possible (54, 60). Many authors feel nasotracheal intubation is the preferred procedure when endotracheal intubation is necessary (16, 48), because the tube is more easily secured to the face, cannot be bitten, and does not increase salivation (48). This route also appears better tolerated by the patient, with fewer patients attempting self-extubation. Some feel that even with a swollen epiglottis, nasotracheal intubation is not difficult to do. Schuller and Birch showed that 85% of patients with epiglottitis were intubated without difficulty and nasotracheal intubation was possible in all patients with epiglottitis in their series (73). Others also have supported this contention (7, 87). Nasotracheal intubation is the only procedure by which endotracheal intubation can be performed in the patient who is sitting upright.

Indications

1. Decreased patency of the oral airway due to neoplasm, inflammatory disease, or neurogenic disturbances.
2. Inability to open the mouth, markedly retruded mandible, and previous head and neck surgery; all of which make oral intubation difficult with a laryngoscope (5, 72).
3. Mandibular fractures and extensive maxillofacial deformities.
4. Alert and conscious patient who requires endotracheal intubation, e.g., asthmatic or chronic obstructive pulmonary disease (COPD) with exacerbation.
5. Possible or actual cervical spine injury, possible or actual herniated disk, poor mobility of the cervical spine (5, 72), or chronic atlantoaxial dislocation, e.g., rheumatoid arthritis.
6. Postradiation fibrosis of the neck (51).
7. Patient who requires endotracheal intubation but who cannot lie supine (severe asthma with respiratory distress).

Contraindications

1. Severe nasal or maxillofacial fractures.

Equipment

Same as for endotracheal intubation
Magill forceps
Topical anesthetic spray
    4% cocaine
    2% Xylocaine® with adrenaline (1:100,000)
    Cotton balls or gauze strips
Lubricant
Xylocaine® jelly

Technique

NOTE

There are essentially three requirements to a successful blind nasotracheal intubation:

1. A well-lubricated tube (31, 50, 92).
2. Topical anesthesia to the nose, pharynx, and larynx (30, 72, 89).
3. Spontaneously breathing patient (72, 92).

Preparatory Steps

1. Select tube. A tube is generally selected which will fit well, but not loosely into the nose. In the adult male a size 7.5 or 8.0 may be passed,

while in the female a size 7 is generally selected (92).

2. Lubricate tube. Lubricate the tube with lidocaine jelly.

3. Anesthetize the nose, pharynx, and larynx.

    a. In the awake, spontaneously breathing patient, Pedersen uses the following method (63): Anesthetize the nose with a spray of 4% cocaine, followed by cotton plugs impregnated with cocaine and instilled into the nostril with a bayonet forceps. These are left in place for 5 minutes. Cocaine reduces the risk of bleeding as well as shrinks the nasal membranes.

Nasopharyngeal analgesia is achieved by spraying the back of the throat. The nasotracheal tube is then passed, and one listens for good breath sounds through the tube. When good breath sounds are heard, ask the patient to take some deep breaths and compress the spray simultaneously, anesthetizing the larynx (Fig. 2.20). As the patient coughs, the anesthetic is dispersed over the nasopharynx.

Alternate Method

A method advocated by several authors (30, 51, 92) is the following: Spray the nasal passage with 4% cocaine and then pack

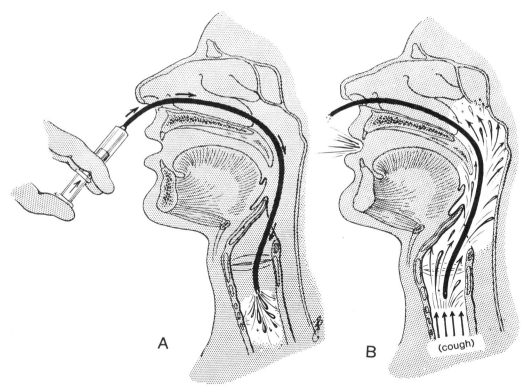

Figure 2.20. Method for anesthetizing the posterior pharynx and glottis. When good breath sounds are heard, ask the patient to take a deep breath and compress the spray simultaneously containing the cocaine solution. *A.* Nasotracheal instillation of cocaine is shown. Notice the firm control of the syringe barrel to prevent expulsion during coughing. *B.* Dissemination of cocaine by coughing, with resultant oropharyngeal anesthesia. (Reprinted with permission of Journal of Thoracic Surgery. Starzl, T. E., A simple method for the induction of topical laryngo-tracheobronchial anesthesia. 37:652. Copyright © 1959, C.V. Mosby Company.)

with cocaine-moistened cotton as above. Then block the internal branch of the superior laryngeal nerve bilaterally as follows: The superior cornu of the thyroid cartilage is palpated at the lateral extent of the thyroid membrane. The fingertip is placed on the cornu of the thyroid cartilage at the site at which the thyroid and hyoid meet laterally. This is the site of the injection (Fig. 2.21). With a 22 gauge needle and a 5 ml syringe filled with 2% lidocaine, insert the needle at your fingertip until the thyroid membrane is felt. One feels a resistance at this point. Then instill 2 ml of anesthetic solution. If unable to feel this membrane, advance the needle until air is aspirated into the syringe and then withdraw; as you withdraw back into the tissue, inject the solution. Perform the same

procedure on the opposite side. Lastly, anesthetize the tracheal mucosa with 2 ml of lidocaine injected through the cricothyroid membrane and into the trachea. At this point the pack is removed from the nose.

   b. In the unconscious, spontaneously breathing patient: Spray the nostril and the posterior pharynx with a 4% cocaine spray. This reduces epistaxis and shrinks the mucosa (89). The maximum dose is 3 mg/kg.

4. Position the patient's head and select the nostril to enter. Nasotracheal intubation can be done in the recumbent or sitting position, e.g., asthmatic in respiratory distress (92), whichever is more comfortable. Often, endotra-

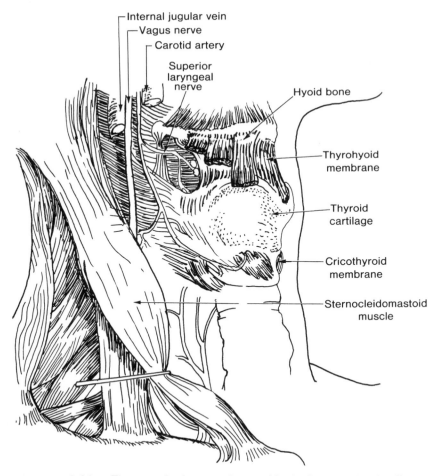

Figure 2.21.   The superior laryngeal nerve block. See text for details.

cheal intubation by this route is easier with the patient sitting since the head can be manipulated easier (54).

Inspect the nose and select the side with the freer airway without nasal obstruction from septal deviation or congested membranes (72). The optimal position of the head for nasotracheal intubation is the sniffing position (54, 72); excessive extension of the neck causes the tube to enter the anterior commissure, and excessive flexion causes it to enter the esophagus. With the patient lying, the head can be supported by a small pillow or folded towel to achieve this optimal position (50, 53, 63, 92).

Procedural Steps

1. Insert the tube through the nose. Insert the tube through the nose with the bevel facing the nasal septum, introducing the tube along the floor of the nose into the hypopharynx (72). When the pharynx is reached, the tube should be rotated into its normal position.

   When a patient is on anticoagulants or may develop a problem with nasal bleeding from other causes, Fry (28) advocates the following after shrinking the nasal membranes with cocaine: The digit is cut off a size 8 glove. The tip is then excised and a slit placed longitudinally. After lubricating both the inside and outside of the "digit," introduce it along the floor of the nostril with a bayonet forceps, leaving part of the glove protruding so that it can be held with a hemostat. When introducing the nasotracheal tube, pass it through the inside of the "digit." This prevents the tip of the tube from striking against and irritating the nasal membranes as the tube passes.

2. Advance the tube into the hypopharynx and trachea.

NOTE

It is often helpful in passing the tube to tilt the patient's head laterally a small amount to the side of the nasal cavity which is being used (51, 63).

Advance the tube into the hypopharynx and listen for breath sounds over the portal (Fig. 2.22). Locate that point at which the breath sounds are heard *maximally* over the portal. From here onward, movement of the tube must be bold and rapid because a slow moving tube is easily deflected from its course (50, 63). The tube should be in the hypopharynx in a position where breath sounds are maximally audible. When the tube is in its proper position, the patient is usually comfortable. With the tube held in the right hand and the left hand palpating the larynx (to stabilize it and "feel" the tube entering), quickly pass the tube during the terminal instances of exhalation or the onset of inhalation. When the trachea is entered, the patient often coughs briskly (92).

NOTE

Often one may think he is hearing breath sounds over the portal when the tube is in fact in the esophagus due to respirations around the tube from the contralateral nostril. If this is a problem, close this nostril (50) and assess respiration.

NOTE

If airflow stops during the advancement of the tube, it may be easily passed into the esophagus without meeting any obstruction. In this case, withdraw the tube until airflow is again audible, then rotate the tube slightly to the right or left and advance it again with the neck rotated slightly to the right or left and with the neck slightly extended. In a patient with a deviated septum, it may be impossible to align the tube tip with the epiglottis, and blind nasotracheal intubation may be unsuccessful (29). Esophageal intubation can be differentiated from the tube entering the vallecula or pyriform sinuses because when the vallecula or pyriform sinuses are entered the breath sounds cease and one is unable to advance the tube further. If one enters the vallecula or pyriform, flex the neck until the tube passes the epiglottis

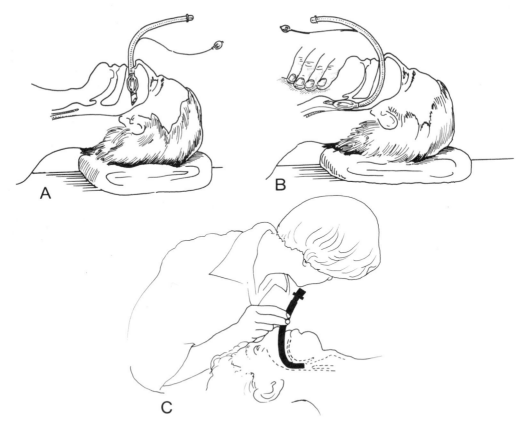

Figure 2.22.   In the supine patient the neck should be flexed as shown in *A*. Insert the tube into the nares and advance it past the nasopharynx. As it passes the nasopharynx and into the oropharynx, a ''give'' will be felt. The larynx can be gently displaced posteriorly with one hand (*B*). The tube is advanced until *maximum breath sounds* are audible through it. The physician should listen over the orifice of the tube for this point. The tube is then passed rapidly during the very beginning of inspiration or terminal instance of exhalation (*C*).

and then place the neck in neutral position and advance the tube (92). The endotracheal tube can be deflected laterally or in an anterior-posterior direction. Lateral deflection can be ascertained by looking into the pharynx through the oral cavity after the tube has been passed into the pharynx. Anterior and posterior deflection can be similarly ascertained. Lateral deflection is corrected by rotating the tube until the breath sounds are heard loudest, and the tube is passed successfully. When (due to septal deviation or other anatomic aberrations) the tube cannot be rotated from its lateral course, three alternatives are available:

A. A Magill forceps, a specially shaped forceps, can be used once the nasotracheal tube is at the level of the oropharynx (Fig. 2.23). In this situation, one uses the laryngoscope to visualize the epiglottis and the glottic opening (when possible) and guides the tube with the Magill forceps during inspiration as an assistant pushes the distal end of the tube (50). Alternately, one may pass the tube with the Magill forceps; however, this is more difficult.

B. When one cannot deviate the tube, another alternative is to pass the endotracheal tube over a nasotracheal

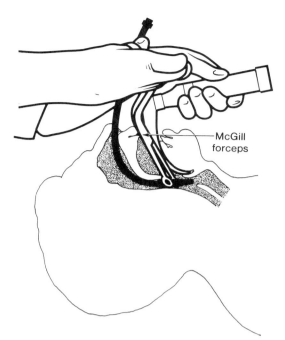

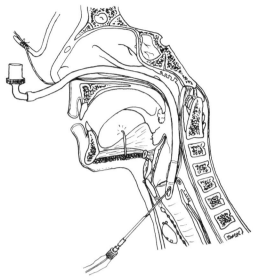

Figure 2.23. The use of the McGill forceps to aid in passing a nasotracheal tube into the trachea.

Figure 2.24. The use of a 14 gauge intracath inserted through the cricothyroid membrane to aid in passage of a nasotracheal tube in difficult patients. The position of the intracath after urethral catheter has been passed to pull the catheter through the nose. By keeping the catheter taut, the nasotracheal tube can be threaded as shown into the trachea. (Reprinted with permission of Anesthesia and Analgesia 46:234. Copyright © 1967, International Anesthesia Research Society.)

suction catheter which has been previously passed. The nasotracheal suction catheter is used to direct the tip of the endotracheal tube while it is passed (63, 84). Alternately, a long, 14 gauge intercath can be passed through the cricothyroid membrane as shown in Figure 2.24 and the nasotracheal tube passed with the catheter used as a guide.

C. A technique which is especially useful in children is to use a copper wire bent to form a hook which is then used as a guide to help pass the tube. The dimensions of the hook are a 6 to 8 inch long handle with the bottom bent into a hook about ½ to 1 inch long (Fig. 2.25). This forms a rectangular hook. After intubating the nose and exposing the larynx, the tip of the nasotracheal tube is then visualized in the oropharynx. The copper wire is then inserted into the mouth, with the hook portion placed gently against the posterior pharyngeal wall. An assistant then advances the

nasotracheal tube until the tip overrides the hook. By lifting the wire while the assistant advances the nasotracheal tube, it can be directed into the larynx with the aid of a laryngoscope. This method is especially useful when a Magill cannot be introduced easily without obstructing vision, e.g., in a child.

NOTE

Pressing down on the larynx with the left hand will displace the glottic opening posteriorly and permit passage of the tube through the glottis when recurrent esophageal intubation occurs. Also, slight extension of the neck from the neutral position will assist in avoiding recurrent esophageal intubation.

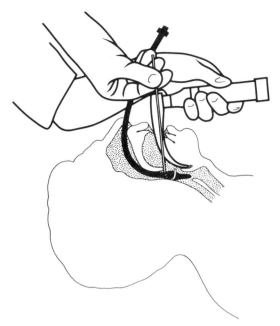

Figure 2.25. The use of a hook to aid in passage of a nasotracheal tube is shown. See text for details.

3. Inflate the endotracheal cuff and secure the tube.
4. Auscultate bilaterally to insure that the endotracheal tube has not entered the right main stem bronchus.

Complications

1. Nasal bleeding. Always look into the nostrils with a nasal speculum and determine which nostril is more dilated. The nares must be free of polyps and should not have a deviated septum, and the tube should be introduced through the more dilated side. Nasal bleeding is the most common complication of this procedure. The method indicated by Fry (28) (stated above) is probably the best preventive measure for the patient who is predisposed to this condition. Usually the bleeding will stop and no treatment is indicated; however, in some cases in which continuous bleeding is a problem and tamponade by the tube does not occur, the tube may have to be removed and an alternate site selected with nasal intubation. Some cases may have minor bleeding, but this bleeding may compromise the airway in a patient with severe respiratory distress; therefore, Fry's method is strongly encouraged.
2. Laryngeal spasm. This is an uncommon complication. If it cannot be relieved, attempted passage of the endotracheal tube may cause injury to the vocal cords, and cricothyroidotomy should be selected (16).
3. Esophageal intubation. The aforementioned techniques should aid in reducing this problem. If, after attempting all modifications to avoid esophageal intubation, there is still difficulty, then alternate routes for endotracheal intubation should be selected.
4. Retropharyngeal insertion. Retropharyngeal insertion has been described as a complication occurring from nasotracheal intubation (85).

Esophageal Obturator Airway (EOA)

Advantages

1. Easier to perform than endotracheal intubation.
2. Maintains as good a level of PO_2 as one obtains with endotracheal intubation.
3. Avoids the complication of gastric distension associated with bag valve mask devices.

Disadvantages

1. Does not provide complete airway control.
2. One is unable to suction the patient with this airway in place.
3. Depends on a tightly fitting mask with little air leak to provide good ventilation.
4. Associated with very high incidence of gastric regurgitation once EOA is removed.
5. Hypercarbia is more prominent than with endotracheal intubation.

Indications

1. Respiratory arrest with no equipment or personnel capable of endotracheal intubation.
2. In the arrest victim who has vomited in a situation where suction is not available or is too inadequate so that endotracheal intubation can be performed.

Contraindications

1. Conscious patient (use only in unconscious patients).
2. Should not be used in children under 16 years of age.
3. Do not use in patients with obstructive esophageal disease.
4. Do not use in caustic ingestion.
5. Do not use for more than 2 or 3 hours.
6. Functioning tracheal stoma.
7. Pharyngeal or laryngeal airway obstruction.

Equipment

Esophageal obturator airway. This airway is 15 inches long and is open at the top and blind at the bottom. Holes are located near the upper end to allow for the egress of air into the pharynx. A total of 16 holes, each 3 mm in diameter are located in this tube. A special mask is used with this device (Fig. 2.26).
50 cc syringe
K-Y jelly

Technique

Preparatory Steps

1. Check the cuff and tube and connect the esophageal tube to the face mask.
2. Set the syringe at 35 cc mark so as not to overinflate or underinflate. Overinflation can cause esophageal rupture, a complication associated with a very high mortality rate. Underinflation can result in regurgitation of vomitus, if vomiting occurs with aspiration.
3. Lubricate the tube.

Procedural Steps

1. Hyperventilate the patient.
2. Position the patient's head in a neutral position. Sometimes, slight flexion may facilitate insertion but NEVER hyperextend.
3. Grasp the lower jaw and tongue with the thumb and forefinger of the left hand and lift the jaw straight up (Fig. 2.27A).
4. Insert the tube while the patient's head is maintained in a neutral position or slight flexion. Grasp the tube below the mask portion and insert it from the right side of the mouth. Advance until the mask is well-seated on the face (Fig. 2.27B and C).
5. Ventilate and auscult both lung fields.

CAUTION!

Step 5 must be done before inflation of the cuff, because if the tube is in the trachea and the cuff is inflated, severe tracheal damage may result.

CAUTION!

The cuff must be below the level of the carina. If the cuff is at or above the level of the carina, it will compress the posterior

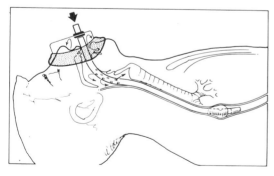

Figure 2.26. Schematic presentation of the EOA tube. Note the special mask which is used with this device. Air blown into the proximal end exits via small holes and is forced down the trachea as the other routes are occluded. (Reprinted with permission of Chest 69:68, Copyright © 1976.)

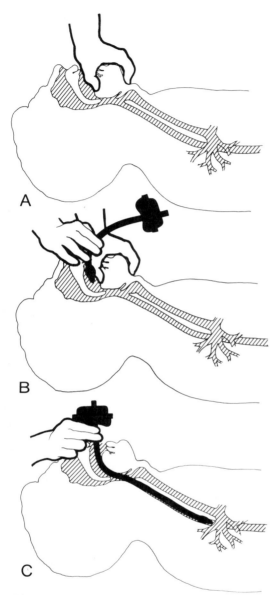

Figure 2.27. The technique of inserting the esophageal obturator airway is shown. See text for discussion.

membrane portion of the trachea and lead to obstruction. The best way to insure against this problem is to pass the tube all the way.

6. Inflate the cuff with 35 cc of air.
7. With the cuff inflated, check again for breath sounds.

CAUTION!

If the chest does not rise or no breath sounds are heard, the tube may be in the trachea. If so, or if in doubt, remove the tube after deflating the cuff and repeat the procedure.

Aftercare

1. Remove the tube only when the patient is conscious and breathing spontaneously or an endotracheal tube is in place. To remove:
   a. Turn head to side and have good suction available since vomiting is common.
   b. Deflate the cuff and remove.

Complications

1. Obstruction of trachea by compression of inflated cuff against membranous portions of trachea (see procedural step 5).
2. Tracheal intubation. This complication is due to hyperextension of the neck. Always keep the neck in the neutral or slight flexion position.
3. Rupture of the esophagus. This complication is due to excessive inflation of the cuff or retching by the patient. This complication is associated with a high mortality rate. If suspected, obtain a chest radiograph looking for mediastinal emphysema or subcutaneous emphysema. Suspect this complication if the patient develops palpable subcutaneous emphysema on examination of the neck.
4. Vomiting and regurgitation upon extubation of the patient.
   a. Prevention and treatment
      1) *Do not* remove tube or deflate the cuff until an endotracheal tube is in place or the patient is conscious with spontaneous respirations. Regurgitation is an extremely common problem on removal of the EOA. If the patient awakens during resuscitation and the EOA is in place, turn him on his side and/or preferably in the prone position and proceed to deflate the cuff and extubate the patient.

2) Should vomiting occur, suction the patient immediately and treat as one would an aspiration.

ESOPHAGEAL GASTRIC TUBE AIRWAY (EGTA)

After removal of the esophageal airway, the patient frequently vomits secondary to gastric distension. Because of this complication, the EGTA was developed to maintain the airway while simultaneously decompressing the stomach during resuscitation. The EGTA is similar to the EOA, with the exception that it has an additional portal on the mask which permits passage of a gastric tube to decompress the stomach. The technique of insertion is similar to the EOA except that a gastric tubing is inserted while ventilating the patient. This permits decompression of the stomach while resuscitation is ongoing.

TRACHEOTOMY

Cricothyroidotomy

The cricothyroid membrane is recommended as an ideal area for performing an emergency laryngotomy by many authors (11, 12, 15, 32, 58, 59, 61). It is the authors' opinion that the cricothyroid membrane puncture is the safest and simplest method for establishing a satisfactory airway under adverse conditions. Even the most skilled surgeon would be unwise to attempt emergency tracheostomy when cricothyroid membrane puncture would admirably control the crisis (59). The largest study was conducted by Brantigan and Grow in 1975. They performed 655 cricothyroidotomies, both electively and in emergency situations, and found an extremely low incidence of complications, much lower than that reported with tracheostomy (12).

When critical airway obstruction presents to the emergency center, an orderly plan of action is essential—otherwise irreversible brain damage or death may ensue shortly. The four basic steps are: 1) recognition of the obstruction; 2) maneuvers to relieve obstruction, e.g, Heimlech maneuver; 3) artificial ventilation (mouth-to-mouth, bag, mask, etc.) to relieve ob-

struction; and 4) diagnosis of persistent obstruction and treatment by the establishment of an emergency surgical airway by cricothyroidotomy (59).

Indications

1. Any situation in which a standard endotracheal or nasotracheal intubation cannot be performed.
   a. Excessive oropharyngeal or nasopharyngeal hemorrhage.
   b. Massive regurgitation.
   c. Massive congenital or traumatic deformities of oropharynx or nasopharynx.
   d. Complete airway obstruction such that endotracheal intubation is impossible, e.g., foreign body and maneuvers which open the airway are unsuccessful.
2. Cervical spine fracture suspected or proven in patient who needs an airway but in whom nasotracheal intubation is unsuccessful or contraindicated.
3. Unsuccessful attempts at endotracheal intubation in patient in whom inordinate delay would result in cerebral anoxic damage.

Contraindications

1. Fracture or serious injury to the larynx or cricoid cartilage, in which case a tracheostomy should be performed.

Equipment

#11 blade
scalpel
trousseau dilator
plastic tracheostomy tube (Silex^R or Portex tracheostomy tubes)
   Standard endotracheal tube can be used.
   The size of the endotracheal tube is dependent on the age of the patient and size of the trachea. In general, one can insert a size 6, 7, or 8 tube in the adult. The tube is cut to the proper size once in place.
small curved hemostats
prep solution
1 dozen 4 × 4 gauze pads
scissors
10 cc syringe

tracheal suction catheter
skin hook

Technique

NOTE

There are currently devices on the market which can be inserted through the cricothyroid membrane with relative ease and which provide an excellent airway through which the patient can be ventilated. These devices will not be discussed here.

1. Position the patient in the recumbent or semirecumbent position. This position is not absolutely necessary.
2. Locate the cricothyroid membrane by placing the thumb and middle finger around the larynx; the middle finger should be walked down the thyroid notch toward the trachea until an indentation is felt between the cricoid and thyroid cartilages (Fig. 2.28). This indentation is the cricothyroid membrane (Fig. 2.29).
3. Infiltrate the skin and subcutaneous tissue with lidocaine.
4. Hold the larynx and locate the cricothyroid membrane with the left hand in the manner noted in step 2 (Fig. 2.30).
5. Make a transverse incision through the membrane with a single motion (Fig. 2.31) (12, 61).

NOTE

The scalpel should be held between the thumb and index finger in such a way that only the tip of the blade can enter the trachea during the initial stab incision.

CAUTION!

The esophagus is located behind the cricoid cartilage. If the blade is not held in such a manner that will keep one from going too deeply, then the esophagus may be perforated. It is for this reason that the

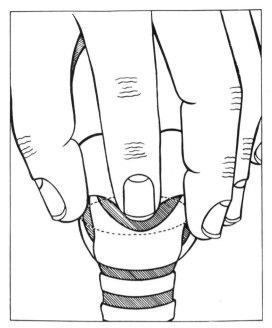

Figure 2.28.   Drawing showing the larynx stabilized between the left thumb and middle finger. The tip of the index finger is inserted over the cricothyroid membrane. To puncture the membrane a #11 scalpel and blade is directed along the nail of the index finger and through the membrane in one step. (Reprinted with permission of J.A.M.A. 174:1934. Copyright © 1960, American Medical Association.)

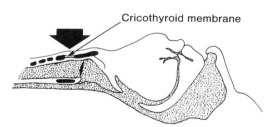

Figure 2.29.   The indentation of the cricothyroid membrane is shown.

authors advocate this somewhat unorthodox method of holding the scalpel when making the initial incision.

6. Carry the incision a few millimeters laterally until resistance is met, or about 1 cm, and turn the scalpel and blade 180 degrees and carry the in-

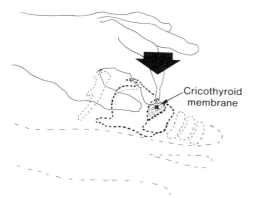

Figure 2.30.   Hold the larynx as shown in Figure 2.28, with the index finger placed over the cricothyroid membrane.

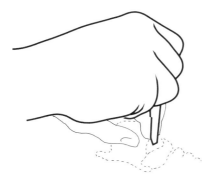

Figure 2.31.   A transverse incision is made after puncture through the membrane with a single step. The scalpel should be held between the thumb and index finger in such a manner that only the tip of the blade can enter the trachea to the depth desired. This prevents penetration too deeply and perforation into the esophagus during the initial stab incision (not shown above). After this the hand can be placed in the position shown above for extending the incision transversely across the membrane.

cision laterally again but in the opposite direction. Again resistance will be noted at the lateral edge of the incision. The length of the incision will be large enough to just pass the endotracheal tube, approximately 1.5 to 2.0 cm.

7. Place the curved hemostat or the Trousseau dilator through the incision and open the instrument perpendicular to the incision (Fig. 2.32).

8. Insert the tracheostomy or endotracheal tube and ventilate the patient.

NOTE

In some patients one may find that upon insertion of the Trousseau dilator or hemostat the larynx displaces posteriorly upon attempting to insert the tracheostomy or endotracheal tube, making insertion difficult. When this occurs, a skin hook should be inserted through the cricothyroidotomy incision and the larynx uplifted to aid in stabilizing the larynx in position while passing the tracheostomy tube.

9. The endotracheal tube will of course be too long and should be cut to an appropriate length and the adapter attached to the cut end. Inflate the cuff of the tube.
10. Ventilate the lungs and auscult to ensure proper tube placement.

Complications

1. Esophageal perforation.
   Prevention and treatment: see step 5 in technique.
2. Subcutaneous emphysema.
   a. Prevention and treatment
      1) One should not carry the incision beyond that needed to pass the tracheostomy or endotracheal tube. A laterally placed incision which requires sutur-

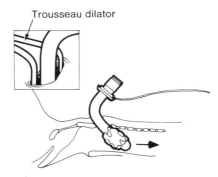

Figure 2.32.   The Trousseau dilator or curved hemostat is used to open the cricothyroid membrane vertically (see insert above). The Pyrex^R tube is then inserted as shown above.

ing around the tube is prone to subcutaneous emphysema.
2) No treatment is indicated.
3. Hemorrhage
  a. Prevention and treatment
    1) This complication will not be encountered if one does not make his incision too wide. Occasionally a small vessel is found crossing the cricothyroid membrane which causes significant bleeding and this may require ligation.
    2) Treat this complication with simple pressure unless a major vessel is bleeding in which case ligation is indicated.

Tracheostomy

When airway obstruction is secondary to acute injuries to the larnyx or trachea, tracheostomy may be indicated (26, 36, 41, 48, 74, 79, 88); however, overall, this procedure has been replaced by cricothyroidotomy.

Indications

1. Acute injuries to the larynx and trachea.
2. Similar to those of cricothyroidotomy.

Contraindications

NOTE

In the authors' opinion, tracheostomy is no longer regarded as the procedure of choice in emergency airway management in which the traditional "emergency tracheostomy" is indicated. Cricothyroidotomy is currently regarded as the procedure of first choice in emergency medicine. While it is beyond the sccpe of this text to discuss the controversies relating to the use of one technique over another, it is the authors' feeling that this is a vital topic which deserves some discussion. The emergency tracheostomy, even in the most skilled hands, can be a time-consuming and difficult procedure due to the very nature of the situation which makes it an emergency rather than an elective procedure. Brantigan and Grow (12) settled this issue during a large series in which they performed over 600 cricothyroidotomies and showed that the complications often thought to be associated with this technique do not, in fact, occur. The reader is urged to read this classic study. One can go so far as to say that the burden of proof lies distinctly on any individual who feels tracheostomy is as simple to perform as and possesses distinct advantages over cricothyroidotomy.

Equipment (38, 58)

#10 blade and scalpel
#11 blade and scalpel
Preparation cup and iodinated solution
10 cc syringe
18 and 25 gauge needles
8 small curved hemostats (5½ inch)
Tracheostomy tube with inflatable cuff (plastic tube preferable)
  size of the tube should be 6, 7, or 8 for the average adult
7 towels and towel clips
2 dozen 4 × 4 gauze pads
3-0 catgut and 4-0 silk
2 Allis forceps
Mastoid retractor
2 small rakes
2 skin forceps
2 tissue forceps without teeth
Suture scissors and curved scissors
Needle holder
Kocher forceps
1 medium tracheal dilator
Frazier suction tip and suction tubing
2-0 and 3-0 catgut
3-0 nylon suture

Technique (38, 48, 58, 70)

Preparatory Steps

1. Place the patient in the recumbent or semirecumbent position.
2. Hyperextend the neck with a folded sheet placed behind the scapula. This hyperextension is obviously not done when one suspects a fracture of the cervical spine.
3. Prep and drape the patient. The patient should be prepped and draped

to expose the area bordered by the manubrium, root of the neck, supraclavicular space, and chin.

Procedural Steps

1. Choose the incision. This choice is dependent on the degree of urgency. In the emergency situation the vertical incision is usually preferred; however, a description is given of both methods.

    a. Vertical incision—requires minimal dissection

    —associated with less bleeding

    —affords more rapid access to the trachea

    —avoids the superficial veins

    —easier to perform in the patient with a short neck

    —heals cosmetically worse than the transverse incision

    Transverse incision—heals cosmetically better

    — takes more time

    — associated with more bleeding

    —requires more dissection

    b. Vertical incision: Make a midline incision using the 10 blade and carry the incision from the cricoid cartilage to the suprasternal notch (Fig. 2.33).

    Transverse incision: Carry the incision from the point approximately one fingerbreadth below the cricoid cartilage, making an incision approximately 6 cm long.

2. The incision should extend through

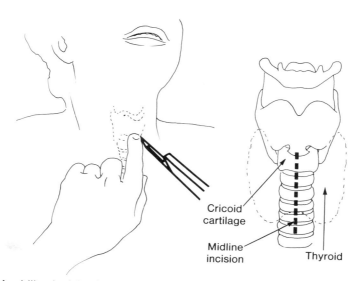

Figure 2.33. A midline incision is made vertically using a #10 blade, extending from the cricoid cartilage to the suprasternal notch. See text for details.

the skin, subcutaneous tissue, and platysma.

3. Vertical incision: Continue through the medial raphe and dissect between the anterior strap muscles until the pretracheal fascia is reached.

CAUTION!

Hemorrhage is a major complication occurring in this step. One must stay in the midline to avoid this potentially lethal complication.

Transverse incision: Separate the platysma from the anterior strap muscles until 4 to 5 cm of the medial raphe is exposed and incise the raphe transversely.

4. Retract the wound edges with the mastoid retractor or small rakes (Fig. 2.34A).

5. Palpate the tracheal and cricoid cartilage. Locate the thyroid isthmus and retract the isthmus upward. The authors find it easier to retract the thyroid inferiorly and hook the cricoid superiorly. Use blunt dissection with small curved hemostat to separate the thyroid isthmus from the trachea.

6. Place 2 small clamps on the isthmus, one on each side, and divide the isthmus. Later one can suture these divided edges with silk (Fig. 2.34B).

7. Locate the second through the fourth rings (Fig. 2.34C).

CAUTION!

Avoid the first ring, as incision of this area causes subglottic stenosis.

8. Make a vertical incision through the third and fourth rings.

NOTE

One can make a window in the trachea through the third and fourth rings as shown (Fig. 2.34D). While this is perfectly

acceptable, it again is more time-consuming in the emergency situation.

9. Suction the tracheal secretions.
10. Insert the tracheal tube and obturator. Sizes 6, 7, or 8 in the adult, smaller in the child (Fig. 2.34D).
11. Remove the obturator and inflate the cuff.

CAUTION!

The tube should fit comfortably in the trachea and not obstruct the carina.

Aftercare

1. Tie in place with umbilical tape around the neck.
2. Approximate the muscles with chromic catgut. To avoid subcutaneous emphysema, do not close the subcutaneous tissue.
3. Close the skin loosely. Dress the wound with 4 × 4 inch gauze.

Complications

1. Mediastinal emphysema.
2. Outer tube coughed out, causing severe mediastinal and subcutaneous emphysema. To prevent this complication:
   a. Secure the tube in place.
   b. Observation.
3. Hemorrhage. Stay within the midline to avoid vessels which lie laterally.
4. Subglottic stenosis. This can be prevented by using the second through fourth tracheal rings.
5. Obstruction of the carina.
6. Erosion into major vessels or the trachea. Erosion into major vessels of the neck or through the trachea is a late complication. It can be avoided by the use of low pressure within the endotracheal tube cuff and periodic deflation when prolonged intubation is necessary. Periodic deflation will avoid pressure necrosis of the mucosa lining the trachea. This complication, due to its late occurrence, is not a problem in the emergency center. However, the emergency physician

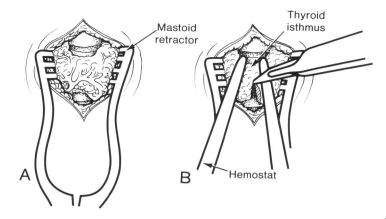

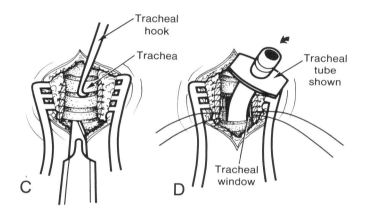

Figure 2.34. Performance of an emergency tracheostomy. See text for discussion.

may see such a patient when called in the middle of the night to the intensive care unit due to major bleeding around a tracheostomy tube previously placed.

Tracheostomy in the Patient with Massive Neck Swelling

A modified technique for emergency tracheostomy in the patient with massive neck swelling has recently been introduced (79a). The patient who has massive neck swelling secondary to hematoma, subcutaneous emphysema, or hemorrhage may present with unpalpable landmarks. The hematoma may deviate the trachea and make it difficult to establish the midline. Such patients often require emergency tracheostomy within a matter of minutes. Using traditional methods of establishing an airway through a tracheos-

tomy or cricothyroidotomy in such patients often is frought with considerable hemorrhage and loss of time trying to identify structures in the distended neck.

The hyoid bone serves to anchor the trachea and larynx superiorly to the mandible, tongue, and base of the skull. The structure is rarely injured during massive neck trauma. It provides an ideal point upon which to place traction to stabilize the trachea and larynx for a tracheotomy. Since the body of the hyoid is a midline structure, by attaching an instrument to it and retracting superiorly and anteriorly, one can pull the trachea and larynx forward as well as stabilize them so that no motion occurs during an emergency tracheotomy. To perform this procedure, measure the distance from the angle of the mandible to the point of the chin as shown in Figure 2.35 (line A). Measure half the

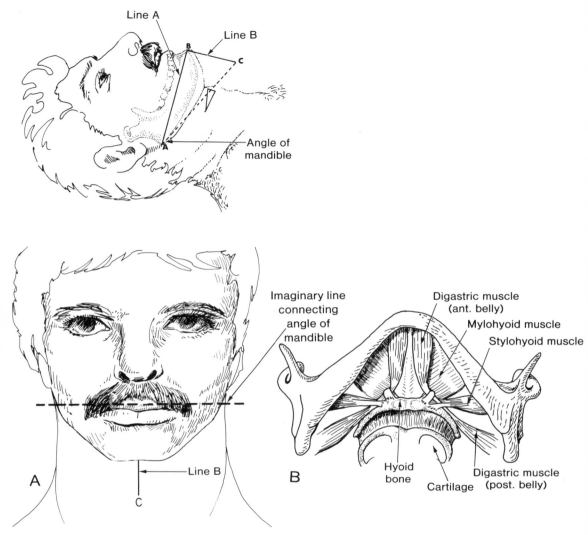

Figure 2.35.   Measuring the distance from the angle of the mandible to the tip of the chin (point A to point B) and measuring down from the tip of the chin inferiorly (point B to point C), one half of the distance from the angle of the mandible to the chin. See text for details.

distance of this line down the anterior aspect of the neck from the midpoint of the chin inferiorly (line B). The ratio of line A (Fig. 2.35) to line B is 2 to 1. The point at which a #11 blade should be inserted is at the end of line B (point "C"). Direct the #11 blade posteriorly, remaining in the midline and angling the tip as if going toward the angle of the mandible (Figs. 2.35A and 2.36). The hyoid bone will be reached at various depths, depending

on the amount of swelling and fat deposition in the anterior neck. Insert a skin hook alongside the tract established by the #11 blade and grasp the hyoid by hooking the skin hook underneath as shown in Figure 2.37. Retract the hyoid superiorly and anteriorly as shown by the arrow. Since the hyoid will have been grasped in the midline, retracting it superiorly will pull forward the larynx and the trachea. Make an incision inferiorly from the point of the

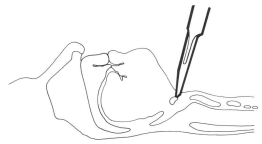

Figure 2.36. Insert a scalpel blade at the point identified (point C) at the end of line B (see Figure 2.35A) and aim the tip of the blade toward the imaginary line connecting the angles of the mandible. The hyoid bone will be reached.

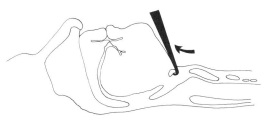

Figure 2.37. Insert a skin hook alongside the scalpel in the puncture site and tract made by the #11 blade and grasp the hyoid, lifting it upward and superior as shown above.

skin hook through the puncture site of the #11 blade, remaining in the midline as shown in Figure 2.38. Since the skin hook is grasping the body of the hyoid in its midpoint, an incision can be easily planned which will remain in the midline even though the patient may have a hematoma which distracts the perception of the midline. Identify the cricothyroid membrane and make a transverse incision through that membrane (Fig. 2.38). Insert a standard Pyrex tracheostomy tube through the cricothyroid membrane as one would routinely do for performing a cricothyroidotomy (Fig. 2.39). Finally, close the incision and connect the patient to a bag valve mask device.

ANCILLARY PROCEDURES

Percutaneous Transtracheal Catheter Ventilation

Percutaneous transtracheal catheter ventilation (PTV) is a useful procedure in

treating a patient who needs ventilation and oxygenation and in whom one cannot place an endotracheal tube for various reasons. It requires very little skill to perform and the material necessary is available in any emergency center. The procedure achieves good ventilation of the lungs within seconds with adequate oxygenation. One can continue CPR with chest compression while performing this procedure. Studies have demonstrated a tendency toward carbon dioxide retention (21, 22) and poor alveolar washout; however, one is able to achieve PO_2 of 300 torr and PCO_2 of 40 torr using this technique. The disadvantages are that it does not safeguard against aspiration. The catheter does not provide for complete control of the patient's airway. One is unable to suction through this device. Ventilation through this device should generally not be continued for more than 1 to 2 hours. The feeling that dangerously high pressures are needed to ventilate adequately through these catheters (9) has been proven wrong

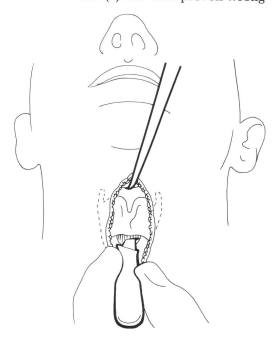

Figure 2.38. Make an incision from the skin hook downward to just above the suprasternal notch. Enter the cricothyroid membrane with a #11 blade. See text for details.

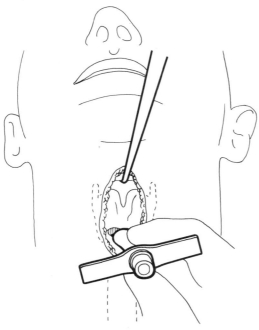

Figure 2.39. Insert the tracheostomy tube through the cricothyroid membrane. See text for details.

(49, 82). With a 16 gauge needle or larger, one can, with oxygen pressures of 50 lbs/sq in, have enough force to inflate the lung and supply a tidal volume (42, 81, 82).

Indications

1. A patient with respiratory arrest in whom one is unable to perform endotracheal intubation for whatever reason.

Equipment

Ordinary flow meter
Oxygen providing 50 lbs/sq in from ordinary wall oxygen source
Standard oxygen tubing
14 gauge Angiocath®
3-way plastic stopcock

While some authors have recommended a more complex setup with a hand operated release valve and other equipment this is not necessary (21, 29, 43, 80). Levinson (49) modified the PTV device described so that it could be assembled from parts found in any hospital emergency

center. The oxygen is provided by a 50 lb/sq in wall oxygen source coupled to an ordinary flow meter.

Technique

Preparatory Steps

1. Assemble device. To assemble the device, a side hole is cut near the distal end of a length of standard oxygen tubing. A standard three-way plastic stopcock made for intravenous tubing is attached to the oxygen tubing. The flow meter attached to the wall oxygen source is set at wide open (flush) position which provides a high flow rate necessary for PTV.

Procedural Steps

1. Identify the cricothyroid membrane.
2. Place the patient in a recumbent or semirecumbent position.
3. Prep the patient with the neck slightly extended.

NOTE

While extension of the neck is desirable, it is not essential to performance of this procedure.

4. Stabilize the larynx with the thumb and middle finger and place the index finger over the cricothyroid membrane.
5. Pass the needle at a 45 degree angle and cannulate the trachea through the cricothyroid membrane (Fig. 2.40).

CAUTION!

The posterior wall of the trachea is membranous below the cricoid cartilage and the esophagus lies posterior to it. One must stop passing the needle the moment air is aspirated into the syringe, to avoid perforation of the esophagus.

6. Attach the catheter to the oxygen tubing.
7. Turn on the oxygen to flush position if not already done.
8. With the thumb placed over the side

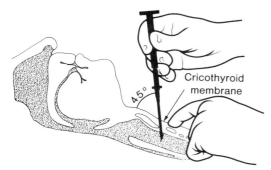

Figure 2.40. Percutaneous transtracheal catheter ventilation. The needle is inserted into the cricothyroid membrane at a 45 degree angle, directed inferiorly. See text for discussion.

hole cut in the oxygen gubint, a jet of pressurized air is delivered. Removal of the thumb permits oxygen to escape through the side hole and allows exhalation passively.

NOTE

An oxygen flow rate of approximately 50 lb/sq in is provided with a flow meter attached to a wall oxygen source set at the flush position (wide open). One can achieve a gas flow rate of 800 ml/sec with the standard oxygen tubing connected to a 14 gauge Angiocath®. All ventilations will be with 100% O_2. The physician can direct this oxygen flow intermittently into the trachea with his thumb over the portal of the three-way valve inserted between the oxygen tubing and the 14 gauge Angiocath®. A 1 second jet of O_2 followed by 4 seconds of an expiratory phase in which the O_2 is permitted to escape achieves good ventilation (21).

Complications

1. Subcutaneous emphysema (21, 29, 80). This may be caused by incorrect catheter placement and is a very common problem. The O_2 escapes into the subcutaneous tissue.
2. Mediastinal emphysema (29, 80).
3. Coughing. This may occur with each ventilation jet in a conscious patient (21).
4. Hemorrhage at site of needle puncture (21, 29).
5. Esophageal or mediastinal puncture if needle passed too far (21, 29).
6. Tracheal mucosal damage (21). This is due to the high pressure jets of oxygen and is not usually a problem. It becomes a problem when high pressure O_2 is permitted to continue striking the mucosa too many times.
7. Kinking of catheter (21). This may occur as the catheter enters the neck. If this is a problem, a larger catheter may have to be used.
8. Pneumatocyst (21). A pneumatocyst is a collection of air which occurs around the trachea, usually within a fascial plane, which is secondary to the high pressures of O_2 being delivered through the catheter. This is particularly prone to occur with improper use of the catheter and displacement. The pneumatocyst can be drained by simple needle aspiration.

Bronchoscopy

There are situations in the emergency center when rigid bronchoscopy is necessary. The procedure is easy to perform and may be lifesaving.

Indications

1. Massive hemoptysis. Bronchoscopy permits identification of the site of bleeding (55). Hemoptysis which is massive has a high mortality rate (18). Eighty-seven percent of patients with massive hemoptysis have a history of previous pulmonary bleeding, and over one half die without surgical intervention (18). In patients who have more than 600 ml of bleeding in 16 hours, the mortality related to the rate of bleeding exceeds 75%. As will be noted below, one may tamponade the bleeding when it is massive by instilling a temporary pack through the bronchoscope. Massive hemoptysis is a definite indication for rigid bronchoscope, since flexible fiberoptic instruments become cloudy when in contact with blood (47). The airway is better controlled and packing can be

placed, which cannot be performed through the fiberoptic bronchoscope (55).

2. Foreign body retrieval. While the flexible instrument is more useful here (47, 91), one can use the rigid bronchoscope in an acute emergency.

3. Massive aspiration. The bronchoscope can be used to remove large particulate matter to permit adequate ventilation.

Equipment

The following list is for emergency center bronchoscopy.

Rigid bronchoscope with light source
Adrenaline (1:1000)
Medicine cup
Small sterile gauze ball sponges
Sterile saline
Jackson bronchoscopic sponge carrier
Suction
Oxygen source
Fogarty balloon catheter
4% cocaine solution
2% lidocaine with epinephrine.

Technique

For Massive Hemoptysis

1. Place the patient in the Trendelenburg position with the head in the sniffing position by placing a folded towel under the head.
2. Light sedation is recommended.
3. Apply topical anesthesia with 4% cocaine spray to the pharynx and instill 2% lidocaine through the cricothyroid membrane. If needed, perform a block of the internal branch of the superior laryngeal nerve as indicated in the section on anesthesia for nasotracheal intubation (page 60).
4. Insert the bronchoscope after hyperextending the head at the atlanto-occipital joint (Fig. 2.41).
5. Remove blood and maintain the airway.
6. Once a site of bleeding has been identified, the topical application of epinephrine with pressure is used to temporarily control bleeding.
7. If bleeding continues, one of two

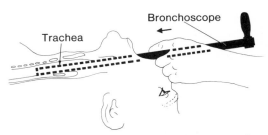

Figure 2.41. Insert the bronchoscope after hyperextending the head at the atlanto-occipital joint as shown. See text for details.

methods may be used for control (39, 55, 75, 91). Under extreme circumstances, passage of a gauze pack through the bronchoscope into the involved bronchus may be necessary for temporary control of bleeding. The sponge is applied with Jackson forceps and should be soaked with adrenaline. Irrigate the bronchus with 10 ml aliquots of sterile saline.

Alternately, the scope may be placed into the uninvolved main stem bronchus to maintain and isolate the airway. In one study with massive hemoptysis involving 10 patients who refused surgery, a balloon tipped catheter was placed and left for 24 hours and then deflated and this worked quite well (75). A Fogarty balloon catheter can be passed through the bronchoscope and the balloon inflated to obstruct bleeding from a secondary bronchus.

NOTE

Not all patients will tolerate isolation of one lung.

Transtracheal Aspiration

Transtracheal aspiration of tracheobronchopulmonary secretions in patients with lower respiratory tract disease is superior to expectorated sputum specimens for both Gram staining and culture of specimens (44, 62, 67). Transtracheal aspiration is a simple bedside procedure that should be used in cases of complicated disease of the lower respiratory tract in which sputum has not been produced or in which examination of expectorated sputum has been uninformative (44). A comparison of cultures obtained by the bronchoscope and by transtracheal aspiration indicated that the latter is more reliable (62). In one large study involving 154 patients (67), the diagnosis of bronchopulmonary infection caused by anaerobic bacteria could not have been made without transtracheal aspiration. Gram stain of transtracheal aspirates provided prompt and accurate bacteriologic diagnosis in more than 90% of cases, while Gram stains of expectorated sputum were nonspecific (67).

Technique

The patient should be supine with the neck hyperextended by a pillow placed beneath the shoulders. Cleanse the anterior aspect of the neck over the cricothyroid membrane with isopropyl alcohol. Raise an intradermal wheal over the cricothyroid membrane with 1% lidocaine injected through a 23 gauge needle. A 14 gauge intracath needle is then passed through this membrane and is directed at a 45 degree angle in a caudad direction with the bevel up. An 8 inch polyethylene catheter is threaded into the trachea. The 14 gauge needle is then quickly withdrawn. Two to 5 ml of sterile 0.9% saline is injected and then aspirated. Invariably a paroxysm of coughing is evoked. At this instant, suction is applied through a 10 ml syringe attached to the catheter. The catheter then is removed and pressure is applied for 3 to 5 minutes to assure hemostasis.

Complications

When this procedure is performed properly, reported complications are uncommon but include subcutaneous and mediastinal emphysema which may be extensive in some patients (44, 67).

Pulmonary Aspiration and Nasotracheal Suctioning

A number of misconceptions exist about nasotracheal suctioning, proper methods to maintain an airway, and immediate treatment of aspiration.

Drainage of foreign matter from the lungs in the prone position is as unlikely as in the supine position since the trachea remains horizontal in both positions. The optimal position in which an unconscious person who is not in need of resuscitation should be placed in bed is in the lateral position, maintained with pillows behind him (6, 69). The foot of the bed can be raised 6 to 9 inches (6) for optimal drainage. When aspiration does occur, suction should be performed to remove the fluid aspirate, and the patient should be optimally oxygenated. Diagnostic and therapeutic bronchoscopy with a flexible fiberoptic scope can be performed. If one sees material that cannot be removed through the fiberoptic scope due to size, insert a rigid bronchoscope and remove the material. With the aid of the fiberoptic scope, one can determine the location of foreign particles better. When aspiration occurs, roll the patient to the right side so the material remains in the dependent lung (71). Clear the mouth and pharynx and suction the patient. Bronchial lavage with normal saline solution after endotracheal intubation has been advocated by some (71). This lavage has been shown to decrease the risk of pulmonary edema following aspiration (44). Five to 10 ml of sterile saline solution are injected by syringe into the endotracheal tube, followed by immediate suction and oxygenation, and this is repeated until aspirated fluid is clear (56, 71). Lavage using large volumes of fluid increases the spread of acid and the extent of lung damage and is ineffective in neutralizing the acid reaction in pulmonary aspiration. A volume of saline equal to the volume of acid secretions will raise the hydrochloric acid pH from 1.6 to only 1.8 (56). This also increases the airway resistance and causes a fall in the lung compliance and PO_2; thus, lavage with large volumes of fluid is contraindicated.

Data available shows that using a straight plastic catheter and varying the head position does not help guide the catheter into the desired bronchus (35, 45). The catheter enters the right side in most patients regardless of the head position (35, 45). The best method to increase the likelihood of left main stem catheterization is to use a curved tip catheter (4, 35, 45).

References

1. Akinyemi, O.O., Complications of guided blind endotracheal intubation. Anaesthesia 34:590, 1979.
2. Alonso, W.A., Caruso, V.G., Roncace, E.A., Minibikes: A new factor in laryngotracheal trauma. Ann. Otol. Rhinol. Laryngol. 82:800, 1973.
3. Alonso, W.A., Pratt, L.L., Zollinger, W.K., et al., Complications of laryngotracheal disruption. Laryngoscope 84:1276, 1974.
4. Anthony, J.S., Sieniewicz, D.J., Suctioning of the left bronchial tree in critically ill patients. Crit. Care Med. 5:161, 1977.
5. Aro, L., Takki, S., Aromaa, U., Technique for difficult intubation. Br. J. Anaesth. 43:1081, 1977.
6. Atkinson, W.J., Posture of the unconscious patient. Lancet
7. Battaglia, J.D., Lockhart, C.H., Management of acute epiglottis by nasotracheal intubation. Am. J. Dis. Child. 129:334, 1975.
8. Behrman, R.E., James, L.S., et al., Treatment of the asphyxiated newborn infant. J. Pediatr. 74:981, 1969.
9. Bougas, T.P., Cook, C.D., Pressure-flow characteristics of needles suggested for transtracheal resuscitation. N. Engl. J. Med. 262:511, 1960.
10. Boutros, A.R., Arterial blood oxygenation during and after endotracheal suctioning in the apneic patient. Anesthesiology 32:114, 1970.
11. Boyd, A.D., Romita, M.C., Conlan, A.A., et al., A clinical evaluation of cricothyroidotomy. Surg. Gynecol. Obstet. 149:365, 1979.
12. Brantigan, C.O., Grow, J.B., Cricothyroidotomy: Elective use in respiratory problems requiring tracheotomy. J. Thorac. Cardiovasc. Surg. 71:72, 1976.
13. Browne, D.R.G., A guide to tracheal tubes. Anaesthesia 24:620, 1969.
14. Butler, R.M., Moser, F.H., The padded dash syndrome: Blunt trauma to the larynx and trachea. Laryngoscope 78:1172, 1968.
15. Caparosa, R.J., Zavatsky, A.R., Practical aspects of the cricothyroid space. Laryngoscope 67:577, 1957.
16. Chandra, P., Blind intubation. Br. J. Anaesth. 38:207, 1966.
17. Conrardy, P.A., Alteration of endotracheal tube position. Crit. Care Med. 4:8, 1976.
18. Crocco, J.A., Rooney, J.J., Fankushen, D.S., et al., Massive hemoptysis. Arch. Intern. Med. 121:495, 1968.
19. Davenport, H.T., Rosales, J.K., Endotracheal intubation of infants and children. Can. Anaes. Soc. J. 6:65, 1959.
20. DeVore, J.S., Resuscitation of the newborn. Clin. Obstet. Gynecol. 19:607, 1976.
21. Dunlap, L.B., A modified, simple device for the emergency administration of percutaneous transtracheal ventilation. J.A.C.E.P. 7:42, 1978.
22. Fell, T., Cheney, F.W., Prevention of hypoxia during endotracheal suction. Ann. Surg. 174:24, 1971.
23. Finster, M., Resuscitation of the newborn. Acta Anaesth. Scand. Supp. 37:86, 1970.
24. Finucane, B.T., Kupshik, H.L., A flexible stilette for replacing damaged tracheal tubes. Can. Anaesth. Soc. J. 25:153, 1978.
25. Fitchett, V.H., Pomerantz, M., Butsch, D.W., et al., Penetrating wounds of the neck. Arch. Surg. 99:307, 1969.
26. Fitchett, V.H., Pomerantz, M., Penetrating wounds of the neck. Arch. Surg. 99:307, 1969.
27. Forbes, J.A., Croup and its management. Br. Med. J. 1:389, 1961.
28. Fry, E.N.S., Letter to the editor. Can. Anaesth. Soc. J. 24:144, 1977.
29. Furgurson, J.E., Meislin, H.W., Airway problems in the trauma victim. Top. Emerg. Med. 1:9, 1979.
30. Gaskill, J.R., Nasotracheal intubation in head and neck surgery. Arch. Otolaryngol. 86:115, 1967.
31. Gold, M.I., Buechel, D.R., A method of blind nasal intubation for the conscious patient. Anesth. Anal. 39:257, 1969.
32. Gonzalez, S., A new instrument for uncomplicated emergency cricothyrotomy, South Med. J. 69:309, 1976.
33. Goodman, L.R., Conrardy, P.A., Laing, F., et al., Radiographic evaluation of endotracheal tube position. Am. J. Roentgenol. 127:433, 1976.
34. Gutgesell, H.P., Tacker, W.A., Energy dose for defibrillation of children. Pediatrics 58:898, 1976.
35. Haberman, P.B., Green, J.P., Archibald, C., et al., Determinants of successful selective tracheobronchial suctioning. N. Engl. J. Med. 289:1060, 1973.
36. Harris, H.H., Tobin, H.A., Acute injuries of the larynx and trachea in 49 patients. Laryngoscope 80:1376, 1970.
37. Heinonen, J., Takki, S., Tammisto, T., Effect of the Trendelenburg tilt and other procedures on the position of endotracheal tubes. Lancet 1:850, 1969.
38. Hemenway, W.G., The management of severe obstruction of the upper air passages. Surg. Clin. North Am. 41:201, 1961.
39. Hiebert, C.A., Balloon catheter control of life-threatening hemoptysis. Chest 66:308, 1974.
40. Hogg, C.E., Airway emergencies. Int. Anesthesiol. Clin. 10:13, 1972.
41. Holinger, P.H., Schild, J.A., Pharyngeal, laryngeal and tracheal injuries in the pediatric age-group. Ann. Otol. 81:538, 1972.
42. Jacobs, H.B., Emergency percutaneous transtracheal catheter and ventilator. J. Trauma 12:50, 1972.
43. Jacoby, J.J., Hamelberg, W., Ziegler, C.H., et al., Transtracheal resuscitation. J.A.M.A. 162:625, 1956.
44. Kalinske, R.W., Parker, R.H., Brandt, D., et al., Diagnostic usefulness and safety of transtracheal aspiration. N. Engl. J. Med. 276:604, 1967.
45. Kirimli, B., King, J.E., Pfaeffle, H.H., Evaluation of tracheobronchial suction techniques. J. Thorac. Cardiovas. Surg. 59:340, 1970.
46. Lambert, G.E., McMurry, G.T., Laryngotracheal

trauma: Recognition and management. J.A.C.E.P. 5:883, 1976.

47. Landa, J.F., Indications for bronchoscopy. Chest 73, 1978.

48. Lazoritz, S., Saunders, B.S., Bason, W.M., Management of acute epiglottitis. Crit. Care Med. 7:285, 1979.

49. Levinson, M.M., Scuderi, P.E., Gibson, R.L., et al., Emergency percutaneous transtracheal ventilation (PTV). J.A.C.E.P. 8:396, 1979.

50. Lewis, I., Endotracheal anaesthesia. Br. Med. J. 2:630, 1937.

51. Liew, R.P.C., A technique for naso-tracheal intubation with the soft Portex tube. Anesthesiology 28:567, 1973.

52. Lumpkin, J.R., Airway obstruction. Top. Emerg. Med. 2:15, 1980.

53. Magill, I.W., Endotracheal anesthesia. Am. J. Surg. 34:450, 1936.

54. Magill, I.W., Macintosh, R.R., Hewer, C.L., Lest we forget. Anaesthesia 30:476, 1975.

55. McCollum, W.B., Mattox, K.L., Guinn, G.A., et al., Immediate operative treatment for massive hemoptysis. Chest 67:152, 1975.

56. McCormick, P.W., Immediate care after aspiration of vomit. Anaesthesia 30:658, 1975.

57. Milstein, J.M., Goetzman, B.W., The Heimlich maneuver as an aid in endotracheal intubation of neonates. Pediatrics 60:749, 1977.

58. Nahum, A.M., Immediate care of acute blunt laryngeal trauma. J. Trauma 9:112, 1969.

59. Nicholas, T.H., Rumer, G.F., Emergency airway—A plan of action. J.A.M.A. 174:98, 1960.

60. Oh, T.H., Motoyama, E.K., Comparison of nasotracheal intubation and tracheostomy in management of acute epiglottitis. Anesthesiology 46:214, 1977.

61. Oppenheimer, R.P., Airway ... Instantly. J.A.M.A. 230:76, 1974.

62. Pecora, D.V., A comparison of transtracheal aspiration with other methods of determining the bacterial flora of the lower respiratory tract. N. Engl. J. Med. 269:664, 1963.

63. Pedersen, B., Blind nasotracheal intubation. Acta Anaesth. Scand. 15:107, 1971.

64. Penlington, G.N., Endotracheal tube sizes for children. Anaesthesia 29:494, 1974.

65. Redding, J.S., Tabeling, B.B., Parham, A.M., Airway management in patients with central nervous system depression. J.A.C.E.P. 7:401, 1978.

66. Richardson, W.R., Thoracic emergencies in the newborn infant. Am. J. Surg. 105:524, 1963.

67. Ries, K., Levison, M.E., Kaye, D., Transtracheal aspiration in pulmonary infection. Arch. Intern. Med. 133:453, 1974.

68. Ruben, H.M., Elam, J.O., Ruben, A.M., et al., Investigation of upper airway problems in resuscitation: I. Studies of pharyngeal x-rays and performance by laymen. Anesthesiology 22:271, 1961.

69. Safar, P., Escarraga, L.A., Chang, F., Upper airway obstruction in the unconscious patient. J. Appl. Phys. 14:760, 1959.

70. Salem, J.E., Intubation of conscious patients with combat wounds of upper respiratory passageway in Vietnam. Oral Surg. 24:701, 1967.

71. Salem, M.R., Anesthetic management of patients with "a full stomach": A critical review. Anesth. Anal. 49:47, 1970.

72. Salem, M.R., Mathrubhutham, M., Bennett, E.J., Difficult intubation. N. Engl. J. Med. 295:879, 1976.

73. Schuller, D.E., Birch, H.G., The safety of intubation in croup and epiglottis. Laryngoscope 84:33, 1975.

74. Seed, R.F., Traumatic injury to the larynx and trachea. Anaesthesia 26:55, 1971.

75. Selecky, P.A., Evaluation of hemoptysis through the bronchoscope. Chest 73:741, 1978.

76. Shapiro, S.L., Emergency airway for acute laryngeal obstruction. Eye, Ear, Nose, Throat Month. 49:35, 1970.

77. Sheely, C.H. II, Mattox, K.L., Beall, A.C., Jr., Management of acute cervical tracheal trauma. Am. J. Surg. 128:805, 1974.

78. Shim, C., Fine, N., Fernandez, R., et al., Cardiac arrhythmias resulting from tracheal suctioning. Ann. Intern. Med. 71:1149, 1969.

79. Shumrick, D.A., Trauma of the larynx. Arch. Otolaryngol. 86:109, 1967.

79a. Simon, R.R., Brenner, B.E., Emergency tracheostomy in the patient with massive neck swelling. (Submitted for publication.)

80. Smith, R.B., Transtracheal ventilation during anesthesia. Anesth. Anal. 53:225, 1974.

81. Smith, R.B., Babinski, M., Klain, M., et al., Percutaneous transtracheal ventilation. J.A.C.E.P. 5:765, 1976.

82. Spoerel, W.E., Narayanan, P.S., Singh, N.P., Transtracheal ventilation. Br. J. Anaesth. 43:932, 1971.

83. Stark, D.C.C., Biller, H.F., Aspiration of foreign bodies: Diagnosis and management. Int. Anesthesiol. Clin. 15:117, 1977.

84. Tahir, A.H., A simple manoeuvre to aid the passage of a nasotracheal tube into the oropharynx. Br. J. Anaesth. 42:631, 1970.

85. Tintinalli, J.E., Complications of nasotracheal intubation. Ann. Emerg. Med. 10:142, 1981.

86. Todres, I.D., Rogers, M.C., Methods of external cardiac massage in the newborn infant. J. Pediatr. 86:781, 1975.

87. Tos, M., Nasotracheal intubation in acute epiglottis. Arch. Otolaryngol. 97:373, 1973.

88. Urschel, H.C., Razzuk, M.A., Management of acute traumatic injuries of tracheobronchial tree, Surg. Gynecol. Obstet. 136:113, 1973.

89. Verrill, P.J., Anaesthesia in upper respiratory obstruction. Br. J. Anaesth. 35:237, 1963.

90. Wallace, C.T., Cooke, J.E., A new method for positioning endotracheal tubes. Anesthesiology 44:272, 1976.

91. Wilson, H.E., Control of massive hemorrhage during bronchoscopy. Dis. Chest 56:412, 1969.

92. Zuck, D., A technique for tracheo-bronchial toilet in the conscious patient. Anaesthesia 6:226, 1951.

93. Zwillich, C.W., Pierson, D.J., Creagh, C.E., et al., Complications of assisted ventilation: A prospective study of 354 consecutive episodes. Am. J. Med. 57:161, 1974.

Bibliography

1. Agosti, L., Modification of Magill's intubating forceps (letter). Anaesthesia 31:574, 1976.
2. Ashworth, C., Williams, L.F., Byrne, J.J., Penetrating wounds of the neck: Reemphasis of the need for prompt exploration. Am. J. Surg. 121:387, 1971.
3. Bearman, A.J., Device for nasotracheal intubation. Anesthesiology 23:130, 1962.
4. Bergen, R.P., Lost or broken teeth. J.A.M.A. 221:119, 1972.
5. Berman, R.A., A method for blind oral intubation of the trachea or esophagus. Anesth. Anal. 56:866, 1977.
6. Boyles, J.H., Lacerations of the larynx. Arch. Otolaryngol. 87:114, 1968.
7. Coghlan, C.J., Blind intubation in the conscious patient. Anesth. Anal. 45:290, 1966.
8. Coldiron, J.S., Estimation of nasotracheal tube length in neonates. Pediatrics 41:823, 1968.
9. Curtin, J.W., Holinger, P.H., Greeley, P.W., Blunt trauma to the larynx and upper trachea. J. Trauma 6:493, 1966.
10. Ducrow, M., Throwing light on blind intubation. Anaesthesia 33:827, 1978.
11. Eross, B., Nonslipping, nonkinking airway connections for respiratory care. Anesthesiology 34:571, 1971.
12. Evans, J.A., Fundamentals of infant resuscitation. Int. Anesth. Clin. 11:141, 1973.
13. Foster, C.A., An aid to blind nasal intubation in children (letter). Anaesthesia 32:1038, 1977.
14. Gaskill, J.R., Gillies, D.R., Local anesthesia for peroral endoscopy. Arch. Otolaryngol. 84:94, 1966.
15. Harris, H.H., Ainsworth, J.Z., Immediate management of laryngeal and tracheal injuries. Laryngoscope 75:1103, 1965.
16. Harris, H.H., Tobin, H.A., Acute injuries of the larynx and trachea in 49 patients. Laryngoscope 80:1376, 1970.
17. Hey, V.M.F., Relaxants for endotracheal intubation: A comparison of depolarizing and non-depolarizing neuromuscular blocking agents. Anaesthesia 28:32, 1973.
18. Holinger, P.H., Johnston, K.C., Factors responsible for laryngeal obstruction in infants. J.A.M.A. 143:1229, 1950.
19. Jacobs, H.B., Needle-catheter brings oxygen to the trachea. J.A.M.A. 222:1231, 1972.
20. Kerr, M., Pre-lubrication before nasal intubation. Br. J. Anaesth. 40:632, 1968.
21. LeMay, S.R., Penetrating wounds of the larynx and cervical trachea. Arch. Otolaryngol. 94:558, 1971.
22. Lynn, H.B., van Heerden, J.A., Tracheostomy in infants. Surg. Clin. North Am. 53:945, 1973.
23. Mattila, M.A.K., Heikel, P.-E., Suutarinen, T., et al., Estimation of a suitable nasotracheal tube length for infants and children. Acta Anaesthesiol. Scand. 15:239, 1971.
24. Meltzer, S.J., Auer, J., Continuous respiration without respiratory movements. J. Exp. Med. 11:622, 1909.
25. Morch, E.T., Saxton, G.A., Gish, G., Artificial respiration via the uncuffed tracheostomy tube. J.A.M.A. 160:864, 1956.
26. Munnell, E.R., Fracture of major airways. Am. J. Surg. 105:511, 1963.
27. Nilsson, R.K., Brendstrup, A., Fixation of nasotracheal tubes. Lancet 2:260, 1973.
28. Olson, N.R., Miles, W.K., Treatment of acute blunt laryngeal injuries. Ann. Otol. Rhinol. Laryngol. 80:704, 1971.
29. Pecora, D.V., Brook, R., A method of securing uncontaminated tracheal secretions for bacterial examination. J. Thorac. Med. Surg. 37:653, 1959.
30. Pennington, C.L., External trauma of the larynx and trachea. Ann. Otol. Rhinol. Laryngol. 81:546, 1972.
31. Powell, W.F., Ozdil, T., A translaryngeal guide for tracheal intubation. Anesth. Anal. 46:231, 1967.
32. Ripoll, I., Lindholm, C.-E., Carroll, R., et al., Spontaneous dislocation of endotracheal tubes. Anesthesiology 49:50, 1978.
33. Rosen, M., Hillard, E. K., The use of suction in clinical medicine. Br. J. Anaesth. 32:486, 1960.
34. Safar, P., Recognition and management of airway obstruction. J.A.M.A. 208:1008, 1969.
35. Safar, P., Penninckz, J., Cricothyroid membrane puncture with special cannula. Anesthesiology 28:943, 1967.
36. Saha, A.K., The estimation of the correct length of oral endotracheal tubes in adults (letter). Anaesthesia 32:919, 1977.
37. Schellinger, R.R., The length of the airway to the bifurcation of the trachea. Anesthesiology 25:169, 1964.
38. Schwab, J.M., Hartman, M.M., The management of the airway and ventilation in trauma. Med. Clin. North Am. 48:1577, 1964.
39. Seed, R.F., Traumatic injury to the larynx and trachea. Anaesthesia 26:55, 1971.
40. Sellick, B.A., Cricoid pressure to control regurgitation of stomach contents during induction of anaesthesia. Lancet 2:260, 1973.
41. Sheely, C.H., Mattox, K.L., Beall, A.C., Management of acute cervical tracheal trauma. Am. J. Surg. 128:805, 1974.
42. Smith, R.M., The critically ill child: Respiratory arrest and its sequelae. Pediatrics 46:108, 1970.
43. Szold, P.D., Glicklich, M., Children with epiglottitis can be bagged. Clin. Pediatr. 15:792, 1976.
44. Wang, K.P., Wise, R.A., Terry, P.B., et al. A new controllable suction catheter for blind cannulation of the main stem bronchi. Crit. Care Med. 6:347, 1978.
45. Yoshikawa, T.T., Chow, A.W., Montgomerie, J.Z., et al., Paratracheal abscess: An unusual complication of transtracheal aspiration.

Anesthesia and Regional Blocks

3

I. The Clinical Pharmacology of Local Anesthetics
  A. Allergic Reactions to Anesthetic Agents
  B. Long-Acting Local Anesthetics
  C. Types of Local Anesthesia
  D. Equipment
II. Head and Neck Blocks
  A. Mental Nerve Block
    1. Indications
    2. Technique
  B. Mandibular Nerve Block
    1. Indications
    2. Technique
  C. Maxillary Nerve Block—Greater Palatine and Nasopalatine Block
    1. Indications
    2. Technique
  D. Supraorbital and Supratrochlear Nerve Block
    1. Indications
    2. Technique
  E. Infraorbital Nerve Block
    1. Indications
    2. Technique
  F. Anesthesia to the Nose
    1. Indications
    2. Technique
  G. Scalp Block
    1. Indications
    2. Technique
  H. Anesthesia of the Ear
    1. Indications
    2. Technique for Block
       of the Auricle
    3. Technique for Block
       of the Auditory Canal
III. Upper Extremity Blocks
  A. Brachial Plexus Block
    1. Indications
    2. Technique
    3. Complications
  B. Median Nerve Block at Elbow
    1. Indications
    2. Technique
  C. Ulnar Nerve Block at the Elbow
    1. Indications
    2. Technique
  D. Median Nerve Block at the Wrist
    1. Indications
    2. Technique
  E. Ulnar Nerve Block at the Wrist
    1. Indications
    2. Technique
  F. Radial Nerve Block of the Wrist
    1. Indications
    2. Technique
  G. Digital Nerve Blocks
    1. Indications
    2. Technique
IV. Lower Extremity Nerve Blocks
  A. Nerve Blocks of the Foot
    1. Posterior Tibial Nerve Block
    2. Sural Nerve Block
    3. Saphenous Nerve Blocks
    4. Superficial Peroneal
       Nerve Block
    5. Anterior Tibial Nerve Blocks
    6. Block of the Great Toe
    7. Blocks of the Toes other
       than the Great Toe
V. Blocks of the Torso and Other Areas
  A. Block of the Intercostal Nerves
  B. Transvaginal Pudendal Nerve Block
  C. Block of the Penis
  D. Urethral Anesthesia
  E. Infiltration Anesthesia for Cesarean Section
  F. Anesthesia of the Surface of the Cornea and Conjunctiva
  G. Hematoma Block for Reduction of a Fracture
  H. Intravenous Regional Analgesia

THE CLINICAL PHARMACOLOGY OF LOCAL ANESTHETICS

Two general types of local anesthetics currently exist: ester compounds (procaine, cocaine and tetracaine) and amide compounds (mepivacaine, bupivacaine, lidocaine). Ester anesthetics are hydrolyzed by pseudocholinesterase in the serum, whereas amide type compounds are metabolized in the liver. The only local anesthetic agent excreted unchanged in the urine is cocaine (10). The mechanism of action of local anesthetics is a decrease in the rate of rise of depolarization of the action potential such that after excitation of the cell, depolarization does not reach threshold for firing; thus, a propagated action potential fails to occur (10).

All local anesthetic agents are vasodilators due to a relaxant effect on smooth muscle. Only cocaine produces immediate vasoconstriction preceded by a brief period of vasodilation. This vasoconstriction is due to inhibition of uptake of catecholamines by cocaine (10). Vasoconstrictors are often added to local anesthetics, e.g., lidocaine, to diminish bleeding in a wound. Vasoconstrictors are less effective subcutaneously than intradermally because the blood supply is more abundant intradermally (4). Thus, local anesthetics containing epinephrine should be injected intradermally. Effective vasoconstriction is obtained using the dilution of 1:100,000 of epinephrine.

In using local anesthetics, aspiration is essential before all injections as some of the nerves being blocked course with the major vessels. In most regional nerve blocks, paresthesias are desirable to elicit before infiltration of an anesthetic solution; however, when resistance is encountered to injection combined with a paresthesia, it is likely that one is depositing the anesthetic solution intraneurally. Thus, when paresthesia is elicited, the needle must be withdrawn 1 or 2 mm before the deposition of the agent to avoid injection into the nerve fiber itself. The clinical uses, concentrations, onset and duration of action and maximum single doses of common local anesthetics are listed in Table 3.1.

Lidocaine is currently the most commonly used local anesthetic in most emergency centers. Lidocaine toxicity involves an initial excitement, apprehension, disorientation, nausea and vomiting which are often prodromal signs of convulsions. Frequently this prodrome is overlooked or the symptoms are termed hysteria by physicians who are unaware of the hazards of local anesthesia. The severity and duration of the convulsions vary with the nature of the drugs used, the quantity and rapidity of absorption, and the susceptibility of the patient. Large quantities of lidocaine infused intravenously rapidly may cause fleeting convulsive manifestations which may quickly be followed by severe central nervous system collapse. This reaction is characterized by coma, areflexia, apnea, and circulatory collapse. The cardiovascular responses of lidocaine toxicity involve myocardial depression as well as vasodilation. Local anesthetics also may slow conduction in the myocardium. For more extensive discussion see Chapter 9: "Plastic Surgery, Principles and Techniques."

Allergic Reactions to Anesthetic Agents

There is a high incidence of allergic reactions with ester-type local anesthetics. The incidence of allergic reactions to lidocaine is extremely low. Procaine, an ester-type local anesthetic, is hydrolyzed by pseudocholinesterase in the serum. This reaction results in the formation of p-aminobenzoic acid and diethylamino-alcohol. p-Aminobenzoic acid will competitively inhibit sulfonamide antibiotics (10). In patients who are allergic to lidocaine, an amide compound, e.g., procaine, can be safely used for local anesthesia.

Long-Acting Local Anesthetics

Bupivacaine is a long-acting local anesthetic in common use today. In a review of 2,077 cases by Moore et al. (21), the onset of action of this drug was within 4 to 10 minutes and the maximum analgesic was achieved within 15 to 30 minutes. When the drug was used for peripheral nerve blocks, 0.25 and 0.5% were satisfactory in most cases. An inadvertent intravenous injection of 100 ml of bupivacaine occurred twice in their series without any untoward sequelae (21).

Types of Local Anesthesia

Local infiltration is the production of analgesia by direct infiltration of the wound. This type of local anesthesia is probably the most commonly used in the emergency center. Its disadvantages are that it distorts the wound margins and is more painful at the site of injury than peripheral nerve block or other types of anesthesia.

Field block anesthesia is the production of regional anesthesia by creating a wall of anesthetic around the operative field by local infiltration around the wound site.

Regional nerve block is regional anesthesia produced by directly injecting around the nerve or nerves supplying the area with sensation. This type of anesthesia is the type on which this chapter will concentrate. The following factors make regional nerve block anesthesia the procedure of choice (6) for a number of procedures performed in the emergency center: 1) it does not increase or cause tissue anoxia, 2) the complications of general anesthesia are avoided, and 3) it does not disturb the wound edges. Regional nerve block anesthesia is commonly used for repair of extensive lacerations as it avoids multiple injections and the use of large volumes of local anesthetics (22). It is particularly useful in situations in which local infiltration produces much pain, such as abscesses and arthrocentesis for acute arthritis.

There is little evidence that topical anesthetics are of any value on unbroken skin (10). They are of value on broken skin and on mucous membranes as is discussed in the chapter on plastic surgery procedures.

To avoid intravascular injection, one must be certain to aspirate before the deposition of any anesthetic agent (8). The authors prefer injection during advancement rather than withdrawal of the needle, as this produces less pain for the patient as one advances the needle. This facilitates deposition in the correct line and plane. All blocks used in this chapter are those with easily recognized landmarks. We have purposely omitted those blocks which are more difficult to perform and are of little value in the emergency center.

Equipment

The equipment needed for regional nerve block anesthesia will not be discussed separately and includes the following:

1% lidocaine without epinephrine
1% lidocaine with epinephrine
2% lidocaine with epinephrine
0.25% bupivacaine (when a long-acting anesthetic agent is desired)
4% and 10% cocaine solution
Assortment of needles. 23,25 gauge and 18 gauge (for drawing up the anesthetic solution). The lengths should be 1½"–3".
Syringes; 10, 20, 30 cc.
Iodinated prep solution
4 × 4 gauze (1 dozen)
Sterile towels
Sterile gloves

HEAD AND NECK BLOCKS

Mental Nerve Block

The mental nerve is a branch of the inferior alveolar nerve, which in turn is a branch of the mandibular division of the fifth cranial nerve. It exits from the mental foramen which is directly below the level of the second premolar and inside the lower lip at its junction with the lower gingiva called the inferior sulcus (Fig. 3.1). This nerve supplies sensation to the skin and mucous membranes of the lower lip (Fig. 3.2).

Indications

Repair of lacerations of the lower lip.

Technique

While the extraoral route has been described, the authors prefer the intraoral route for anesthetizing this nerve because it is less painful to the patient and easier to perform. The nerve is blocked as it

Table 3.1.   Local Anesthetic Agents Concentrations and Clinical Uses (4)

Agent	Concentration and Clinical Use	Onset and Duration of Action	Maximum Single Dose (mg)	Comments
AMIDES				
Lidocaine (Xylocaine[R])	0.5–1.0% for infiltration or IV 1.0–1.5% for peripheral nerve 4.0% for topical	Rapid onset. Short to intermediate duration (60–120 min)	300 plain 500 adrenaline	Excellent spreading ability. Wide range of applications.
Prilocaine	0.5–1.0% for infiltration or IV block 1.0% for peripheral nerve	Slower onset. Short to intermediate duration (60–120 min)	400 plain 600 adrenaline	0.5% is choice for intravenous block. Most rapidly metabolized and safest of all amide type agents. Doses in excess of 600 mg produce significant amounts of MetHb. Therefore avoid doses above 600 mg and repeated doses. Good choice in outpatient block. Not suitable for obstetrics.
Mepivacaine (Carbocaine[R])	1.0% for infiltration 1.0–1.5% for peripheral nerve	Slower onset. Intermediate to longer duration (90–180 min)	300 plain 500 adrenaline	Duration slightly longer than equal dose of lidocaine, and blood levels not as sensitive to inclusion of adrenaline as lidocaine; thus may be useful if adrenaline not desirable.
Etidocaine	0.5% for infiltration 0.5–1.0% for peripheral nerve	Rapid onset. Long duration (4–8 hrs)	200 plain 300 adrenaline	Capable of producing profound motor block. Useful in postoperative pain management by peripheral blocks.
Bupivacaine (Marcaine[R])	0.25– for infiltration 0.5% for peripheral nerve 0.25– 0.5%	Slow onset. Long duration (4–8 hrs)	175 plain 250 adrenaline	Favored for obstetric nerve blocks because of minimal fetal effects. Excellent for postoperative analgesia because of minimal motor block.

ESTERS

Drug	Concentration	Dose (mg)	Onset/Duration	Comments
Procain (Novocain^R)	1.0% for infiltration	500 plain 600 adrenaline	Slow onset. Short duration (30–45 min)	Indicated where history of malignant hyperpyrexia (MH). Ideal for skin infiltration. Very rapidly metabolized.
Chloroprocaine	1.0–2.0% as for procaine	600 plain 750 adrenaline	Rapid onset. Short duration.	Drug of choice for obstetric and outpatient neural blockade. Metabolized four times more rapidly than procaine.
Amethocaine (Tetracaine^R)	0.5–1.0% for topical 0.1–0.2% for infiltration and peripheral nerve	100 approx.	Slow onset. Long duration.	May be useful alternative if amides contraindicated (e.g., MH). Metabolized four times more slowly than procaine.
Cocaine	4.0–10.0% for topical	150 approx. (1.5 ml of 10% or 4 ml of 4%)	Slow onset. Medium duration.	Topical use only. Addictive. Indirect adrenoceptor stimulation. No evidence that 10% solution more effective than 4%. Patients sensitive to exogenous catecholamines should receive topical lidocaine rather than cocaine.
Benzocaine	0.4–5.0% for topical only. Usually dispensed in admixture with other therapeutic ingredients related to site of application.	No information	Rapid onset. Short duration.	Occasionally dispensed in urethane solution. Urethane is a suspect carcinogen and should not be used.

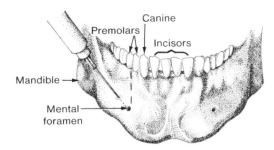

Figure 3.1. The mental foramen through which the mental nerve exits lies directly below the level of the second premolar.

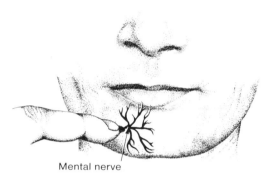

Figure 3.2. The mental nerve supplies sensation to the skin and mucous membranes of the lower lip.

exits from the mental foramen (18). The left index finger is used to palpate the point where the nerve exits from the mandible. The needle is inserted at the inferior sulcus of the mouth and directed toward the foramen. While the site of insertion of the needle has been described to be between the apices of the bicuspid (18), in the authors' experience it has been easier to retract the lower lip with the thumb of the left hand and insert the needle at the level of the canine directing it to the mental foramen (Fig. 3.3). The needle point is directed at the foramen and 2 ml of lidocaine with 1:100,000 aqueous epinephrine is injected. The same is performed on the opposite side to achieve complete block of the lower lip (Fig. 3.4). As the solution is injected, vigorous shaking of the lower lip will decrease the pain of injection. This procedure gives excellent anesthesia and block is usually complete. When the foramen cannot be palpated, then inject about

0.5 cm below the second premolar and massage the area to achieve good distribution.

Mandibular Nerve Block

The mandibular nerve contains both sensory and motor fibers. The sensory branches include the auriculotemporal nerve, which courses anterior to the external auditory meatus and innervates the skin of the temple as well as that of the external auditory canal and a portion of the pinna. The lingual nerve runs between the ramus of the mandible and the medial pterygoid bone and supplies sensation to the anterior two thirds of the tongue. The

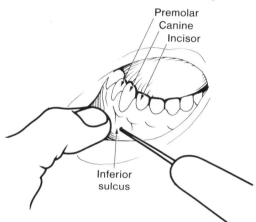

Figure 3.3. Retract the lower lip with the thumb of the left hand and insert the needle at the level of the canine, directing it toward the mental foramen.

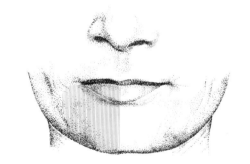

Figure 3.4. Infiltration provides anesthesia for one half of the lower lip. Bilateral infiltration of the mental nerve will provide good anesthesia for the entire lower lip.

inferior alveolar nerve courses through the mandibular foramen and transverses the mandibular canal, supplying sensation to the teeth, gums, and lower jaw. This third division of the mandibular nerve branches to form the mental nerve, which innervates the lower lip.

Indications

1. Repair of gingival and oral lacerations along the mandible.
2. Reduction of displaced or avulsed teeth of the lower jaw.

Technique

Complete block of the sensory distribution of the mandibular nerve is achieved by injecting the anesthetic solution proximal to the division of the nerve into its sensory branches. The site of injection is the mandibular sulcus on the inner surface of the ramus. This blocks the inferior alveolar and lingual nerves. Palpate the retromolar trigone with the patient's mouth partly opened (Fig. 3.5). Insert a needle at the apex of the pterygomandibular raphe and advance it to the ramus of the mandible and the muscles over the internal surface of the ramus. A point of resistance will be felt against the posterior wall of the ramus and will halt further advancement of the needle. At this point, 2 ml of anesthetic solution (lidocaine with epinephrine) are deposited here and another 2 ml are deposited as the needle is withdrawn.

Maxillary Nerve Block—Greater Palatine and Nasopalatine Block

The maxillary nerve is entirely sensory. It exists through the foramen rotundum and enters the pterygopalatine fossa, where it divides. The sensory nerves which are of importance to the emergency physician are the posterior nasal branches which supply the mucous membrane lining the posterior inferior portion of the nasal cavity. One of these branches, the nasopalatine nerve, courses forward and downward along the nasal septum to exit through the incisive foramen and supplies sensation to the anterior part of the hard palate and the adjacent gums. The greater palatine nerve is another important branch of this nerve and supplies sensation to the posterior two thirds of the palate. The infraorbital nerve, a branch of the maxillary nerve, supplies sensation to the malar region and side of the nose and upper lip.

Indications

1. Repair of injuries involving the face over the sensory distribution of the nerve.
2. Reductions of displaced or avulsed superior incisors.
3. Repair of lacerations involving the palate.

Technique

Individual branches of this nerve are anesthetized, rather than the entire nerve.

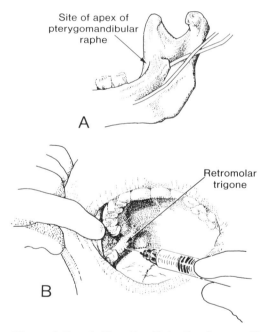

Site of apex of pterygomandibular raphe

A

Retromolar trigone

B

Figure 3.5.   A. The site of injection for mandibular nerve block is shown. The injection site is on the inner surface of the ramus of the mandible. This can be found by locating the retromolar trigone, which lies behind the third molar. The needle is inserted at the apex of the pterygomandibular raphe or apex of the trigone B. Advance the needle to the ramus of the mandible on the inner surface and inject 2 ml of anesthetic solution.

There is no indication for block of the maxillary nerve in the emergency center. Those individual divisions which are blocked will be discussed below.

The *nasopalatine nerve* is blocked by injecting 1 cc of 1% lidocaine with epinephrine at the point where the nerve exits from the anterior midline of the hard palate, behind and between the upper incisors. This provides anesthesia to the anterior one third of the palate and the adjacent gingiva.

The *greater palatine nerve* is blocked by injecting 1 cc of 1% lidocaine with epinephrine at the site where the nerve exits from the greater palatine foramen. This is just medial to the third molar, anterior to the junction of the soft and hard palate. This anesthetizes the posterior two thirds of the palate and gingiva (Fig. 3.6).

Supraorbital and Supratrochlear Nerve Block

The supraorbital and supratrochlear nerves emerge through notches or depressions at the upper border of the orbital ridge about 2.5 cm from the midline, after which they are distributed to the forehead and the scalp (Figs. 3.7 and 3.8). The depression of the supraorbital notch as it exits from the upper border of the orbit is easily palpated.

Indications

1. Extensive lacerations of the forehead.
2. Debriding abrasions of the forehead and removal of particles of dirt or glass.

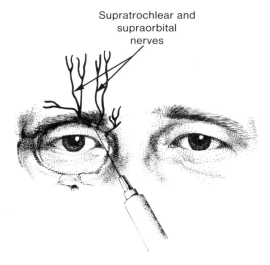

Supratrochlear and supraorbital nerves

Figure 3.7.   The supraorbital and supratrochlear nerves emerging through the notches at the upper border of the orbital ridge.

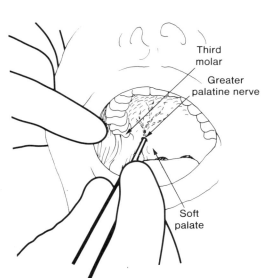

Third molar

Greater palatine nerve

Soft palate

Figure 3.6.   Block of the greater palatine nerve. See text for discussion.

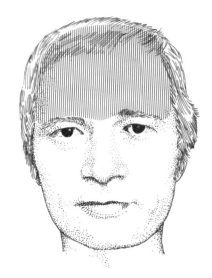

Figure 3.8.   The supraorbital and supratrochlear nerves supply sensation to the forehead and scalp as far back as the coronal suture.

Technique

These nerves are easily blocked by palpating the supraorbital ridge with the index finger of the right hand until the notch is palpated just medial to the midpoint of the eyebrow (Fig. 3.9). This marks the point where the supraorbital nerve exits. The supratrochlear nerve exits just medial to this point. The nerves can be blocked by one of two methods. A 23 gauge, 1.5 inch needle attached to a 3 ml syringe filled with 1% lidocaine with epinephrine is inserted and directed by the index finger of the left hand towards the notch palpated above (Fig. 3.9). This is the site of injection. Paresthesias do not have to be elicited. A site approximately 0.5 to 1 cm medial to this point is also infiltrated to anesthetize the supratrochlear nerve.

An *alternate method* has been described which assures infiltration of all the branches of the nerves. A line of anesthetic solution is deposited horizontally, extending across both supraorbital ridges (Fig. 3.10).

Infraorbital Nerve Block

The infraorbital nerve exists along the infraorbital ridge at a point directly below

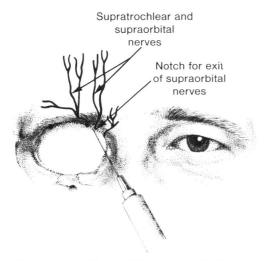

Supratrochlear and supraorbital nerves

Notch for exit of supraorbital nerves

Figure 3.9. Block of the supraorbital and supratrochlear nerves is performed by inserting the needle just beneath the supraorbital ridge and directing it to the notch where the supraorbital and supratrochlear nerves emerge.

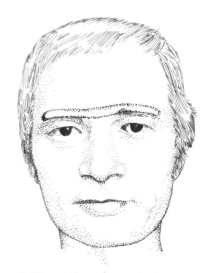

Figure 3.10. A line of anesthetic solution can be deposited horizontally to block all the branches of the supraorbital and supratrochlear nerves.

the exit of the supraorbital nerve superiorly. The site of exit can be palpated as a depression or foramen just inferior to the infraorbital ridge (Fig. 3.11). This nerve supplies sensation to the infraorbital region of the cheek and the lateral aspect of the nose and upper lip (Fig. 3.12).

Indications

1. Extensive lacerations of the malar area of the upper lip.
2. Drainage of facial abscess in the cheek.
3. Debridement of abrasions of the cheek.

Technique

While two methods are described in the literature, one intraorally and the other extraorally, the authors prefer the intraoral route as it is less painful and easier to perform (18). A 23 gauge, 1½ inch needle attached to a 5 ml syringe is filled with 1% lidocaine with epinephrine. Infiltrate the site of injection on the mucous membrane with a 25 gauge needle and lidocaine. This site is at the buccogingival fold just medial to the canine tooth of the maxilla on the side to be blocked. The needle is inserted at this point and advanced to the infraor-

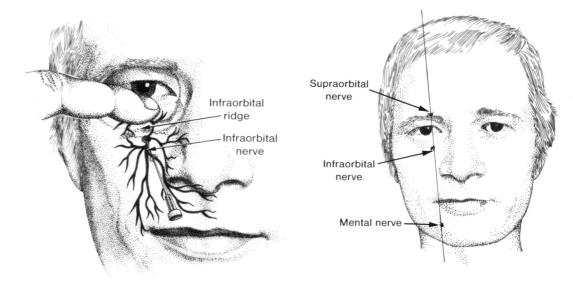

Figure 3.11. *A.* The infraorbital nerve courses through a foramen which lies inferior to the infraorbital ridge. *B.* In many patients in whom an infraorbital nerve block is desirable but in whom the malar area is markedly swollen, one cannot palpate or find the infraorbital foramen. In such cases a line may be extended from the supraorbital notch to the mental foramen and this will traverse the infraorbital foramen.

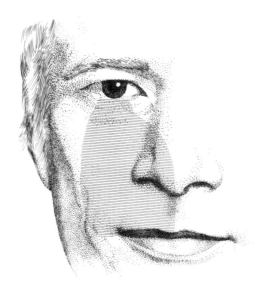

Figure 3.12. The sensory distribution of the infraorbital nerve.

bital foramen, guided by the index finger of the left hand externally. One to 2 ml of anesthetic solution is infiltrated at this point, and anesthesia usually is complete within 5 minutes. Vigorous shaking of the upper lip will decrease the pain of injection. With a bilateral block, good anesthesia can be obtained for the entire upper lip. The injection in this method does not have to be exactly at the foramen.

Alternate Technique

An alternate method has been described (11) which is extraoral. The lateral nasal sulcus 1 cm from the ala of the nose is the site of injection (Fig. 3.11). The needle inserted here is advanced upward and laterally, guided by the index finger of the left hand palpating the depression of the infraorbital ridge. At 0.5 cm below the infraorbital ridge, 1 to 2 ml of anesthetic solution is injected.

Anesthesia to the Nose

The sensory innervation of the nose is provided by branches of the first and second divisions of the fifth cranial nerve. The anterior ethmoidal arises from the first (ophthalmic) division within the orbit and reenters the skull by passing through the anterior ethmoidal foramen on the medial wall of the orbit. It then courses down through the cribriform plate and innervates the anterior third of the nasal septum and the lateral walls in the upper nasal cavity. The posterior two thirds of the septum and the lateral walls inferiorly and posteriorly receive supply from the sphenopalatine nerve arising from the sphenopalatine ganglion of the maxillary division of the fifth.

Indications

1. Nasal lacerations.
2. Nasal fracture reduction.
3. Epistaxis.
4. Drainage of a septal hematoma or abscess.

Technique

Two techniques have been described for anesthetizing the nose. When anesthesia is required for reduction of nasal fractures, further steps are needed to provide adequate anesthesia than when intranasal mucosal anesthesia is indicated. These will be discussed separately.

***Modified Sluder's Technique* (9, 20).** A nasal tampon is dipped into a solution of 1:1000 epinephrine and the excess fluid is removed by squeezing the tampon between the fingers. Then dip the tampon into 10% cocaine and again remove the excess. Place this tampon between the turbinates and the septum and leave it in place for 5 minutes. Remove this tampon from the nose, and the membranes are now maximally shrunken. Now wind a small amount of cotton onto the end of a metal applicator and moisten with 1:1000 epinephrine, press this dry and dip into cocaine flakes. The applicator is then passed into the nose at the angle between the middle and posterior thirds of the middle turbinate and septum until it reaches the face of the sphenoid sinus (Fig. 3.13). A second applicator is placed in the cleft of the nose at a point between the anterior end of the middle turbinate and the septum until it comes to rest on the inferior surface of the cribiform plate. The first applicator provides anesthesia to the sphenopalatine ganglion and the second to the anterior ethmoids.

These applicators must be left in place

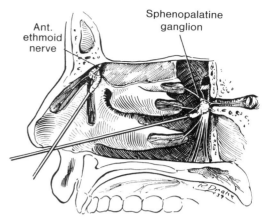

Figure 3.13. Cotton-tipped applicator is in the position to anesthetize the anterior ethmoid nerve and the nasal branches of the sphenopalatine ganglion. (Reprinted with permission of Mousel, L.H., Anesthesia for operations about the head and neck. Anesthesiology 2:61–73, 1941.)

for at least 10 minutes. This procedure provides excellent anesthesia for all intranasal procedures.

Moffetts Technique. This is not the authors' preferred procedure. It is indicated when one is dealing with an uncooperative patient or a child who will not permit placement of applicators into the proper position. The technique requires no applicators and so is less traumatic. Lying supine and with the head tilted as far back as possible, the patient is in the optimal position for blocking these nerves to the nose. Two milliliters of anesthetic solution are deposited into the nostril with a dropper so that it reaches the site of the anterior ethmoidal nerve. To anesthetize the sphenopalatine nerve, the patient's head is tilted slightly forward. The solution used is 4 or 10% cocaine and this is permitted to remain in the nose for 10 minutes. Both nostrils are anesthetized at the same time.

Additional anesthesia required for reduction of nasal fractures

In addition to the intranasal blocks indicated above, the following nerves should be blocked for nasal fracture reduction:

1. The infraorbital nerve (technique described elsewhere) (Fig. 3.14).

2. Infratrochlear nerve. This nerve courses just above the inner canthus of the eye (Fig. 3.14). It is blocked with a 1½ inch needle passed just laterally to the bridge of the nose and superior to the inner canthus. One to 2 ml of 1% lidocaine with epinephrine is instilled at this site.

3. The external nasal nerves are anesthetized by inserting a needle from the inside of the nose, exiting just above the superior rim of the lateral cartilage. This is shown in Figure 3.14 and in needle *A* in Figure 3.15. The needle continues upward over the lateral portion of the nasal bone, diagrammatically represented in needle position *B* in Figure 3.15. To anesthetize the external nasal nerve which courses at the junction of the lateral cartilage with the nasal bone (Fig. 3.14), the anesthetic solution is deposited as the needle is withdrawn.

4. Additional anesthetic is then injected submucosally into the membranous nasal septum and into the area of the nasal spine. Infiltration around the anterior nasal spine will block the anterior alveolar nerves.

Scalp Block

Almost the entire nerve supply to the scalp is superficial (Figs. 3.16 and 3.17). Anteriorly the supraorbital and supratrochlear nerves, which are terminal branches of the first division of the fifth cranial nerve, reach the forehead through a depression in the superior bony ridge of the orbit. They supply the scalp as far as the crown of the head, supplying innervations to both the forehead and the front of the scalp. Laterally the auriculotemporal nerve, a branch of the mandibular division of the fifth cranial nerve, passes beneath the parotid gland to reach the temporal fossa posterior to the superficial temporal artery where it supplies innervation to the temporal aspect of the scalp. A small area between these two nerves is innervated by the zygomaticotemporal nerve, a branch of the maxillary nerve. The posterior scalp is supplied by the

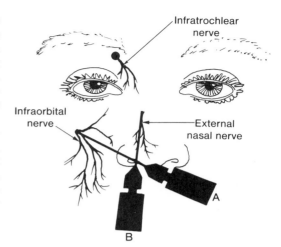

Figure 3.14. To completely anesthetize the nose for reduction of nasal fractures and for complex repairs one must anesthetize the infratrochlear, infraorbital and external nasal nerves as shown and described in the text.

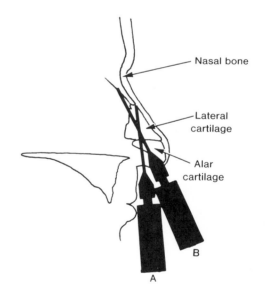

Figure 3.15. The technique of anesthetizing the external nasal nerve is shown. Needle "A" is inserted from inside the nose and emerges from above the lateral cartilage between that cartilage and the nasal bone. The needle then continues upward over the lateral portion of the nasal bone as represented by position "B," and the anesthetic solution is then deposited as the needle is withdrawn. See text for details.

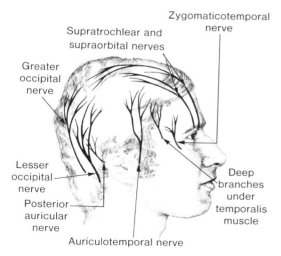

Figure 3.16.   Nerve supply to the scalp. See text for discussion.

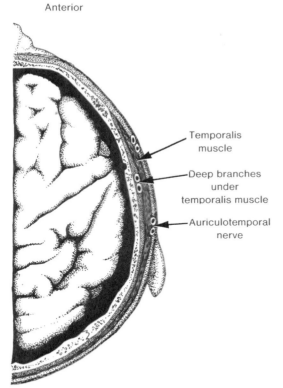

Figure 3.17.   Portions of the sensory nerve supply to the scalp over the temporal region lie deep to the temporalis muscle. See text for discussion.

greater and lesser occipital nerves, which are branches of the first through the third cervical roots after they pierce the erector spinae muscle and become superficial as they cross the occipital ridge. These nerves supply the posterior scalp as far anteriorly as the vertex and laterally to the mastoids (6, 9).

Indications

This block is useful when repairing extensive lacerations of the scalp.

Technique

Using a 3 inch, 22 gauge needle, intradermal and subcutaneous local infiltration with 0.5 to 1% lidocaine with epinephrine is carried out circumferentially around the scalp. The temporal regions may require extra anesthetic to be deposited deep to the temporalis muscle because of the depth of the nerves in this area. A "cap" of analgesia is produced over the head above the line of infiltration (Fig. 3.18).

When only a portion of the scalp needs to be anesthetized (anterior or posterior portion), specific nerves may be blocked. The supraorbital and supratrochlear nerve blocks providing anesthesia for the anterior portion of the scalp and forehead were discussed earlier in this chapter. When a posterior nerve block is indicated, this can

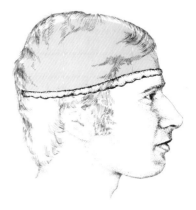

Figure 3.18.   A cap of anesthesia is deposited circumferentially around the scalp for complex lacerations of the scalp as shown. In addition to this, the deep branches which lie beneath the temporalis muscle must be anesthetized as shown in Figure 3.17.

be provided by anesthetizing the greater occipital nerve as it courses through its hiatus along the superior aspect of the trapezius muscle where it attaches to the base of the occiput (Fig. 3.19A). In performing this block, paresthesias should be elicited. Alternatively, a line of anesthesia may be deposited subcutaneously at the base of the occiput, at the level of the external occipital protuberance which can be palpated along the occipital bone (Fig. 3.19B). This block will provide anesthesia to the greater occipital nerve, lesser occipital nerve branches, and the third occipital

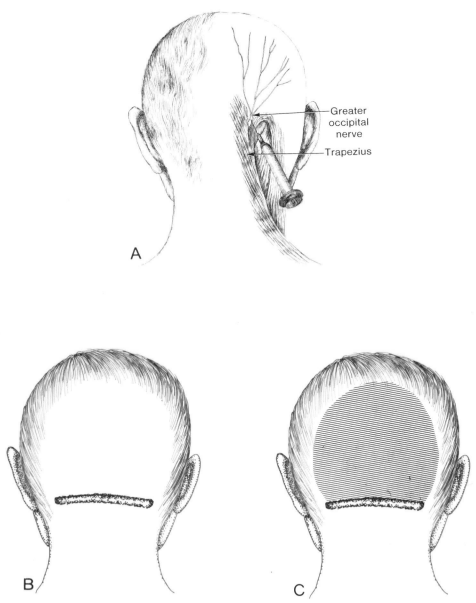

Figure 3.19.   *A*. Block of the greater occipital nerve. *B*. Alternately, a line of anesthetic can be deposited subcutaneously at the base of the occiput, at the level of the external occipital protuberance. *C*. The area of anesthesia provided by this block is shown. See text for discussion.

nerve (Fig. 3.19C). The amount of anesthetic solution required is approximately 10 cc of 1% lidocaine with epinephrine.

Anesthesia of the Ear

Four nerves are of importance in considering anesthesia to the ear. The innervation of the auricle is mainly via the *great auricular nerve* which is a branch of the cervical plexus. It becomes subcutaneous posterior to the midpoint of the sternocleidomastoid muscle from which it runs directly toward the ear. This nerve supplies the medial portion of the auricle and the lower and peripheral portion of the lateral aspect of the ear by the anterior branch. The auriculotemporal nerve, a branch of the mandibular nerve, supplies the anterior-superior portion of the lateral surface of the auricle. This nerve courses immediately in front of the external auditory canal. The *auricular branch of the vagus* nerve supplies innervation to the concha (Fig. 3.20) as it emerges through the tympanomastoid fissure just anterior to the mastoid process and behind the external meatus.

The external auditory meatus is innervated by two of the previously discussed nerves: the auriculotemporal nerve and the auricular branches of the vagus nerve. The auriculotemporal nerve gives off a branch to the canal and supplies the skin of the superior, anterior, and inferior boundaries of the canal as well as the tympanic membrane. The auricular branch of the vagus innervates the skin of the inferior and posterior walls of the auditory canal. Another nerve supplying sensation to the ear is the tympanic nerve, which is a branch of the glossopharyngeal nerve and innervates the middle ear.

Indications

1. Lacerations of the ear. In patients with extensive lacerations of the ear, it is difficult to provide anesthesia by local infiltration of the wound edges due to the close apposition of the skin to the cartilaginous surface. Block of the greater auricular nerve and auriculotemporal nerve provides adequate anesthesia to repair the wound in the majority of cases. In lacerations extending posterior to the ear, one may find it necessary to block the lesser occipital nerve which supplies innervation to the skin behind the ear. This will be discussed below.

2. Irrigation of the ear and removal of impacted cerumen. In patients with otitis externa and in patients who have cerumen impacted close to the tympanic membrane, block of the ear canal may be necessary to adequately cleanse the canal of debris for topical antibacterials to work adequately or to dislodge a particle of cerumen without discomfort.

3. Myringotomy. Myringotomy requires anesthesia of the canal and tympanic membrane. This anesthesia may be difficult to accomplish; the techniques described below relate the procedures specifically.

4. Foreign body removal. Removal of foreign bodies, particularly in children, may be difficult without adequate anesthesia of the external auditory canal.

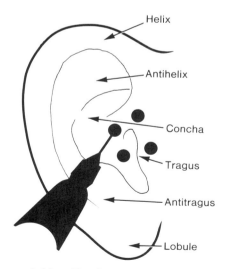

Figure 3.20. The four-quadrant block for anesthetizing the auditory canal. See text for discussion.

Labels in figure: Helix, Antihelix, Concha, Tragus, Antitragus, Lobule

Technique for Block of the Auricle

Deposit a line of anesthetic solution subcutaneously in the sulcus behind the auricle, extending semicircularly from the inferior to the superior pole (Fig. 3.21). This blocks the greater auricular nerve and the lesser occipital nerve supplying much of the external ear. The auriculotemporal nerve is then blocked by deposition of 5 ml of solution just anterior to the cartilaginous tragus (Fig. 3.20), at the point where the zygomatic arch meets the tragus. This is easily palpable with the index finger and is marked with an X in Figure 3.21. The success rate of this block is approximately 60 to 70% in the authors' experience.

Technique for Block of the Auditory Canal

Inject 1 ml of 2% lidocaine with epinephrine at the points indicated in Figure 3.20. This four-quadrant block is used to anesthetize the ear canal. This generally provides adequate anesthesia of the ear canal and tympanic membrane for foreign body removal and irrigation. For myringotomy, one may have to spray or instill several drops of anesthetic into the ear canal and leave it in place for 5 to 10 minutes. This block is usually incomplete in its effective-

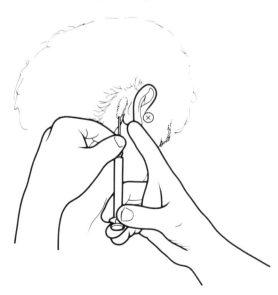

Figure 3.21. Subcutaneous infiltration in a semicircle behind the ear and this, accompanied by a block of the auriculotemporal nerve anteriorly (see text for discussion) will provide anesthesia for the auricle.

ness when compared with other blocks. With large foreign bodies entrapped near the tympanic membrane, the patient may need general anesthesia or ionotophoresis.

UPPER EXTREMITY BLOCKS

Brachial Plexus Block

This is one of the most widely used nerve blocks. It produces anesthesia of the arm and forearm and hand for virtually any procedure necessary in this region. There are two approaches described in the literature, the supraclavicular approach and the axillary approach (3, 8, 25, 26). The axillary approach is the procedure of choice in the emergency center (1–3, 7, 12, 14, 19). The supraclavicular approach is fraught with hazards, especially pneumothorax and trauma to the great vessels (3, 8). The advantage of the supraclavicular approach is that anesthesia is achieved in 10 to 15 minutes, whereas by the axillary route a good block is not achieved for 30 minutes. In addition, the musculocutaneous or axillary nerve may not be adequately blocked with this approach (3).

The brachial plexus is formed by the anterior primary rami of the lower four cervical and the greater portion of the first thoracic nerves. The plexus emerges from the lateral border of the anterior and middle scalene muscles. As it emerges from this region it carries with it an investing fascial sheath from the paravertebral fascia which completely encircles the plexus. This investing sheath is called the axillary sheath. This sheath is composed of tough fibrous connective tissue extending laterally to a little beyond the pectoralis minor. Regardless of the level (interscalene, supraclavicular or axillary) at which this sheath is encountered to block the brachial plexus, an effective block of the brachial plexus is possible since the anesthetic will remain within the sheath.

Indications

1. Repair of extensive lacerations of the forearm, arm, or hand.
2. Reduction of fractures of the forearm, elbow, and hand.
3. Debridement of extensive abrasions

to the upper extremity with (e.g., abrasions with embedded dirt, resulting from a motorcycle accident).

4. Reduction of dislocations of the elbow and wrist.

Technique

Preparatory Steps

1. The patient is positioned supine, with the arm on the side to be injected held at 90 degrees of abduction and externally rotated.
2. Rotate the head to the opposite direction.
3. The operator stands at the side which is to be injected.
4. Prep and drape the axilla.
5. Locate landmarks.
   a. Palpate the humeral insertions of the latissimus dorsi posteriorly and the pectoralis major anteriorly (Fig. 3.22). Draw a vertical line between these two points. Bisect the line and mark the point. This point lies directly over the brachial artery which can be palpated in all but the very obese (1, 3).
   b. When the axillary artery is easily palpable, the above procedure is not necessary. The point of maxi-

mum pulsation of the axillary artery is the only landmark.

6. Calculate amount of anesthetic necessary for adequate block. All of the solutions should be 1% lidocaine with 1:200,000 epinephrine at approximately 0.33 ml/kg.
   - 80 kg male = 25 to 30 ml
   - 70 kg = 20 to 25 ml
   - 40 to 60 kg = 15 to 20 ml
   - 25 to 30 kg = 14 to 20 ml

A 25 gauge, 5 cm needle attached to a 20 to 30 cc syringe is used.

Procedural Steps

1. Palpate the axillary artery with the index finger of the left hand.
2. Insert the needle at a right angle to the skin alongside the palpating finger, which is placed at the point of maximum pulsation or the region indicated in step 5 above (Fig. 3.23).
3. When the needle is properly placed, the pulsation of the artery is transmitted to the needle and one may feel a give as the axillary sheath is entered.
4. Inject the anesthetic solution directly into the sheath after aspiration to be

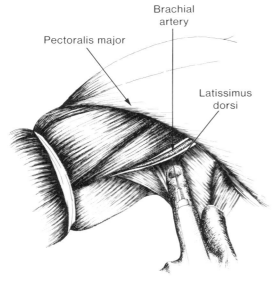

Figure 3.22.   Brachial plexus block. See text for discussion.

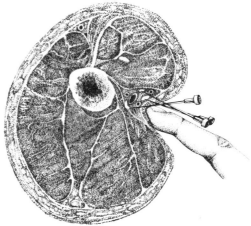

Figure 3.23.   Insert the needle at a right angle to the skin alongside the palpating finger, which is placed over the point of maximum pulsation of the axillary artery. When the needle is within the sheath which encloses the axillary artery and brachial plexus, the needle will "pulsate." At this point, aspirate and inject the anesthetic solution within the sheath.

certain one is not in the lumen of the artery.

NOTE

Sometimes the musculocutaneous nerve is not reached and patchy anesthesia is achieved on the radial side of the forearm. A tourniquet should be placed high on the arm or the blood pressure cuff inflated to between systolic and diastolic at about the level of insertion of the deltoid (Fig. 3.22). This effectively limits the spread of the solution, causing distention of the sheath and permitting an effective block (8).

Complications

1. Intraarterial puncture and a small hematoma in the sheath are the only complications of significance. This produces little difficulty if aspiration is performed and a small gauge needle is used.

Median Nerve Block at Elbow

The median nerve courses in the arm medially and is included in the large neurovascular sheath which contains the brachial artery. In the antecubital fossa the nerve courses laterally to the brachial artery and is covered by the aponeurosis of the biceps muscle.

Indications

1. Repair of lacerations over the sensory distribution of the nerve in the hand and forearm.
2. Debridement of abrasions in the distribution of the nerve to the forearm and hand.

Technique

The landmark for blocking this nerve is the brachial artery and the nerve is best blocked on the ulnar side of this artery. The medial condyle of the humerus and the tendon of the biceps form two additional landmarks for locating the nerve. Place the patient in the supine position, with the arm abducted and the forearm extended. Moisten an applicator with iodine and place it in the antecubital fossa.

Next ask the patient to flex the arm to an angle of 90 degrees. A transverse line results which is at the same level as a line drawn between the two epicondyles. The nerve lies superficially here and can be palpated in some thin individuals. One can feel the tendon of the biceps by flexing and extending the forearm with the hand in supination. The brachial artery is medial to the tendon, and the nerve is medial to the artery and superficial at the level of the line drawn (Fig. 3.24). An intradermal wheal is raised medial to the artery, a needle is introduced through the skin and fascia, and paresthesia is sought. Inject 5 ml of 1% lidocaine at this site in a fanwise fashion (31).

Ulnar Nerve Block at the Elbow

The ulnar nerve courses along the medial aspect of the arm and in the distal one third perforates the medial intermuscular septum to enter the extensor compartment of the forearm. In doing so it passes behind the posterior aspect of the medial epicondyle of the humerus. The nerve can be easily palpated in this area, usually without difficulty. Almost everyone has at some time or another struck their "funny bone"; the paresthesias elicited are those from the ulnar nerve.

Indications

1. In repairing injuries over the sensory distribution of the nerve.

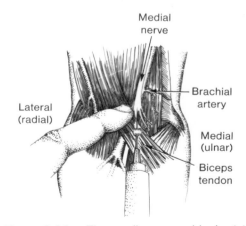

Figure 3.24. The median nerve block at the elbow. See text for discussion.

2. To augment an inadequate brachial plexus block. The fibers of C8 and T1 are often difficult to block.

Technique

Place the patient in the lateral prone position on the side opposite the one to be injected. The elbow should be flexed at 90 degrees. The landmarks are the groove between the medial condyle of the humerus and the olecranon process, particularly in the obese patient in whom palpation of the nerve behind the medial epicondyle may be difficult (Fig. 3.25). Palpate the nerve and grasp the skin and subcutaneous tissue above this groove with the thumb and index finger of the left hand. After raising an intradermal wheal in the skin grasped, introduce a 25 gauge, 1½ inch needle in the direction of the nerve (Fig. 3.25). The injection should ideally be 1 to 2 cm above its position in the groove behind the epicondyle. This avoids the possibility of neuritis which may result from injection at the epicondyle. Paresthesias should be elicited and 3 to 5 ml of 1% lidocaine introduced at this site (2, 3).

Median Nerve Block at the Wrist (3, 8, 22)

The median nerve courses between the superficial and deep flexor tendons supplying the digits. At the level of the proximal wrist crease, the nerve courses superficially to lie immediately radial to the tendon of the palmaris longus (Fig. 3.26). In patients who do not have a palmaris longus, the median nerve courses between the flexor carpi radialis and the flexor superficialis tendons. The landmarks for performing a median nerve block at the wrist are the tendons of the palmaris longus and the flexor carpi radialis. The nerve

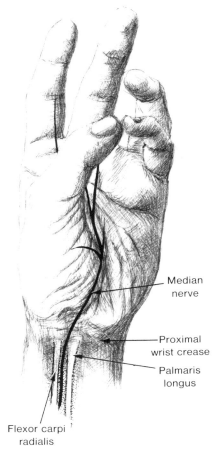

Figure 3.26. The median nerve block at the wrist. At the level of the proximal wrist crease, the nerve courses superficially and lies immediately radial to the tendon of the palmaris longus. See text for discussion.

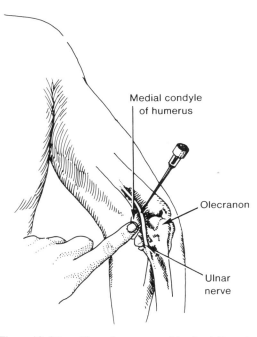

Figure 3.25. The ulnar nerve block at the elbow. See text for discussion.

lies deep to the tendon of the palmaris longus on its radial side; however, while the tendon of the palmaris longus is superficial, all other flexor tendons and the nerve itself lie deep to the flexor retinaculum.

Indications

1. Lacerations of the hand over areas supplied by the median nerve.
2. Removal of foreign bodies in the hand.

Technique

To perform the block, locate the palmaris longus and the flexor carpi radialis tendons by asking the patient to oppose the thumb and small finger while flexing the wrist against resistance as shown in Figure 3.26. In patients who are missing the palmaris longus, locate the flexor carpi radialis and the flexor digitorum superficialis tendons by having the patient make a fist and flex the wrist against resistance (Fig. 3.27). Mark the palmaris longus and the flexor carpi radialis tendons. The point of injection is immediately radial to the palmaris longus tendon at the level of the proximal skin crease of the wrist (Fig. 3.27). Insert a 23 gauge, 1½ inch needle through the skin at right angles to the tendon. One may feel the resistance of the flexor retinaculum. The nerve lies deep to

the retinaculum and, unless the nerve is palpated, it is difficult to appreciate the depth for infiltration. Insert the needle approximately 0.5 cm beyond the retinaculum and attempt to obtain paresthesias in the hand which indicate that nerve has been touched by the needle point. At this point, inject 2 ml of 1% lidocaine. If paresthesias are not elicited, inject approximately 5 ml of 1% lidocaine in an in-and-out fashion to spread the anesthetic throughout the area.

Ulnar Nerve Block at the Wrist

The ulnar nerve divides into a palmar and dorsal branch approximately 5 cm proximal to the wrist (8, 22). The ulnar artery accompanies the palmar branch of the nerve (Fig. 3.28). The dorsal branch is

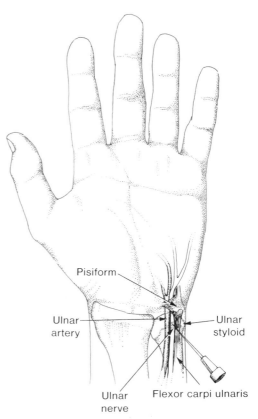

Figure 3.28. The ulnar nerve block at the wrist. The ulnar artery and ulnar nerve course beneath the flexor carpi ulnaris tendon. See text for discussion.

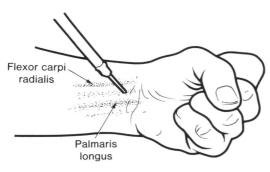

Figure 3.27. Locate the flexor carpi radialis by having the patient make a fist and flex the wrist against resistance as shown. The point of injection is immediately radial to the palmaris longus tendon at the level of the proximal skin crease of the wrist. See text for discussion.

entirely sensory and courses beneath the tendon of the flexor carpi ulnaris to reach the dorsal aspect of the wrist and supplies sensation to the ulnar side of the dorsum of the hand. The palmar branch is a mixed nerve and continues along the tendon flexor carpi ulnaris to divide on the radial side of the pisiform bone into a superficial and a deep branch. The superficial branch is entirely sensory and supplies sensation to the ulnar side of the palmar portion of the hand and to the fourth and fifth fingers.

Indications

1. Lacerations of the hand over areas supplied by the ulnar nerve.
2. Removal of foreign bodies in the hand.

Technique

Landmarks for an ulnar nerve block at the wrist are similar to those for the median nerve block except that the tendon of the flexor carpi ulnaris is used. Palpate the tendon of the flexor carpi ulnaris at the level of the styloid process of the ulna (Fig. 3.28). The flexor carpi ulnaris can be easily identified at its attachment to the pisiform bone by palpating the pisiform and asking the patient to flex the wrist against resistance, which makes the tendon stand out. Insert a 23 gauge, 1½ inch needle perpendicular to the skin on the radial side of the flexor carpi ulnaris tendon at the level of the proximal skin crease (3, 8). The palmar branch lies superficial to the flexor retinaculum and the injection should be subcutaneous. Paresthesias should be sought before injection and one should then inject 2 ml of 1% lidocaine. To anesthetize the dorsal branch of the ulnar nerve a subcutaneous wheal is deposited, similar to that used for radial nerve block in the wrist (see Figure 3.30). This wheal should extend subcutaneously from the dorsal aspect of the wrist on the ulnar side to the tendon of the flexor carpi ulnaris on the palmar aspect of the wrist. A band of anesthetic solution then extends from the flexor carpi ulnaris tendon posteriorly to the middle of the dorsal aspect of the wrist on its ulnar border. This method should provide good anesthesia for both the dorsal and the palmar branches of the ulnar nerve (3, 8, 22).

Radial Nerve Block of the Wrist

The radial nerve accompanies the artery alongside the brachioradialis muscle in the forearm. Approximately 7 cm proximal to the wrist joint, the superficial branch passes laterally beneath the tendon of the muscle and goes to the dorsal aspect of the wrist. At this point the nerve breaks up into superficial rami to supply the radial side of the dorsum of the hand with sensation. At the level of the skin crease of the wrist, all the sensory branches of the radial nerve are superficial (8).

Indications

1. Extensive lacerations involving the hand. It is unusual to do a radial nerve block as an isolated procedure and usually this block accompanies the ulnar and median nerve blocks to provide complete anesthesia of the hand in dealing with extensive lacerations.
2. Removal of foreign bodies from areas of the hand supplied by the radial nerve.

Technique

Inject approximately 10 ml of anesthetic solution (1% lidocaine) subcutaneously in a band along the radial side of the wrist at the level of the proximal skin crease. Begin the injection at a point just lateral to the radial artery (Fig. 3.29), extending dorsolaterally to the midportion of the dorsal aspect of the wrist (2, 22) (Fig. 3.30).

Digital Nerve Blocks

The digital nerves lie in pairs on either side of the phalanges; two on the ulnar and two on the radial aspect. The nerves of the digits are easily blocked at the base of the involved digit.

Indications

1. Lacerations involving isolated fingers.
2. Applying a skin graft or rotating a flap in a patient with an amputation of a fingertip.

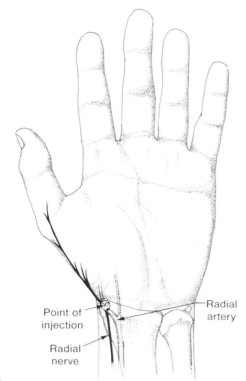

Figure 3.29. Block of the radial nerve at the wrist. Begin the injection at the point shown above just lateral to the radial artery.

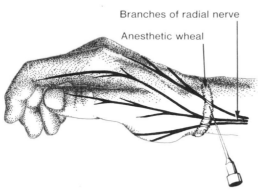

Figure 3.30. Deposit a subcutaneous wheal of anesthesia in a semicircular fashion as shown to block all branches of the radial nerve.

3. Procedures requiring removal of a nail or repair of a nailbed of an isolated finger.
4. Reduction of an interphalangeal joint

dislocation or a fracture of the phalanx.
5. Complex repairs involving the individual digits.

Technique

It is difficult to reach the nerves on both sides of the bone by a single injection at the midpoint; thus, two separate needle insertions are made (Fig. 3.31) (2, 8). No attempt is made to elicit paresthesias. Infiltrate superficially with 1 ml of 1% lidocaine and deeply, almost to the bone, on both sides of the proximal phalanx on the involved finger at the base so that a half-ring block is made.

The pressure from the anesthetic solution in this small area may obstruct blood flow to the digit and for this reason the authors prefer a metacarpal block of the digital nerves in the web space. This is performed by inserting a needle along each side of the finger at the interdigital fold in the web space, as shown in Figure 3.32. The needle is advanced approximately 0.5 cm and 1 ml of local 1% lidocaine is deposited (3). A bilateral block on both sides of the finger at this level provides good anesthesia for all procedures involving the finger. When using this procedure for blocking the index finger or the little finger, a half-ring wheal of anesthesia must be deposited on the radial border of the index finger or the ulnar border of the little

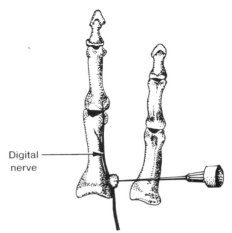

Figure 3.31. Digital nerve block. See text for details.

finger, respectively, to provide adequate anesthesia. When blocking the thumb, a circumferential block must be used as the thumb is supplied by multiple branches of the radial nerve as well as branches from the median nerve which are difficult to anesthetize with one or two injection sites.

LOWER EXTREMITY NERVE BLOCKS

Nerve Blocks of the Foot

Nerve blocks of the foot are commonly used in the emergency center when deal-

ing with extensive lacerations involving the foot, particularly the sole, and when a deep exploratory procedure is needed for the removal of a foreign body (17). A number of nerves supply the foot and these will be discussed separately (Fig. 3.33).

POSTERIOR TIBIAL NERVE BLOCK

The posterior tibial nerve is located along the medial aspect of the ankle, coursing between the medial malleolus and the Achilles tendon (3, 6, 17) (Fig. 3.34). The nerve accompanies the posterior tibial artery, lying just posterior and slightly deep to the artery. The nerve courses between

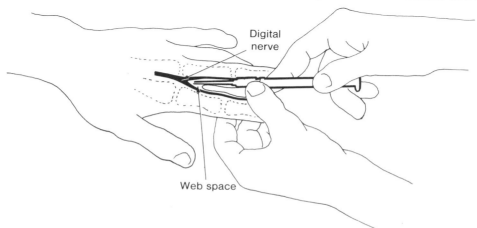

Figure 3.32. Block of the digital nerve in the web space. See text for discussion.

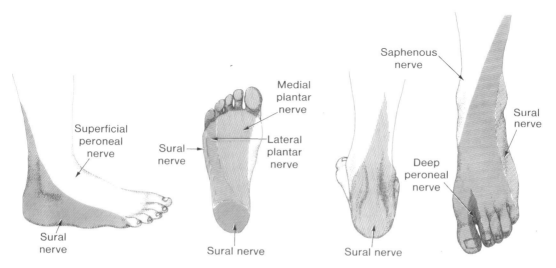

Figure 3.33. The sensory nerve supply to the foot.

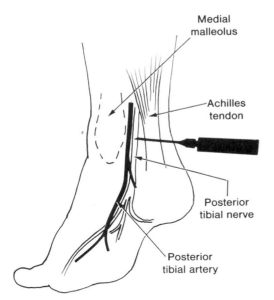

Medial malleolus

Achilles tendon

Posterior tibial nerve

Posterior tibial artery

Figure 3.34.   Posterior tibial nerve block. The nerve accompanies the posterior tibial artery and lies slightly deep and "lateral" to the artery.

the tendons of the flexor digitorum longus and the flexor hallucis longus muscles and is covered by the laciniate ligament. The nerve divides into a medial and lateral plantar branch and these supply sensation to the sole of the foot.

Technique (3, 6, 8, 17, 22)

Locate the base of the medial malleolus and the Achilles tendon, as these serve as landmarks for the injection. Place the patient in a prone position when doing the procedure. Palpate the posterior tibial artery and insert a 23 gauge, 2 inch needle perpendicular to the skin just lateral to the Achilles tendon at the level of the upper border of the medial malleolus. Direct the needle immediately lateral and posterior to the artery and advance it until it touches the tibia (Fig. 3.35A). Attempt to elicit paresthesias by moving the needle medially and laterally. When paresthesias are elicited in the sole, inject 5 ml of 1% lidocaine. If paresthesias are not elicited, inject 10 ml of solution along the posterior border of the tibia while the needle is slowly withdrawn. Anesthesia usually occurs in 5 to 10 minutes when paresthesia is elicited and in 20 to 30 minutes when paresthesia

is not elicited. Almost the entire sole can be anesthetized with this block, with the exception of the proximal area which is supplied by the sural nerve and the lateral portion.

SURAL NERVE BLOCK

The sural nerve is a cutaneous nerve which becomes subcutaneous distal to the middle of the leg and courses along with the short saphenous vein behind the lateral malleolus to supply sensation to the posterior lateral aspect of the ankle and heel and the lateral plantar aspect of the foot and fifth toe (Fig. 3.33). This nerve passes in the subcutaneous tissue just lateral to the Achilles tendon.

Technique

This nerve is usually blocked along with blocking the posterior tibial nerve when complete anesthesia is desired for procedures performed at the heel of the foot. The landmarks for marking the sural nerve are the Achilles tendon and the outer border of the lateral malleolus. The patient should be placed in the prone position. A 23 gauge, 1½ inch needle is introduced just lateral to the Achilles tendon, at a level of 1 cm above the lateral malleolus (Fig. 3.35B). The needle is directed toward a spot 1 cm superior to the malleolus of the fibula, and 5 ml of 1% lidocaine are infiltrated as the needle is moved in a fanwise fashion within the subcutaneous tissue between the lateral malleolus and the Achilles tendon.

SAPHENOUS NERVE BLOCKS

The saphenous nerve runs parallel to the saphenous vein in the subcutaneous tissue on the anteromedial aspect of the ankle (22). It is one of the superficial nerves supplying the anterior aspect of the foot and is a sensory branch of the femoral nerve, becoming subcutaneous at the lateral side of the knee joint (Fig. 3.35C).

Technique

The patient should be placed in the supine position, with a sandbag or pillow under the calf to relax the foot in a plantar flexed posture (17). The nerve can be blocked by infiltrating the anesthetic so-

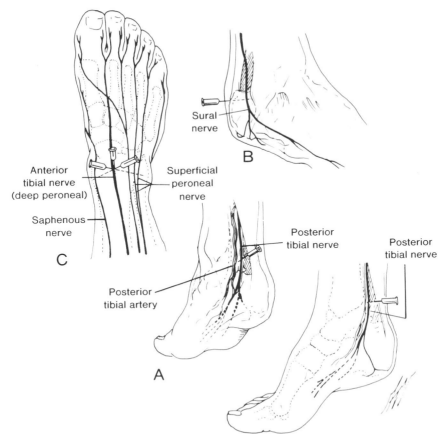

Figure 3.35. The technique of posterior tibial, sural, and anterior tibial nerve block is demonstrated. See text for details. (Reprinted with permission of Locke, R.K., Locke, S.E., Nerve blocks of the foot. JACEP 5:701, 1976.)

lution subcutaneously along a line extending from the medial malleolus to the tendon of the extensor hallucis longus (Fig. 3.36). Mark a line circumscribing the ankle, approximately 1 cm above the base of the medial malleolus. At a point on the line just medial to the extensor hallucis longus tendon, insert a 1½ inch, 23 gauge needle perpendicular to the skin until it reaches the tibia, then slightly withdraw the needle and inject a small amount (2 cc) of anesthetic solution, followed by a subcutaneous injection toward the malleolus.

SUPERFICIAL PERONEAL NERVE BLOCK

The superficial peroneal nerve runs subcutaneously along the dorsum of the foot, after piercing the fascia along the anterior aspect of the lower leg. It has a wide area of distribution, supplying the entire dorsum of the foot except for the small area between the first and second toe which is innervated by the anterior tibial nerve (Figs. 3.33 and 3.35C).

Technique

The superficial peroneal nerve is blocked by injecting 5 to 10 ml of 0.5% lidocaine subcutaneously in a line from the anterior border of the tibia to the lateral malleolus. This block and that of the saphenous nerve can often be performed from one injection site, as shown in Figure 3.35 and 3.36 (17).

ANTERIOR TIBIAL NERVE BLOCK (DEEP PERONEAL NERVE BLOCK)

The deep peroneal nerve is largely muscular in its innervation; however, it does

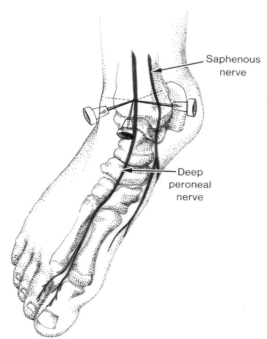

Figure 3.36. The saphenous, deep peroneal nerve blocks. See text for discussion.

supply sensation to the area between the first and second toes (Fig. 3.33). The origin of the nerve is the medial branch of the lateral popliteal nerve after it crosses the neck of the fibula. It passes deep to the flexor retinaculum at the ankle and emerges toward the base of the first and second toes, supplying a small area between these toes (8). The nerve is usually blocked when procedures are performed in the region of its sensation (3, 6). The deep peroneal nerve lies between the tendons of the tibialis anterior and the extensor hallucis longus.

Technique

A 2 to 3 cm needle is inserted dorsally on the foot, midway between the medial and lateral malleoli (Figs. 3.35C and 3.36). In less than 1 cm depth the anterior aspect of the tibia is encountered, and at this point 3 to 4 ml of 0.5% lidocaine solution is deposited which will spread between the flexor tendons and the bone (8). Paresthesias occasionally may be elicited. Alternately, when the extensor hallucis longus muscle or the tibialis anterior can be iden-

tified, they serve as excellent landmarks for the point of injection. With the patient supine, insert the needle lateral to the tendon of the tibialis anterior until the tibia is encountered. Withdraw the needle approximately 3 mm and inject 5 ml of 1% lidocaine into this area. Some authors have suggested that, in addition, the needle should be withdrawn and directed laterally between the extensor hallucis longus and extensor digitorum longus tendons until the tibia is encountered and additional anesthetic solution should be deposited here (3).

BLOCK OF THE GREAT TOE

To anesthetize the great toe, one must block the base of the toe circumferentially by depositing anesthetic solution subcutaneously.

A 1½ inch, 25 gauge needle attached to a 10 cc syringe containing 1% lidocaine without epinephrine is inserted at the anterior lateral portion of the toe (point A, Fig. 3.37) and is directed medially in the

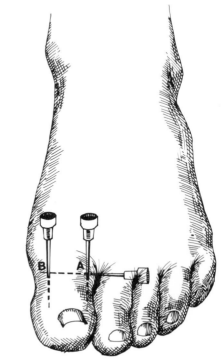

Figure 3.37. Block of the great toe. See text for discussion.

subcutaneous tissue. The anesthetic solution is deposited as the needle is advanced, followed by redirecting the needle posteriorly through the same puncture site and additional anesthetic solution is deposited in this area. The needle then is introduced at a second puncture site along the anterior medial portion of the great toe (point *B*, Fig. 3.37) and the anesthetic solution is deposited posteriorly as shown in Figure 3.37. Finally, to complete the circumferential block, the needle is introduced at the base of the toe over the volar aspect, as shown in Figure 3.38, and is directed medially and anesthetic solution is deposited in this portion as well. The block usually takes 5 to 10 minutes to take effect.

BLOCKS OF THE TOES OTHER THAN THE GREAT TOE

To block the remainder of the toes of the foot, anesthetic solution is deposited through one needle puncture at the dorsum of the toes in the midpoint, as shown in Figure 3.39. The needle is inserted at the midpoint of the dorsum of the foot and is directed laterally and medially to the ex-

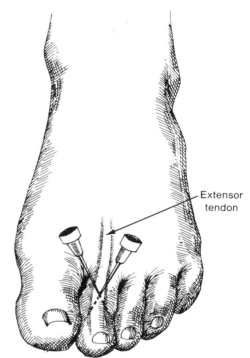

Figure 3.39. Block of the toes other than the great toe. The needle was inserted in the midline dorsally over the extensor tendon and directed to either side of the digit. See text for discussion.

tensor tendon, and 2 ml of 1% lidocaine solution is deposited along both sides of the toes. This technique provides good anesthesia for repairing lacerations of the toes, as well as for removing foreign bodies and dealing with nailbed injuries.

BLOCKS OF THE TORSO AND OTHER AREAS

Block of the Intercostal Nerves

The intercostal nerves course inferior to the ribs along with the intercostal artery and vein. The first six intercostal nerves carry sensation to the chest, while the lower intercostals also carry sensation to the abdomen. The most common occasion necessitating intercostal nerve block in the emergency center is in the patient with rib fractures. This is particularly true in the aged, in whom hypoventilation secondary to pain can result in serious complications, especially respiratory infections. Most of

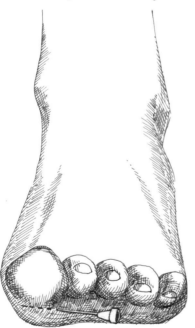

Figure 3.38. Block of the great toe. See text for discussion.

the patients with simple rib fractures who die do so from pneumonia, which has a fairly high incidence in the aged (23). The authors advise that no attempt be made to immobilize the chest mechanically (strapping, taping, rib belts) in the elderly due to this complication. Rib blocks with long-acting anesthetics (Marcaine[R]) provide good anesthesia during the acute phase and permit good respiration and coughing, thus avoiding atelectasis and pneumonia (6, 23).

Indications

1. Rib fractures for pain relief and to permit full inspiration without pain.

Technique

The intercostal nerves can best be blocked in the area of the costal angles posteriorly, just lateral to the lateral border of the erector spinae muscles. This avoids the deep mass of paravertebral muscles in the middle of the back. In the average adult, this is about 3 inches from the midline. The patient should be placed in the sitting position, leaning forward over a pillow placed on his lap with his arms folded. This displaces the scapula laterally, permitting easier palpation of the rib borders. With the index finger of the left hand palpate the rib or ribs to be injected and pull the skin overlying the rib cephalad to tense it (Fig. 3.40). Insert, at a right angle to the skin, a 23 gauge or smaller, long needle attached to a 5 ml syringe filled with Marcaine[R] until it strikes the outer aspect of the rib (9). Cautiously walk the tip of the needle inferiorly until it slips off the edge of the rib, advance the needle 3 mm further (half the thickness of the adult rib), and inject 5 ml of 1% lidocaine (22) (Fig. 3.41). Usually the intercostal nerve above and below the affected rib needs to be blocked to provide good anesthesia for rib pain.

Complications

1. Pneumothorax. Pneumothorax is the most frequent complication reported secondary to intercostal nerve block (9, 22, 23). The use of a small gauge needle and care in avoiding penetrating deeper than the distance indicated

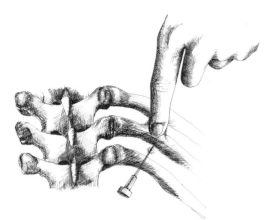

Figure 3.40. The intercostal nerve block. With the index finger of the left hand, palpate the rib to be injected and pull the skin overlying the rib cephalad. Insert the needle at a right angle to the skin and touch the rib.

above should avoid this complication. If coughing is induced, discontinue the injection until the needle is properly placed as coughing often indicates intrapleural penetration. All patients with an intercostal nerve block should have a chest radiograph performed after the procedure.

2. Puncture of intercostal blood vessel with a small hematoma. To avoid this complication, be certain to aspirate before injecting as with all blocks.

3. Cerebrospinal fluid aspiration. This is a rare complication which results from a severely misdirected needle (23). With proper care, this complication should not occur.

Transvaginal Pudendal Nerve Block

The pudendal nerve forms a single trunk 0.5 to 1 cm proximal to the ischial spine (15). It passes posterior to the spine, between the sacrospinous ligament anteriorly and the sacrotuberous ligament posteriorly to enter the lesser sciatic foramen (Fig. 3.42). The pudendal nerve arises from anterior divisions of S2, 3, and 4 and as the nerve crosses the spine of the ischium it courses medial to the internal pudendal vessels to enter the pelvis. Two approaches for anesthetizing the pudendal nerve have been described in the literature: the transvaginal approach (Fig. 3.43) (5, 13,

16, 25) and the percutaneous extravaginal approach (Fig. 3.44) (15). The transvaginal approach is the procedure of choice, as it

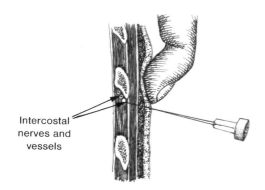

Figure 3.41. The intercostal nerves lie beneath the rib margin, accompanied by the intercostal arteries. The needle should be "walked" cautiously down the rib until it passes just beneath the inferior margin. The anesthetic solution is deposited here. Caution must be exercised not to go too deeply when passing the needle beneath the rib margin.

is simpler to administer the anesthetic agent accurately to the region of the pudendal nerve and thereby reduce the trauma of injection. There are no complications such as infection or hemorrhage with this procedure, and there is no interference with uterine contractile ability (13). The incidence of postpartum hemorrhage is lessened and there is no effect of the anesthetic on the fetus.

In the primiparous patient the injection is withheld until the second stage of labor when there is complete cervical dilatation (5). In the multiparous patient the injection is best withheld until 6 to 8 cm of cervical dilatation (16, 24).

Indications

1. Vaginal delivery. This procedure, when performed properly, provides good anesthesia for vaginal delivery, particularly in the multiparous patient. In the primiparous patient, more complete anesthesia may be

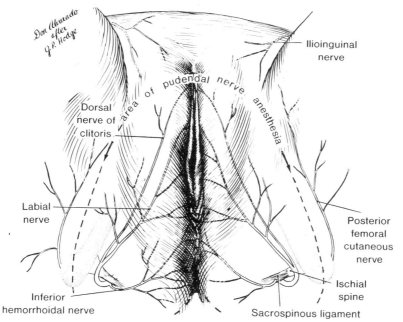

Figure 3.42. The pudendal nerve is shown as it courses from beneath the sacrospinous ligament. The inferior hemorrhoidal nerve and labial nerve are branches of the internal pudendal nerve, as shown. (Reprinted with permission of the publisher from Wilds, P.L., Transvaginal pudendal-nerve block. Obstet. Gynecol. 8:386. Copyright © 1956, American College of Obstetricians and Gynecologists.)

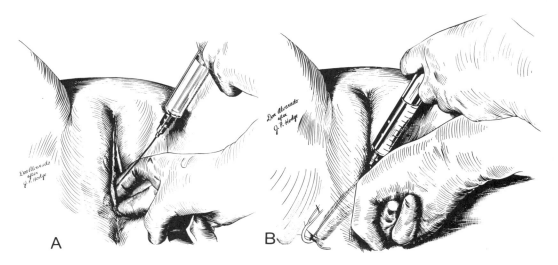

A   B

Figure 3.43.   The transvaginal approach for internal pudendal nerve block. The technique of inserting the needle into the vagina is shown in *A*. The needle tip lies flat against the ball of the index finger during insertion. The sacrospinous ligament is pierced by the needle as shown in *B*. The anesthetic solution is deposited at this site. (Reprinted by permission of the publisher from Wilds, P.L., Transvaginal pudendal nerve block. Obstet. Gynecol. 8:388–389. Copyright © 1956, American College of Obstetricians and Gynecologists.)

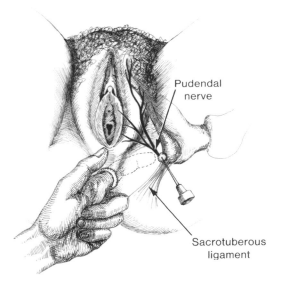

Pudendal nerve

Sacrotuberous ligament

Figure 3.44.   The percutaneous extravaginal approach. See text for discussion.

necessary due to the greater pain experienced during delivery.

Technique

A 6 inch, 20 gauge spinal needle with a 10 ml syringe is used for this procedure.

Alternately a special needle is available with a needle guard which protects against advancing the needle too far. The patient should be prepped for the delivery but no vaginal preparation is necessary. Locate the ischial spines vaginally and hold the needle and attached syringe filled with 1% lidocaine with the tip of the needle pressed flatly against the ball of the index finger so that it is protected by and guided by the finger in its passage through the vagina (5, 24, 25) (Fig. 3.43). Alternately the needle can be held between the index and middle fingers of the left hand (13). With the needle held parallel to the index finger and guided by the finger, it is carried into the vagina to the tip of the ischial spine. The tip of the needle is then passed by lifting the finger and advancing it into the vaginal mucosa overlying the sacrospinous ligament, which is palpated just posterior and medial to the tip of the ischial spine.

NOTE

The most significant limiting factor in this technique is the occasional difficulty in identifying the sacrospinous ligament since it is so thin and relaxed in some multiparous patients at term. When this does occur the needle should be passed just inferior and posterior to the ischial spine (16).

The ligament is infiltrated with 2 to 3 ml of 1% lidocaine, and then the needle pierces the ligament and enters the loose tissue which contains the nerve. At this point the resistance of the plunger decreases and the fluid flows easily. Aspirate before injection to be certain the artery is not entered and deposit the fluid (5 cc) beneath the ligament. Repeat this same procedure on the opposite side.

With the extravaginal approach the point of insertion of the needle is over the ischial tuberosities, as shown in Figure 3.45. The procedure is similar to that of the intravaginal approach with the exception that the physician places his index finger into the rectum as shown in Figure 3.44 and palpates the ischial spine, sacrospinous ligament, and sacrotuberous ligament per rectum. The needle is then directed toward the pudendal nerve and 5 to 10 cc of 1% lidocaine are infiltrated in this site. The procedure is repeated on the opposite side. The area of anesthesia provided by a bilateral pudendal nerve block is shown in Figure 3.46.

Block of the Penis

Block of the penis can be easily performed. Inadequate anesthesia is usually

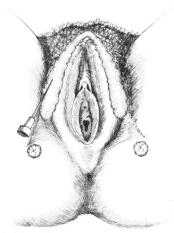

Figure 3.45.   The points of insertion of the needle over the ischial tuberosities are shown by the *X*s.

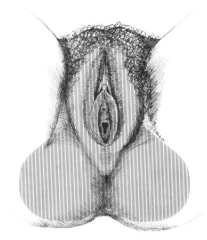

Figure 3.46.   The area of anesthesia provided by a pudendal nerve block is shown.

secondary to poor infiltration of the anesthetic solution.

Indications

1. Penile lacerations.

Technique

With the patient supine, two points are localized above the penis which are the sites of injection. The tubercles of the pubic bone are palpated and the points 0.5 inch caudad and 0.5 inch medial to them are located. These points can be marked, as they are the two superior sites where the needle is to be inserted. The inferior site is on the median raphe of the scrotum at the base of the penis. A 25 gauge, 3 inch needle and 1% lidocaine with epinephrine are used for this block. Vigorous shaking of the penis will decrease the pain of injection. Carefully connect the two superior points with a linear infiltration of anesthetic deposited both intradermally and subcutaneously. Connect the site beneath the penis to the ends of the linear wheal just deposited superiorly, thereby forming a triangle (Fig. 3.47). Again, be careful to deposit the anesthetic both intradermally and subcutaneously. Finally, a ring of anesthetic solution must be deposited around the base of the penis, between the corpora cavernosa and the deep penile fascia (Fig. 3.48), otherwise the small nerve filaments which innervate the posterolateral sides of

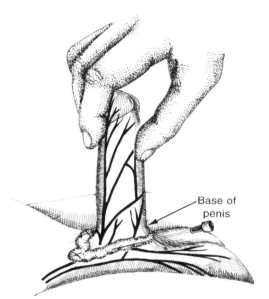

Base of
penis

Figure 3.47. As shown, a subcutaneous wheal of anesthesia is deposited in a triangular fashion at the base of the penis.

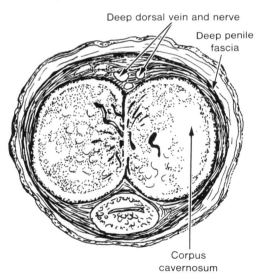

Deep dorsal vein and nerve

Deep penile
fascia

Corpus
cavernosum

Figure 3.48. A ring of anesthetic is deposited around the base of the penis between the corpora cavernosa and the deep penile fascia to anesthetize the small nerve filaments.

the penis and the frenulum will not be anesthetized. This is done by passing the needle through the "points of the triangle" and directing the solution as far as the corpus cavernosum each time, depositing a ring of anesthetic solution at the base of the penis in a fanlike fashion.

Urethral Anesthesia

Urethral anesthesia may be necessary for certain painful procedures involved with catheterization.

Indications

1. Catheterization.
2. Bougienage, if stricture is not too tight.

Technique

Lidocaine gel is used in this procedure. The penis is held firmly in the left hand and a plastic applicator is attached to the tube of lidocaine gel and is inserted into the meatus. Express the gel gently from the tube into the urethra (9). Apply a penile clamp to prevent the gel from running out. Massage the gel backwards into the posterior part of the urethra and leave in place for 5 to 10 minutes for maximum effect.

Infiltration Anesthesia for Cesarean Section

The abdominal wall receives its sensory nerve supply from the lumber nerves and the lower six intercostal nerves. These nerves give off cutaneous branches just lateral to the midline.

Indications

Emergency cesarean section.

Technique

Infiltration between the symphysis pubis to approximately 1 cm above the umbilicus will provide adequate anesthesia. The anesthetic solution should be 0.5% lidocaine with 1:200,000 of epinephrine. Total dose should not exceed 100 ml. A 10 cm needle is used to infiltrate the abdominal wall. The needle should be held parallel to the surface of the skin. The local agent is injected during both insertion and withdrawal of the needle. This raises a wheal linearly parallel to and on both sides of the linea alba. This does not provide complete anesthesia for the patient and may have to be augmented. Nitrous oxide, when available, is a good agent to use.

Anesthesia of the Surface of the Cornea and Conjunctiva

Topical application of anesthetic solutions commercially available (Ophthaine) to the surface of the conjunctiva provides good surface anesthesia for some procedures (9). Two drops should be deposited in the conjunctival sac rather than directly on the cornea. This gives good analgesia for the cornea and conjunctiva but has no effect on any deeper structures (9).

The number of instillations is far more important than the amount administered for each instillation.

Indications

1. Tonometry. This procedure usually requires only one instillation of 2 to 3 drops of anesthetic solution.
2. Corneal foreign body removal. This generally requires repeated instillations, especially if the foreign body is situated in the area of the limbus where the blood vessels rapidly remove the anesthetic agent. Normally the first instillation causes a little pain and blepharospasm. When the discomfort has disappeared, usually within 30 seconds to a minute, a second instillation is made. If this should again cause pain, a third instillation may be necessary.
3. Conjunctival lacerations or foreign body. This requires more frequent instillations, repeated at short intervals. Conjunctival anesthesia is less effective than corneal anesthesia, especially when the conjunctiva is inflamed.

Hematoma Block for Reduction of a Fracture

Infiltration of a fracture hematoma is a useful block for reduction of some fractures, particularly in situations where little manipulation is necessary. The site of the fracture is palpated and the fracture hematoma is punctured with a 21 gauge 1½ inch needle attached to a 10 ml syringe filled with 2% lidocaine without epineph-rine. As the needle enters the hematoma around the fracture, one will be able to aspirate blood into the syringe. At this point the anesthetic solution is injected slowly. Rapid injection may be quite painful. Wait approximately 10 to 15 minutes before proceeding with the reduction. The anesthesia obtained by this method is not comparable to that of nerve block or intravenous regional anesthesia; the latter are the authors' preferred techniques for most fracture reductions. Hematoma block is not recommended for routine use and is only indicated in situations in which time does not permit performance of a regional block.

Intravenous Regional Analgesia

The technique of intravenous regional anesthesia which involves the injection of a local anesthetic into a vein in an extremity after application of a tourniquet proximally was first described by Bier but was largely reintroduced by Holmes (8). No knowledge of anatomy is required to perform this procedure. A suitable vein, preferably on the dorsum of the hand, is essential (8). While this method of anesthesia can be used for both the upper extremity and the lower extremity procedures, intravenous regional anesthesia of the leg is not recommended by some authors (8) due to the total amount of anesthetic needed for good analgesia is large and the risk of cuff deflation is high. Cuff deflation would result in the release of a large volume of anesthesia into the circulation, producing toxicity. In addition, the anterior and posterior tibial vessels lie in the interosseous membrane, and a tourniquet applied beneath the knee would be ineffective in occluding these vessels and keeping the anesthetic from entering the circulation (8). This type of anesthesia is particularly useful for procedures involving the forearm and hand; however, they cannot be used for procedures involving the arm since the greater part of the cuff covers the arm. The primary indications within the emergency center for intravenous regional anesthesia are for soft tissue injuries and reduction of fractures involving the forearm and hand (8, 22).

Technique

Preparatory Steps

1. Collect 40 cc of 0.5% lidocaine without epinephrine in a 50 ml syringe.
2. Locate a suitable vein, preferably on the dorsum of the hand.
3. Begin a standard intravenous infusion in the contralateral arm for an intravenous route in case adverse reactions occur and the administration of emergency drugs becomes necessary (22).

Procedural Steps

1. With the patient in the supine position, place a sphygmomanometer cuff around the upper arm and inflate it to distend the vein distally. Insert a needle into the vein selected and deflate the cuff (8).
2. Exsanguinate the arm with the application of an Esmarch bandage or, if this is impossible due to the nature of the lesion, elevate the arm for a few minutes to allow the blood to drain out of the vessels.
3. After the bandage has been applied, inflate the cuff to approximately 100 mm of mercury above systolic pressure to prevent the arm from refilling with blood (8, 22). The arm is lowered and the bandage is removed.
4. Inject 40 ml of 0.5% lidocaine without epinephrine into the vein. In procedures of the lower extremity, approximately 60 to 80 ml are required for the adult leg. Almost immediately there will be the onset of warmth, tingling, and numbness of the arm. Arm paralysis and analgesia is usually complete after 5 minutes. If analgesia is incomplete after 4 minutes, inject a further 5 to 10 ml of solution into the vein selected. As long as the tourniquet is in place, analgesia is maintained distal to it and one can leave the tourniquet in place for 60 to 90 minutes, permitting enough time to perform most necessary procedures.

CAUTION!

The sphygmomanometer cuff used must be able to maintain pressure without leaking during the entire procedure. If the cuff is not capable of doing so, a large bolus of anesthetic will be released into the circulation and may cause a toxic reaction. A pneumatic tourniquet may be used instead of a sphygmomanometer and is applied to the limb proximal to the side of operation. Clamping the exit tubing with a hemostat may aid in preventing cuff leak.

5. The patient will experience ischemic pain under the tourniquet side in 15 to 20 minutes because this region is not anesthetized. A second tourniquet can be applied distal to the proximal tourniquet (providing the proximal tourniquet is applied high on the arm) and inflated following adequate analgesia, and the proximal tourniquet can then be deflated thus providing anesthesia at the tourniquet site.

The same procedures as indicated above can be performed in the lower extremity.

6. The cuff should be deflated slowly. Repeated deflations and inflations of the cuff limit the amount of analgesic released into the general circulation and reduce the risk of complications. Do not deflate the cuff until 10 minutes after injection of a local anesthetic. Care must be taken to avoid inadvertent deflations (8).

Complications

1. Cardiac irregularities. Due to the absorption of local analgesia after deflation of the cuff, cardiac irregularities such as AV block can occur (8).
2. Transient loss of consciousness and seizures have been reported (8).
3. Due to the rapid delivery of local anesthetic into the circulation following deflation of the cuff, deafness or tinnitus may occur (22).
4. Thrombophlebitis has been reported and the procedure should not be used in patients with peripheral vascular disease.

References

1. Accardo, N.J., Adriani, J., Brachial plexus block: A simplified technic using the axillary route. South. Med. J. 42:920, 1949.

2. Adams, R.C., Regional anesthesia for operations about the neck and upper extremity. Anesthesiology 2:515, 1941.
3. Adriani, J., Local and regional anesthesia for minor surgery. Surg. Clin. North Am. 31:1507, 1951.
4. Adriani, J., The clinical pharmacology of local anesthetics. Clin. Pharmacol. Ther. 1:645, 1960.
5. Atkinson, R.S., Regional analgesia in obstetrics.
6. Bone, J.R., Regional nerve block anesthesia. Anesthesiology 6:612, 1945.
7. Bonica, J.J., Moore, D.C., Orlov, M., Brachial plexus block anesthesia. Am. J. Surg. 78:65, 1949.
8. Bryce-Smith, R., Local analgesia of the limbs. In Lee, J.A., Bryce-Smith, R. (eds.) Practical Regional Anesthesia. Excerpta Medica, Elsevier, 1976.
9. Bryce-Smith, R., Local analgesia of the trunk. In Lee, J.A., Bryce-Smith, R. (eds.) Practical Regional Anesthesia. Excerpta Medica, Elsevier, 1976.
10. Covino, B.G., Local anesthesia. N. Engl. J. Med. 286:975, 1972.
11. Dale, H.W.L., Regional anaesthesia for surgery of the nose and sinuses. Lancet 1:562, 1944.
12. DeJong, R.H., Axillary block of the brachial plexus. Anesthesiology 22:215, 1961.
13. Dugger, J.H., Kegel, E.E., Buckley, J.J., Transvaginal pudendal nerve block: The safe anesthesia in obstetrics. Obstet. Gynecol. 8:393, 1956.
14. Kasdan, M.L., Kleinert, H.E., Kasdan, A.P., Jutz, J.E., Axillary block anesthesia for surgery of the hand. Plast. Reconst. Surg. 46:256, 1970.
15. Klink, E.W., Perineal nerve block. An anatomic and clinical study in the female. Obstet. Gynecol. 1:137, 1953.
16. Kobak, A.J., Sadove, M.S., Kobak, A.J., Childbirth pain relieved by combined paracervical and pudendal nerve blocks. JAMA 183:931, 1963.
17. Locke, R.K., Nerve blocks of the foot. 5:698, 1976.
18. Macht, S.D., Thompson, L.W., Intraoral field block anesthesia for extraoral lesions. Surg. Gynecol. Obstet. 146:87, 1978.
19. Moir, D.D., Axillary block of the brachial plexus. Anaesthesia 17:274, 1962.
20. Monsel, L.H., Regional anesthesia for operations about the head and neck. Anesthesiology 2:61, 1941.
21. Moore, D.C., Fridenbaugh, L.D., Bridenbaugh, P.O., Tucker, G.T., Bupivacaine. A review of 2,077 cases. JAMA 214:713, 1970.
22. Poulton, T.J., Mims, G.R., Peripheral nerve blocks. Am. Family Phys. 16:100, 1977.
23. Rovenstine, E.A., Byrd, M.L., The use of regional nerve block during treatment for fractured ribs. Am. J. Surg. 46:303, 1939.
24. Sadove, M.S., Kobak, A.J., Morch, E.T., Regional analgesia in obstetrics. Med. Clin. North Am. 45:1743, 1961.
25. Wilds, P.L., Transvaginal pudendal nerve block. Obstet. Gynecol. 8:385, 1956.
26. Winnie, A.O., Interscalene brachial plexus block. Anesth. Analg. 49:455, 1970.

Cardiothoracic Procedures

4

PERICARDIOCENTESIS

The only indication for pericardiocentesis within the emergency center is the treatment of cardiac tamponade. Shoemaker lists these criteria for the early diagnosis of cardiac tamponade (48):

1. Progressive increase in central venous pressure (CVP).
2. A CVP of 10 to 12 cm of water is suggestive of early tamponade with compensatory responses.
3. A fall in both CVP and arterial pressure is suggestive of acute tamponade with beginning circulatory deterioration and cardiac arrest being imminent.
4. The presence of Beck's triad (distant heart sounds, neck vein distension, and hypotension) which is a finding late in cardiac tamponade (48). Only one third of the patients have Beck's triad (16); however, 90% of the patients have one or more of the triad (16).

In grade I tamponade, cardiac output and arterial pressure are normal; however, the CVP and heart rate are elevated. In grade II tamponade, the blood pressure is normal or slightly decreased, the CVP is elevated, and the patient has tachycardia. In grade III tamponade, the classic findings of an elevated CVP and a drop in arterial pressure occur (16). A narrowed pulse pressure associated with an elevated CVP is an indication of progressive tamponade and a reliable sign of cardiac tamponade (50).

Pulsus paradoxus is seen in tamponade; however, it also may occur in patients with obesity, asthma, emphysema, and cardiac failure (16). Pulsus paradoxus is defined as an exaggeration of the normal inspiratory fall in blood pressure. In measuring the paradoxical pulse, a blood pressure cuff is slowly deflated until an occasional systolic sound which is synchronous with expiration is audible. Sounds during inspiration are not heard. The cuff then is deflated further until systolic sound is well heard but a sound is only occasionally audible with inspiration. In the normal patient the difference between the two pressures at which these sounds are heard is no greater than 10 mm of mercury; if the difference is greater than 10 mm of mercury, it is considered abnormal. Most patients with cardiac tamponade will have a drop of 20 to 30 mm of mercury or more (16). This absolute figure, however, is not reliable. Patients who have grade III tamponade with a narrow pulse pressure (difference between systolic and diastolic blood pressure) may have a small paradoxical pulse since the paradoxical pulse is a function of the pulse pressure. The ratio of the paradoxical pulse to the size of the pulse pressure is more reliable in indicating tamponade. Paradoxical pulse greater than 50% of the pulse pressure is regarded as abnormal (16).

Venous distension is a late sign in pericardial tamponade. This may be masked by venoconstriction secondary to sympathetic discharge or by hypovolemia. Central venous pressure measurements are more reliable than is the state of venous distension, and a central venous pressure line always should be placed in any patient suspected of tamponade. Most patients with significant tamponade will have an elevated CVP; however, hypovolemia, often present in these patients, changes the intrapericardial pressure-volume curve and will lower the CVP reading at any stage during tamponade compared to the normovolemic state. Thus, the response of the CVP to an infusion of volume is much more reliable as a diagnostic tool than is an isolated CVP reading.

Reliability of Pericardiocentesis

Pericardiocentesis is now considered much less reliable than was previously thought. There is a false negative rate of 20 to 40% (11, 55). In a study performed on patients with stab wounds of the heart, it was found that 96% of the patients had blood in the pericardium. The blood was clotted in 41% of these patients and was partially clotted in another 24% (12). Only 19% of the patients had blood in a fluid state in the pericardium. Thus, pericardiocentesis would be falsely negative as an indicator of hemopericardium in 4 of 5 of these cases. Aspirated blood from the pericardial sac may or may not clot, and thus is not a useful diagnostic sign (52). A negative pericardiocentesis does not rule out pericardial tamponade and with signs of tamponade deterioration in the patient's condition and persistent hypotension, thoracotomy is indicated (7). Many authors feel that pericardiocentesis is unreliable and associated with a high mortality and prefer thoracotomy in many cases (20, 34). Due to the high rate of complications in performing pericardiocentesis, it is recommended that ECG monitoring, defibrillation, and resuscitative equipment be available (41). In one study, 18 of 21 experienced cardiologists and cardiovascular surgeons had seen at least one death from this procedure (25). Even when pericardiocentesis is positive, it is never a definitive treatment even though the aspiration of a small quantity of fluid may result in dramatic improvement in the patient.

Initial Management of Suspected Cardiac Tamponade

For the relatively stable patient in grade I or early grade II cardiac tamponade, volume loading may be used. Distended neck veins do not indicate fluid overload in these patients. Although these patients have right ventricular "failure," pulmonary edema never occurs since right ventricular output is depressed. Even in normovolemic patients, lactated Ringer's solution or whole blood may improve the patient's condition; this is probably the safest initial therapy to gain time for more definitive procedures (16). Another nonsurgical intervention in these patients is the use of sympathomimetic agents. Isoproterenol is the most useful of these agents. Isoproterenol increases the stroke volume and heart rate and reduces the peripheral vascular resistance. Neither digitalis nor epinephrine increases the cardiac output in patients with tamponade, indicating that the reduction in peripheral vascular resistance secondary to isoproterenol is an important factor in its action (16). Therefore, α-adrenergic agents such as metaraminol or levophed should be avoided. Isoproterenol is useful in grade I and grade II tamponade; however, it will

do nothing for grade III patients and may waste precious time.

Indications

1. The diagnosis of cardiac tamponade.
2. Relief of cardiac tamponade.
3. In patients with suspected cardiac injuries who do not respond to replacement of volume (4, 5). If the tap is positive for blood and symptoms are relieved, the patient needs an urgent pericardiotomy (23).

Equipment

Local anesthetic (lidocaine 1%, 10 ml)
25 gauge ⅝ inch and 18 gauge 1½ inch needles
Iodinated prep solution
Sterile field with towels and towel clips
10 ml and 50 ml syringe
2 ¾ inch 18 gauge spinal needle
Alligator clips
Collecting basin
Sterile 4 × 4 sponges
1 inch adhesive tape

Technique

Preparatory Steps

1. Prepare the skin with an iodinated solution in a substernal region and drape the area.
2. Attach the limb leads of the ECG to the patient.
3. Place the patient with the upper portion of the body at a 30 degree elevation.
4. Locate the puncture site.
   a. *Subxyphoid approach*
      In the subxyphoid approach the needle is placed in the angle between the xyphoid process and the left costal arch since the lungs do not cover the heart in this location (47, 50).
   b. *Parasternal approach*
      This approach is not recommended as it places the needle in close proximity to the left anterior descending coronary artery (21).

Procedural Steps

1. Attach an 18 gauge short bevel spinal needle to a 20 ml syringe. Connect an

alligator clip to the base of the needle and the other end to the V-lead of the electrocardiograph (Fig. 4.1).

CAUTION!

One must have a well-grounded ECG machine as small current leakage can cause arrhythmias (16, 41). This should be checked by the technicians.

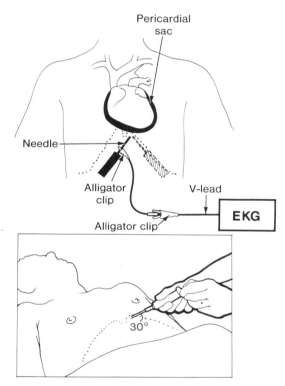

Figure 4.1. Pericardiocentesis. The subxiphoid approach is shown. Attach an alligator clip to the hub of the needle with the other end attached to the V-lead of the ECG. With the needle aimed at the right shoulder, one avoids the coronary arteries. Some physicians prefer to direct the needle toward the tip of the left shoulder. The ECG should be constantly monitored while doing the procedure to determine when the pericardial sac has been entered. See text for discussion. The needle should be passed at a 30 degree angle to the skin.

NOTE

Some authors prefer using a 14 gauge spinal needle with obturator to pass a catheter which may be left in place should blood be aspirated (16). A large polyethylene catheter can be inserted and left in place since reaccumulation of blood within the pericardial sac is likely when the tap is positive in a patient with tamponade (7, 15, 30, 53). This catheter is then left in place en route to the operating room. The pericardial sac then is decompressed periodically before definitive surgery (51).

2. With the V-lead fastened to the metal hub of the spinal needle with an alligator clip, the needle is inserted in the left subxiphoid angle. Aim the needle at the right shoulder or directly cephalid and not the left to avoid injury to the coronary arteries (16, 42). However, the needle may be aimed at the tip of the left shoulder. As the pericardium is entered, a "pop" is often felt.

CAUTION!

When the needle point touches the epicardium, the ECG shows a sudden large current of injury (16, 51). The physician must continuously look at the V-lead connected to the ECG monitor for elevation of the PR or ST segments, depending on whether the auricle or ventricle, respectively, is injured (5, 10, 41, 51). Ventricular asystoles may occur (47). If one does not see any of these electrical patterns, then suspect that the needle is not in the proper place (47). When any of the above patterns are noted, the needle is in contact with the epicardium and should be withdrawn 1 or 2 mm until a normal ECG is noted.

3. With the needle tip in the pericardial sac, aspiration can be performed. If one suspects that the needle is in the heart and time permits, inject fluorescein into the needle and look for a fluorescent "flush" under ultraviolet light under the skin of the eyelid. If the needle is in the cardiac chamber,

the test will be positive (16, 41). Also, ventricular puncture is suggested if the aspirated blood has the same hematocrit as a blood sample from a peripheral vein. When performing the procedure on the alert patient and there is doubt as to the location of the needle, 3 ml of Decholin (sodium dehydrocholate) may be injected. The patient is then asked if he has a bitter taste which indicates ventricular penetration of the needle.

Aftercare

1. Withdraw the catheter and apply a sterile dressing and adhesive tape. Continue ECG monitoring of the patient. All patients who have had pericardiocentesis performed in the emergency center should be admitted to a monitored bed for 24 hours.

Complications

1. Laceration of the myocardium or coronary arteries (16, 25, 41). The left anterior descending artery is especially vulnerable to injury from the advancing needle. The left parasternal approach is especially likely to injure this vessel. Aiming the needle at the right shoulder after entering into the left costosternal angle may avoid injury to this vessel. The patient always should be monitored for any current of injury during advancement of the needle, and aspiration should be performed as the needle is advanced. Most patients with puncture of the myocardium secondary to a needle have no sequelae; the needle is simply withdrawn and the patient is monitored and observed.
2. Pneumothorax (16) and hydropneumothorax (41). All patients with pericardiocentesis should have a follow-up chest radiographs. When a pneumothorax is noted, depending on the size, a chest tube may be indicated.
3. Arrhythmias (5, 10, 16, 41, 47, 51). Asystole has been reported after this procedure (41). Ventricular fibrillation and vasovagal arrest also have been reported (41). If an arrhythmia

occurs, withdraw the needle; if the arrhythmia persists, treat routinely.
4. Pneumopericardium (41).
5. Vasovagal reaction.

THORACOTOMY

The need to perform emergency thoracotomy within the emergency center by an emergency physician has been a debated issue for some time. A number of authors have suggested that immediate thoracotomy performed in the emergency center under specific situations should be the standard of care (6, 7, 15, 18, 26, 31). The authors feel that in patients who have arrested from either penetrating or blunt chest trauma, thoracotomy should be done immediately within the emergency center (38). External cardiac massage is inadequate in massively hypovolemic patients (38). Even if the arrest is due to massive bleeding within the abdomen, temporary occlusion of the descending thoracic aorta diminishes further blood loss and improves the coronary perfusion pressure which aids in resuscitation (38). Thoracotomy has been advocated as a lifesaving maneuver when indicated, and good results occur when thoracotomy is performed properly in the emergency center (43). McDonald reports 25% success with thoracotomies performed in the emergency center by emergency physicians trained in the procedure (28). An 11% long-term survival rate was noted in those patients who came in "dead on arrival" and in whom emergency thoracotomies were performed promptly by emergency physicians. In a study by Mattox et al. the overall survival rate for patients subjected to emergency center thoracotomy was reported as 27%, but the patients who came in "dead on arrival" had a 100% mortality rate (32). This study would indicate that emergency physicians trained in the procedure of emergency thoracotomy, with proper support systems, can anticipate at least as good a success rate as can surgeons.

Pericardiocentesis should be utilized as a diagnostic maneuver and occasionally may be lifesaving, but definitive treatment for cardiac wounds is immediate thoracotomy, preferably in the operating room (33). In critical situations, thoracotomy in the emergency center for control of bleeding, cardiac massage, and the direct repair of cardiac injuries may be lifesaving. The emphasis on conservative therapy for cardiac wounds is clearly disputed by most authors (6, 7, 15, 18, 28, 31).

Patients who arrive in the emergency center in a moribund state (i.e., faint or absent pulses, no audible blood pressure, and distant or absent heart sounds) may have an ultimately good prognosis when thoracotomy is done early, either in the operating room, when time permits, or in the emergency center (26, 40). In summary, the objectives of emergency thoracotomy performed in the emergency center are as follows:

1. Release of cardiac tamponade (32)
2. Control of bleeding and/or suture repair of cardiac or great vessel wounds (32)
3. Internal cardiac massage (32)
4. Cross-clamping of the descending thoracic aorta when necessary (32)

The last two of these four objectives will increase the coronary blood flow and cerebral perfusion and, in some cases, will retard massive abdominal bleeding.

Thoracotomy is not as effective in the emergency center when dealing with massive bleeding in the chest from extracardiac injuries. Here, cardiopulmonary bypass and autotransfusion are good adjuncts until the patient is able to receive definitive care (32). With an autotransfusion, one can infuse up to 2500 ml of blood rapidly into the patient.

The frequency of penetrating wounds to various cardiac stuctures corresponds with the relative surface area of the anterior chest wall; thus, the right ventricle, left ventricle, right atrium, and left atrium are injured in decreasing frequency (53). Studies show that the right and left ventricles are injured in approximately 44% of cases, the left atrium is injured in 7% of cases, and the right atrium is injured in only 4% (12). In 30% of patients, more than one cardiac structure is injured (18, 53). It

is interesting to note that in the majority of cases, clotted blood was found within the pericardium in patients with cardiac wounds, thus dispelling the fallacy that a negative pericardiocentesis (i.e., clotted blood) is a reliable indicator of an uninjured heart. In 40% of patients with cardiac injuries the blood within the pericardial sac was clotted, in 25% of cases the pericardium contained both clotted and nonclotted blood, while in only 20% was the blood entirely unclotted within the sac (12). Patients with cardiac injuries require massive amounts of blood and when the emergency physician knows that such a patient may be coming to his center, he should alert the blood bank. These patients may need up to 63 units of blood, the average being 5 units during the period from arrival in the emergency center to stabilization (32).

Indications

Many of the indications for thoracotomy have been discussed in the introductory section. The most common indications are listed below. In addition the patient must be either unconscious or subjected to general anesthesia.

1. Cardiac arrest in a patient with penetrating or blunt thoracic trauma requires immediate thoracotomy in the emergency center (38).
2. Trauma. Patients who arrive in the emergency center moribund with faint or absent pulses, no audible blood pressure, and distant or absent heart sounds in whom resuscitative efforts prove unsuccessful.
3. Patients with grade III cardiac tamponade in whom pericardiocentesis is unsuccessful in relieving the tamponade and who are deteriorating rapidly.
4. Massive intra-abdominal bleeding with deteriorating vital signs in whom mast suit and other measures are not effective in maintaining the blood pressure. This is usually due to arterial bleeding and proximal aortic occlusion may be lifesaving and can be used only when the patient can be taken to the operating room within 20

to 30 minutes for definitive management (45).

Equipment

#3 Bard-Parker knife handle
#10 and #11 blades
6¾ inch Mayo scissors, curved
8¾ inch Mayo scissors, curved
5½ inch Metzenbaum scissors, curved
10½ inch Masson needle-holder
7 inch Mayo Hegan needle-holder
1 set U. S. Army retractors
Bailey rib contractor
6 inch tissue forceps
10 inch tissue forceps
six 5½ inch Crile forceps
six 6¼ inch Crile forceps
two 8 inch Mayo Pean forceps, curved
one 10 inch DeBakey tangental occlusion clamp
1 Yankouer suction, with finger control
four 5¼ inch Backhaus towel clips
1 Finochietto retractor, 12 inch spread
4 towels
thirty 4 × 4 sponges

Technique

In this section the steps will be divided into preparatory steps, procedural steps, and aftercare. Since the procedural steps will depend on what is found upon performing thoracotomy, three areas will be discussed in the procedural section: cardiac injuries and their repair, open cardiac massage and resuscitation, and cross-clamping of the aorta.

Preparatory Steps

1. The patient should be intubated early in the course, preferably before performing a thoracotomy (50). At the same time as endotracheal intubation is performed, large-bore lines, a Foley catheter, and a nasogastric tube are inserted and blood is obtained for typing (50). Resuscitative efforts will be fruitless unless one is able to reverse hypoxia, acidosis, and hypovolemia.

In moribund or arrested patients, it is critical to treat hypovolemia if resuscitation is to be successful. The most effective means of infusing a large volume of fluid over a short period of time in these patients is to perform bilateral femoral or saphenous vein cutdowns and introduce a polyethylene catheter which has the same dimensions as intravenous tubing. A 14 gauge Angiocath placed centrally through a subclavian or internal jugular cannula is grossly inadequate for infusing the large volumes which these patients require rapidly if one is to have any hope of a successful outcome. These central vein cannulae have too much resistence to flow to provide rapid infusions of fluid.

2. A sandbag should be placed beneath the left scapula and the left arm should be elevated (13). This places the patient in an optimal position for thoracotomy.

Procedural Steps

Site of incision

1. The left anterolateral incision over the fourth or fifth intercostal space, extending from the sternum to the posteroaxillary line (Fig. 4.2) is the one preferred by most authors (6, 18, 31, 32, 34, 50). For emergency center thoracotomy, this site of incision is better than the median sternotomy (6, 34, 50). Left-sided thoracotomy provides easy access to the heart for suturing cardiac injuries, internal cardiac massage, and cross-clamping the aorta. When necessary, the incision may be extended across the sternum to the right side, when dealing with a

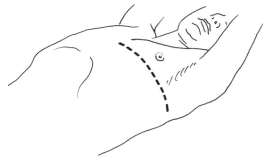

Figure 4.2. Thoracotomy incision. A left anterolateral incision is made over the fourth or fifth intercostal space. See text for discussion.

right-sided injury (21, 32, 50). While some authors prefer a right-sided thoracotomy on obvious right-sided injuries (6, 32), this is not advocated in the emergency thoracotomy. To save time, the area of incision is not prepped in these patients (50). In the female, center the incision in the inframammary fold (13).

2. In a single maneuver, using a #10 blade, incise the skin, subcutaneous tissue, and chest wall muscles (pectoralis). The incision should be carried deeply to the rib cage (Fig. 4.3). This must be done rapidly and preferably in one single step.

3. Using a blunt scissors, enter the chest cavity through the fourth intercostal space and incise the intercostal muscles, using the second and third fingers to separate the pleura of the lung from the chest wall while carrying the incision from the posterior axillary line to the sternum (Fig. 4.4).

4. Insert a rib spreader (Fig. 4.5) and spread it forcefully (13). If necessary, the costochondral junctions may dislocate and, in an elderly patient, ribs may be fractured (13). For adequate visualization in some cases, the sternum may need to be transsected.

5. Any blood in the left side of the chest

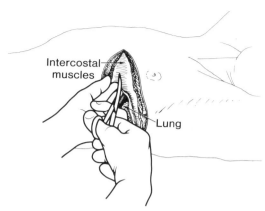

Figure 4.4.   Using the second and third fingers of the left hand to separate the pleura of the lung from the chest wall, insert a blunt scissors at the fourth intercostal space and cut the intercostal muscles along this space from the posterior axillary line to the sternum.

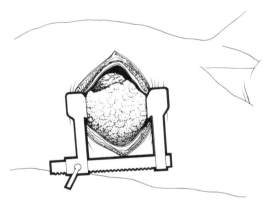

Figure 4.5.   Insert a rib spreader and spread it forcefully apart to expose the thoracic cavity. See text for discussion.

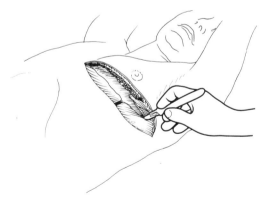

Figure 4.3.   Using a #10 blade on a long handle, the incision is carried with one sweep through the skin, subcutaneous tissue, and chest wall muscles. This should preferably be done in one step as this is an emergency procedure performed when the patient is moribund.

should be evacuated and the pericardium opened widely through a horizontal incision made anterior to the phrenic nerve with the patient supine (Fig. 4.6) (13). The phrenic nerve courses superior to inferior along the lateral aspect of the pericardial sac. In most cases of hemopericardium, clotted blood will be present in the pericardial sac in a larger quantity than liquid blood due to the rapidity of the bleed from the cardiac wound (13). Before the pericardial sac is en-

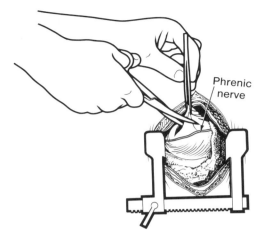

Figure 4.6. Open the pericardial sac through a horizontal incision made anterior to the phrenic nerve.

tered, the hilum should be rapidly inspected for any active bleeding unless the patient has arrested in which case the pericardium should be opened, since open heart massage should be performed as soon as possible.

NOTE

The technique of open cardiac massage and cross-clamping of the thoracic aorta is discussed separately later. It is obvious that these procedures may be necessary before step #5; however, since they are not always part of the step-by-step technique of repairing wounds of the heart, they have been separated from this discussion.

CAUTION!

It must be remembered that when vital signs are restored suddenly after repair of the heart, anesthesia may be needed since the patient may wake up (50).

CARDIAC REPAIR

If when the pericardium is opened the heart is found to be in standstill, one must restore action by doing massage. One may need to place a finger over the wound while performing cardiac massage (13, 50). In hemopericardium the heart often is found to be beating when the pericardium is opened and the clotted blood is removed. Ideally, the bleeding from a ventricular wound should be stopped by placing a finger upon the wound; the patient should be taken to the operating room where the heart wound is repaired, using new instruments and a new drape and sterile scrub (13). Unfortunately, the immediate availability of an operating suite and staff is often not available to the emergency center when the patient arrives, and the physician in the center must perform some basic repairs of cardiac wounds. The discussion below is divided into ventricular repairs, atrial repairs, and hilar and great vessel repairs. A planned anoxic arrest is rarely needed to suture a wound of the heart, with the exception of large posterior wounds (50). While debridement is often recommended when dealing with gunshot wounds of the heart (25b), this is usually not performed when dealing with these cases. Subsequent aneurysm formation in the wall of the heart can be dealt with later should this be a problem. Intermittent occlusion of venous "inflow" can be created by quickly placing a vascular clamp on the vena cava inferior and/or superior, which decreases the chamber size of the heart, and exsanguinating hemorrhage may be controlled for 60 to 90 seconds while suture repair is performed (55). In the absence of severe hypotension, an intravenous drip of trimethaphan can decrease aortic and left ventricular pressure to allow safe closure of the wound in a decompressed chamber (55). By using this method, one can close a large wound in the emergency center without cardiopulmonary bypass. When the wound is too large to close in 60 to 90 seconds or is located on the posterior aspect of the heart, cardiopulmonary bypass is needed (53). Hemorrhage from the very large wounds in a ventricle can be controlled by placing a finger over the cardiac laceration, inserting a loop of suture parallel to the opening on either side of the wound, and then crossing the sutures over one another after removing the finger and asking an assistant to hold the suture ends (11). Definitive repair then can be performed as described below, using horizontal mattress sutures (11). When torrential bleeding is a problem, an alternative method is to use a *Sauerbruch* grip for occlusion of the vena cava. The vena cava is gripped between the ring and middle finger of the left hand which occludes the flow into the heart, causing fibrillation and permitting repair. However, as with the vascular clamps, this cannot be left in place for more than 60 to 90 seconds (35).

CAUTION!

In patients requiring multiple transfusions of bank blood, rapid infusion of cold blood results in lowering of the core temperature, making cardiac resuscitation harder (7). In these patients, warming of the blood should be performed before the infusion. Pericardial and pleural lavage with warm saline may assist in restoring normal cardiac action in such patients (7).

When dealing with a large ventricular wound in which bleeding is difficult to control or a stellate laceration of the ventricle, one can pass a Foley catheter into the wound, inflate the balloon and apply traction to control the bleeding. This is an excellent method to control bleeding while repairing the wound edges.

Ventricular Repair

The best way to stop bleeding from a ventricular wound is by placing a finger over but not in the wound (Fig. 4.7) (8). In the beating heart, it is often difficult to keep a finger on the wound due to movement. One can deal with this problem by placing an apical traction stitch, which is performed by placing a suture at the apex of the heart and holding the suture between the thumb and third finger of the left hand while the index finger is placed over the wound (Fig. 4.8) (8, 9, 21). The apex is selected due to the fact that it is the region farthest from major coronary

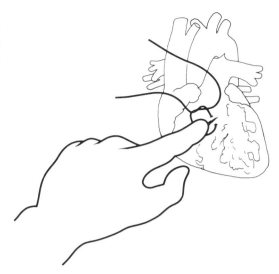

Figure 4.7.   The best way to stop bleeding from a ventricular wound is by placing a finger over but not in the wound. After this a horizontal mattress stitch or simple stitch may be secured across the wound edges to stop the bleeding.

arteries. This apical traction suture is commonly referred to as *Beck's suture.*

In some cases the heart is extremely pliable and soft, and the apical traction suture is not used due to the fact that it may cut through the cardiac apex and require repair later (13, 35, 50). While some authors prefer 3-0 Dacron suture for cardiac wound repair (32), most authors prefer nonabsorbable 2-0 or 2-0 silk wedged on a half-circle atraumatic needle (13, 18, 21, 35). When suturing the ventricle, a suture should be placed 6 mm from the edges of the wound, and the wound closed just tight enough to stop bleeding without strangulating or cutting the myocardium (7, 18, 35). The suture should pass down to but not through the endocardium and should not be tied tightly (13, 21, 35). When dealing with very pliable tissue, one may have to pass several sutures beneath the occluding finger before tying to avoid tearing the myocardium (7, 9, 18, 21). Small wounds of the ventricle are closed with interrupted vertical mattress sutures (18, 53). Those wounds which are larger or near vessels are closed with horizontal

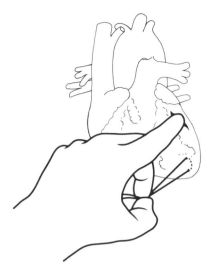

be treated by electively fibrillating the heart for decompression, and intermittent internal massage should be performed while repair is taking place (55). The fi-

Figure 4.8.   In a patient with a beating heart it is often difficult to keep a finger on the wound due to movement. In addition, it is difficult to stabilize the heart to place a suture. An apical traction suture (Beck's suture) can be placed in the apex of the heart, which is relatively avascular, and the suture can be held between the thumb and third finger of the left hand, while the index finger is placed over the wound. See text for discussion.

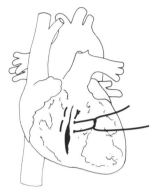

Figure 4.9.   Large wounds of the ventricle are closed with horizontal mattress sutures as shown. When such a large wound extends into the ventricular cavity, the patient usually exsanguinates; however, when a slash laceration from a knife extends through a partial thickness of the heart the patient may be resuscitatable.

mattress sutures (8, 33, 53) (Figs. 4.7 and 4.9). In placing the horizontal mattress suture in a ventricular wound which is adjacent to a coronary artery, the suture can be passed under and adjacent to the artery without incorporating the vessel within the tie (Fig. 4.10B). In wounds with surrounding areas of damaged myocardium, the mattress suture can be reinforced by passing it through Teflon pledgets so that there is no cutting through the damaged heart (25b, 53) (Fig. 4.10A). Some authors have advocated that in large ventricular wounds horizontal strips of Teflon be placed adjacent and parallel to the wound edges and the interrupted mattress pass through these Teflon strips (19) (Fig. 4.10). When dealing with large wounds of the ventricle, horizontal mattress sutures may be placed on either side of the lesion and crossed to stop bleeding temporarily while a definitive repair is performed (Fig. 4.11) (55). Large wounds of the ventricle should

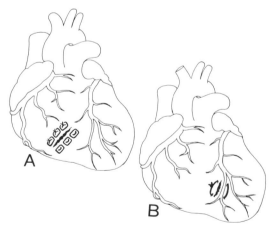

Figure 4.10.   *A.* A mattress suture may be passed across the lacerated myocardium through Teflon pledgets, reinforcing each side to prevent the suture from cutting through weakened myocardium. *B.* When suturing a laceration which is in close proximity to a myocardial vessel, a horizontal mattress stitch is passed beneath the vessel, and the wound is closed as shown above.

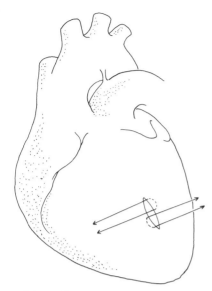

Figure 4.11. When dealing with large ventricular wounds with pronounced bleeding, horizontal mattress sutures may be placed on each side of the lesion and crossed to stop the bleeding temporarily while definitive repairs are performed.

brillation paddles are placed anterior and posterior to the surface of the heart and discharged at 20 watt/sec (Fig. 4.12). The wound then is repaired in the routine fashion (Fig. 4.13).

Coronary Vascular Injuries

Coronary artery wounds are not common injuries. The overall mortality rate is approximately 44% (25b). Some authors have advocated ligating the injured artery despite precipitating a myocardial infarction; the overall survival rate with this method is 90% (25b). When one vessel is injured, a ligature should be placed proximal to the artery, using fine silk (21, 35). One should avoid grasping the bleeding coronary vessel with a hemostat (21). In all cases in which both the right and left main coronary arteries (left anterior descending and circumflex artery) were lacerated, this procedure was fatal (25b). With the advent of aortocoronary bypass, such cases may receive definitive surgery with a better survival rate.

Atrial Repair

In dealing with wounds of the atrium, one cannot place a finger over the wound since the atrial wall is very thin and this will not stop the bleeding. The management of wounds of the atria is divided into three categories depending on the location

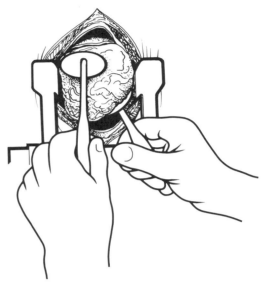

Figure 4.12. The fibrillation paddles are placed anterior and posterior to the surface of the heart and discharged at 20 watt-seconds.

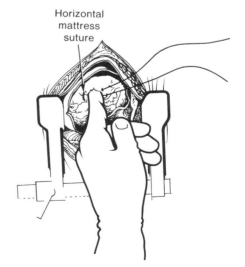

Figure 4.13. After defibrillation is performed, the wound is repaired in the routine fashion.

of the atrial injury: central, marginal, and atrial-caval junction. In dealing with a *central* wound, the bleeding atrial wound can be compressed between the thumb and index finger and then an atraumatic vascular partial exclusion clamp placed around the wound (Fig. 4.14) and the wound repaired (13, 21, 25b, 35, 55). Alternately, small hemostats or allis clamps (21, 35) can be placed on the opposing edges of the wound, uplifted and crisscrossed to control bleeding and approximate the edges while a repair is taking place. Repair of these wounds should be with interrupted fine silk sutures (4-0 or 5-0) which should be tied with care. It is best to avoid passing through the endocardium during suturing since this can result in a mural thrombosis (21, 35). When dealing with a *marginal* atrial wound at the periphery of the atrium, suture ligature of the puncture site is advocated. This is performed similarly to suture ligature for a bleeding vessel. When dealing with a wound near the *atrial-caval junction*, a Foley catheter may be inserted into the laceration for temporary tamponade and repair then carried out (25b). The size of the Foley and amount of air depends on the patient's wound. Usually a 12 or 14 French is adequate.

Atrial Cannulation

When the cardiac chambers are "empty" and devoid of blood upon opening the pericardium, an atrial line can be

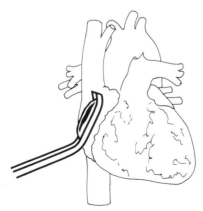

Figure 4.14. An atraumatic vascular partial occlusion clamp is placed around the wound of the atria. See text for discussion.

placed quickly to supply volume directly to the heart. In doing so, the intra-atrial line should consist of either sterilized intravenous extension tubing with the tip cut off or, preferably, sterilized polyethylene tubing the size of intravenous tubing. This permits rapid volume replacement which is desperately needed if the outcome is to be favorable. The right atrial appendage is the preferred site for an intra-atrial line, since this area is usually accessible and thin-walled and will permit blood to pass through the lungs for oxygenation before going into the central circulation, which does not occur with a left atrial line. In performing this procedure, the following technique should be used (Fig. 4.15).

1. Two small hemostats are placed with the tips opposing one another and securing the right atrial appendage. The appendage is uplifted and held separated by these two hemostats by an assistant.
2. A small stab incision is placed with a #11 blade between the opposing tips of the hemostats.
3. The polyethylene tubing or intravenous tubing then is passed through the small opening and a purse-string suture is applied to secure the tubing. Alternately, (authors' preference) a purse-string suture may be applied first in the atrial appendage and then an incision made within the center of the purse-string suture, before tying, and an atrial cannula (sterile polyethylene tubing the size of intravenous tubing) passed. The purse-string secured around the tubing avoids the bleeding which occurs during placement of a suture after the tubing has been passed. One can then take the ends of the suture, after tying the purse-string around the tubing and make a second tie around the polyethylene tubing approximately 1 cm above its entrance into the atrium to secure its position.

Aftercare

1. The patient should be transferred to the operating room for loose closure

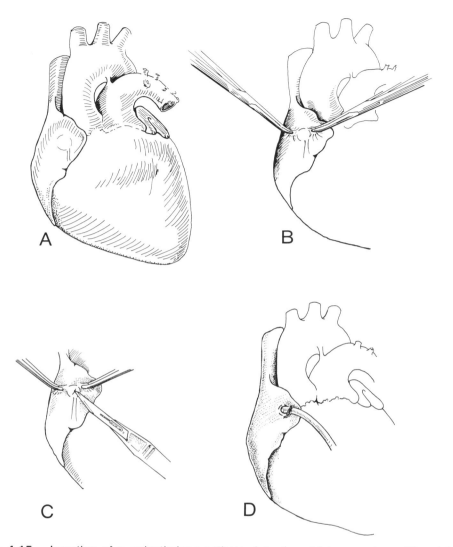

Figure 4.15. Insertion of a polyethylene catheter into the atrial appendage. The right atrial appendage is preferred for this procedure as this permits unoxygenated blood to be passed through the lungs and to become oxygenated. *A.* The authors prefer placing a purse-string suture first around the atrial appendage. *B.* Two small hemostats are placed with the tips opposing one another and securing a piece of the atrial appendage just outside of the purse-string suture. The appendage is uplifted and held separated by these two hemostats by an assistant. *C.* Make an incision with a #11 blade over the center of the purse-string suture. *D.* Pass a polyethylene catheter the size of intravenous tubing through the incision just made and tie the purse-string suture around the tubing, and again 1 cm above to secure it in place.

of the pericardium and chest incision (51). Chest drainage is established by placing two tubes, one thoracostomy tube in the seventh intercostal space at the anterior axillary line and a lower tube placed in the vicinity of the open pericardium; several holes are cut in the tube to aspirate along the entire distance from the pericardium to the chest wall (50). Since the

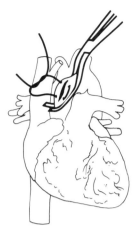

Figure 4.16. A horizontal mattress suture is used to repair a large wound over the great vessel. The repair is performed only after the area is separated by a partial inclusion clamp.

procedure is not sterile, it is recommended that the area be profusely irrigated with saline containing neomycin sulfate or bacitracin and be closed layer-by-layer using catgut for the muscles and silk, steel, or staples for the skin (50). A large pericardial window may be placed posterior to the phrenic nerve, and the anterior pericardiotomy incision can be closed loosely with 4-0 silk after thorough irrigation of the pericardium and pleural cavities (13). Thus, the pericardium is not drained externally; however, the pericardial incision should be closed with widely spaced interrupted sutures of 4-0 silk and a window placed as discussed above to provide an opening into the pleural space for internal drainage. If the wound of entrance or exit is in line with the thoracotomy incision, it is excised before closure (21).

Injuries to the Hilum and Great Vessels

Injuries to the hilum produce significant bleeding which can be initially controlled by grasping the hilum proximal to the bleeding site between two fingers and rotating the hilum (when dealing with large bleeding sites) or by applying a vascular

clamp to the hilum (32). Definitive repair of hilar injuries should be performed by physicians with expertise in this area and must be performed in the operating room. When dealing with wounds to the great vessels such as the aorta, the bleeding from the laceration may be controlled by placing a partial exclusion clamp separating the injured portion from the remainder of the vessel. It is best to repair this injury in the operating room. When this is not possible, smaller wounds may be closed with simple interrupted vertical mattress sutures and larger wounds may be closed with a horizontal mattress suture (Fig. 4.16) (50).

Open Cardiac Massage

Open cardiac massage can be performed by one of two methods: the one-handed or two-handed technique. Using the one-handed technique the heart is grasped in the palm of the hand (Fig. 4.17) and the fingers are wrapped around the heart so that the tips of the fingers and the thumb

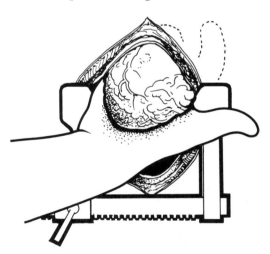

Figure 4.17. The one-handed technique of open heart massage is shown. The heart is grasped in the palm of the hand while the fingers are wrapped around the heart such that the tips of the fingers and the thumb do not protrude into the heart muscle. Massage then is gently performed by wavelike compression, beginning with the small finger and ascending up to the index finger and thumb.

do not protrude into the heart muscle. Massage then is performed gently by a wavelike compression, beginning with the small finger and ascending up to the index finger and thumb. Remember never to press the tips of the fingers or the thumb into the heart tissue, as this may result in perforation of a pliable ischemic myocardium. Massage is performed with the volar surface of the digits and the "pads" of the fingertips rather than the tips of the fingers.

The second technique with which to perform open cardiac massage is by the two-handed technique, in which the heart is compressed between two hands placed on either side of the heart (Fig. 4.18). This provides for more effective cardiac compression than does the one-handed technique.

Intracardiac Injection

This procedure is not commonly indicated in the emergency center as most medications can be given through a central venous line. However, when one is unable to give medications by the normal route, emergency drugs may have to be given through intracardiac injection.

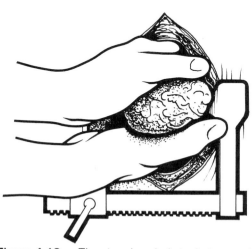

Figure 4.18. The two-handed technique of open heart massage is demonstrated. See text for discussion.

Technique

The technique in performing this procedure is as follows:

1. Prepare the chest wall with an iodinated preparation. The area of prep should be in the precordial region around the fourth intercostal space and from the midclavicular line to the sternum and the xyphoid region.
2. Using a long spinal needle, insert the needle in the left costosternal angle, aspirating while advancing the needle until the ventricular chamber is entered. While the paraxyphoid approach is preferred, when entrance into the cardiac chamber is not possible by this method the needle may be placed through the anterior chest wall in the fourth intercostal space midway between the sternum and the midclavicular line.
3. Medications can be injected through the needle at this point.

Complications

1. Coronary artery injury. This is a less common problem using the paraxyphoid approach. With the anterior approach, the anterior descending coronary artery may be injured.
2. Pericardial hemorrhage and tamponade. This complication may be prevented by using a small gauge spinal needle while performing the procedure and avoiding the anterior approach when possible.

During internal massage, ECG monitoring is obscured; however, the heart can be observed and both atrial and ventricular action noted. The rates of the observed atrial and ventricular activity and their synchronization are as useful as the ECG. Treatment of dysrhythmias should follow standard ACLS protocol. During internal massage, intracardiac injection may be performed with a 22 gauge needle inserted into the left ventricle or, preferably, the atrium. Care should be taken to avoid the coronary vessels. Intramyocardial injection of fluid can result in refractory ventricular fibrillation; therefore, aspiration of blood should be performed before any injection into the heart.

Thoracic Aortic Occlusion

The indications for thoracic aortic occlusion are two: when the heart is empty in the presence of severe hypovolemia and with massive hemoperitoneum which is unresponsive to the usual conservative measures (18a, 25a). Proximal descending thoracic aortic occlusion is effective in patients who have massive hemoperitoneum and in whom the systolic blood pressure is less than 60 and rapid infusion of type specific blood causes no return of pressure (18a). The thoracic aorta should be cross-clamped above the diaphragm. This procedure can be done in the emergency center after all other resuscitative efforts including massive transfusions and the application of a mast suit have failed, and the patient's death is certain (18a).

The aorta must be identified and isolated from the esophagus before cross-clamping. This is best performed by palplating the thoracic vertebral bodies just superior to the diaphragm. The thoracic aorta is the first structure which overlies the vertebral body as one brings his finger anteriorly. Just anterior to the aorta and medial to it courses the esophagus. These structures are difficult to palpate in the hypovolemic patient in whom the thoracic aorta may be collapsed. In these patients the pleura adjacent and anterior to the body of the thoracic vertebras should be opened and separated transversely (in the supine patient). The aorta then can be identified beneath the pleural reflection and separated from the esophagus just proximal to its passage through the diaphragm. A vascular clamp then is used to clamp the aorta (Fig. 4.19). In patients in whom thoracic aortic occlusion was performed, the interval of clamping varied from 7 to 60 minutes (25a). The authors have had complications with clamping, primarily with left ventricular failure. The recommendation is made that if the systolic blood pressure is between 120 and 200 after clamping, the clamp should be removed periodically (25a). The blood pressure should be checked every 30 sec-

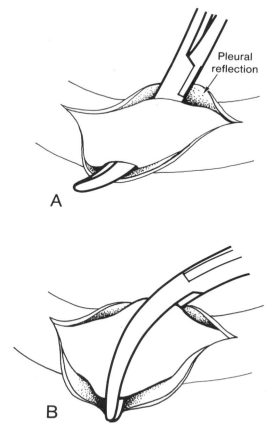

Figure 4.19.   Thoracic aortic occlusion. *A.* The pleural reflection over the aorta and mediastinum is incised longitudinally. A curved Kelly or vascular clamp is then used to separate the aorta from the pleura. *B.* The vascular clamp is gently applied to occlude the aorta. See text for discussion.

onds while clamping is continued. Other complications encountered with thoracic aortic occlusion include ischemic bowel, renal failure, and spinal cord ischemia.

CLOSED THORACOSTOMY (CHEST TUBE INSERTION)

Approximately 300 ml of blood must collect in the pleural space to be visible on chest radiographs (19). A hemothorax with approximately 500 ml of blood in the pleural space can be treated conservatively (29). Pleural resorption of the hemothorax will restore the radiographs to normal within 10 days to 2 weeks. A pure hemothorax usually necessitates the insertion of a posterolateral chest tube. A pure pneumothorax usually requires an anterior chest tube. When the patient has a hemopneumothorax, a posterolateral chest tube is inserted initially; however, both an anterior and a posterolateral tube may be needed to adequately drain these patients (19). Continuous bleeding through the chest tube of more than 200 ml/hr *after* the initial hemothorax has been evacuated is an indication for a thoracotomy to control bleeding (38).

Second chest wounds should be closed rapidly with vaseline gauze dressing and a chest tube should be inserted posterolaterally (5, 19).

Three sites for chest tube insertion have been described in the literature: anterior, posterolateral, and apical posterior. The apical posterior tube is rarely indicated in the emergency center; the one most commonly used in the emergency center is the posterolateral chest tube (1).

Indications

1. Tension pneumothorax. In patients with a tension pneumothorax, needle aspiration of the pneumothorax should be performed first, as this may be lifesaving, and should be followed by an anterior chest tube (29).
2. Hemothorax (19, 38). In patients with a hemothorax, a posterolateral chest tube should be placed.
3. Hemopneumothorax (19, 38). These patients should have a posterolateral chest tube placed; however, they may require an anterior chest tube as well for adequate drainage when there is a persistent pneumothorax.
4. A simple pneumothorax greater than 20%.
5. Penetrating thoracic trauma without evidence of a pneumothorax in patients who may be subjected to positive pressure breathing in the operating room or intensive care unit.

Equipment

Iodinated preparation with sponges

Sterile towels
Local anesthetic
10 ml syringe
18 gauge, 1½ inch needle
25 gauge, ⅝ inch needle
21 gauge, 1½ inch needle
1% lidocaine with epinephrine, 20 ml
#10 scalpel blade with handle
Chest tube (5, 37, 38)
    Adults—28 to 32 French Argyle chest tube
    Children—20 to 24 French Argyle chest tube
    Infant—18 French Argyle chest tube

NOTE

The size of the tube will vary depending on whether one is draining a pneumothorax or a hemothorax. With a pneumothorax, one may use a small size 24 to 28 French tube in the adult. When draining a hemothorax, a size 32 chest tube is preferred.

2 curved Kelly or Rochester-Pean clamps
Serrated plastic connector—"Y" type with one end occluded. This can be used when two chest tubes need to be inserted (37).
Soft plastic connecting tubes ½ inch in diameter and 6 feet long (37).
    In children and infants ¼ inch diameter tube is needed (37).
Pleuravac^R (37) or 3-bottle chest suction set
Adequate suction

NOTE

Suction should be high-volume suction. The vacuum source should be able to deliver 60 cm of water pressure with a flow volume of 15 to 20 liters/min (37). Wall suction provides this amount of negative pressure. When a mobile unit is needed for transport, it should be a high-volume suction unit (Emerson, Sorenson). Do not use low-volume systems (Stedman, Gomco).

Needle holder
Suture scissors

0 Silk suture
2-0 silk suture
Dressing
   Sterile sponges
   Xeroforms[R] gauze dressing
   Antibacterial ointment
   Tincture of benzoin
   Elastoplast tape—3 inch
   1 inch adhesive tape

Technique

Posterior Lateral Chest Tube—Preparatory Steps

1. Select the site for insertion of the chest tube. The fourth intercostal space in the midaxillary line is the best site for insertion (5, 38). While the posterior axillary line is preferred by some authors (19), this insertion causes unnecessary pain for the patients since they must lie on the tube. Some authors prefer the eighth or ninth intercostal space (29); however, in the authors' opinions this is dangerously low, risking intra-abdominal insertion.

CAUTION!

Lower insertion may result in perforation of the liver or spleen due to a high-lying diaphragm (5, 38). The diaphragm may reach as high as the fifth intercostal space in a patient who is supine.

2. Prepare and drape the area.
3. Locally infiltrate an anesthetic solution along the site of the incision, in the subcutaneous tissue, and along the anterior rib margin where the tube will be inserted (Fig. 4.20, inset).

Procedural Steps

1. Make a linear incision along the rib, one interspace below the site of insertion of the tube (Fig. 4.20).
2. Insert a curved clamp and tunnel superiorly to the interspace which is to be entered (Fig. 4.21). Remain on the upper border of the rib in the interspace to be entered to avoid the neurovascular bundle which courses

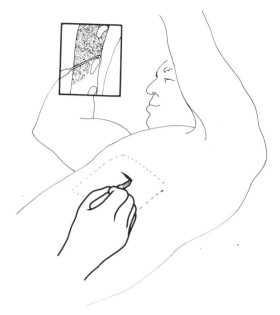

Figure 4.20.   Locally infiltrate 1% Xylocaine® with epinephrine anesthetic solution in the skin and subcutaneous tissue and also along the rib margin as shown in the inset above. Make a linear incision along the rib cage, one interspace below the site of insertion of the tube.

along the inferior margin of the rib within the interspace (38) (Fig. 4.21).
3. Form a small tunnel by separating the clamp to provide for easy access for the chest tube once the puncture is made (Fig. 4.22). The advantage of entering one interspace above the site of puncture is that a flap of skin is formed which prevents air entrance into the thorax upon removal of the chest tube.
4. Gently but forcibly enter the thoracic cage by advancing the closed curved clamp just above the rib margin and puncturing through the intercostal muscles and parietal pleura. Remember to hold the closed clamp close to the upper rib margin (Fig. 4.23). When the thoracic cavity is entered, a gush of air and/or blood will exude through the wound. If the patient is awake, this process will be painful. The curved clamps then are opened to enlarge the puncture site.

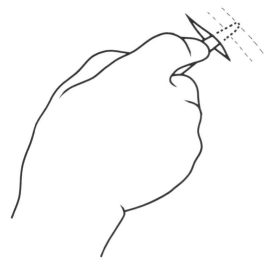

Figure 4.21. Insert a curved clamp and tunnel superiorly to the interspace which is to be entered. Remain on the upper border of the rib and inferiorly in the interspace to be entered.

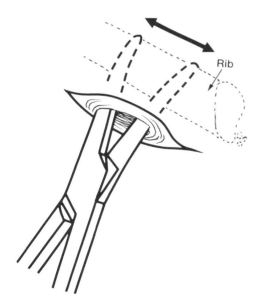

Figure 4.22. Form a small tunnel by opening the clamps to provide easy access to the chest tube.

To open the interspace, do not advance the tips of the clamps any farther than necessary as one may enter the lung tissue itself.

5. Insert the gloved finger into the

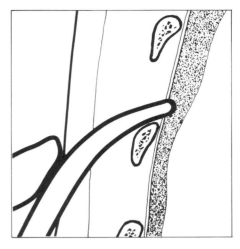

Figure 4.23. Gently but forcibly enter the thoracic cavity by advancing the closed curved clamp just above the rib margin and puncturing the intercostal muscles and parietal pleura. Steady the clamp during insertion by placing the index finger over the curved portion as it exists from the skin. Hold the clamp close to the upper rib margin.

pleural space to prevent inadvertent passage of the chest tube into the lung should unsuspected pleural adhesions be present (5, 19, 38) (Fig. 4.24). If adhesions are felt, with the gloved finger they should be separated away from the lung before insertion of the chest tube.

6. The pleural cutaneous opening should be covered with the hand before the tube is placed into the pleural space. With a curved clamp, grasp the tip of the chest tube and advance it through the skin and into the intercostal puncture site (Fig. 4.25). It may be necessary to hold the puncture site open before advancing the tube, by reinserting the curved clamp and spreading it apart to guide the advancing tube which is passed in the center of the opened clamp. The tube must be advanced so that all of the holes in the chest tube are within the thoracic cavity.

7. Direct the catheter posteriorly, superiorly, and laterally so that the most dependent area is drained (19).

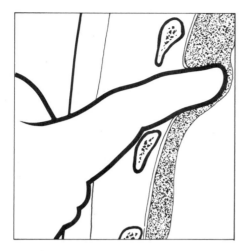

Figure 4.24.   Insert a gloved finger into the pleural cavity to ascertain whether there are any pleural adhesions.

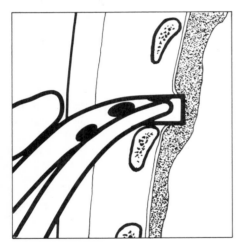

Figure 4.25.   With a curved clamp, grasp the tip of the chest tube and advance it through the skin and into the intercostal puncture site. The tunnel may have to be held open with another curved Kelly clamp to pass the chest tube with this technique, or with the finger.

NOTE

Some authors prefer using a trochar when placing a chest tube rather than using the clamp method indicated above (19). This is dangerous in the authors' opinions as the trochar may inadvertently puncture

the lung tissue, especially when the lung is fixed to the chest wall by adhesions.

NOTE

When adhesions are present, as determined by the finger placed into the pleural cavity, an alternate site should be selected either above or below the original site or an anterior chest tube placed.

8. For drainage, connect the chest tube to an underwater seal with suction at 10 to 15 cm of water pressure (5, 19, 38).

NOTE

Simple underwater seal without suction may be adequate when one is draining only fluid and not air. In the emergency center, usually one is draining both blood and air, and a suction system must be provided. The tip of the tube placed underwater should be 2 cm or less under the surface of the water as positive pleural pressure is needed to displace the fluid from the column before air can escape (3). Dependent position of the tubing may impede the flow of air and is not desirable. Positive pressure equivalent to the vertical elevation of the fluid in the loop of tubing is necessary in order to pass air from the pleural cavity out (Fig. 4.26).

9. A number of methods have been described for securing the chest tube in place. The one listed below is the authors' preferred method.

Pass 0 silk suture into the skin through the subcutaneous tissue at the point marked *A* (Fig. 4.26) as if one is going to close the incision with a horizontal mattress stitch. Come out through the opposite side. Then, wrap the suture around the tube *several times* and tie it securely in place using a one-handed tie as shown in Figure 4.26 B, C, D. Following this, pass the needle through the skin at the point marked *B* as if to complete the horizontal mattress stitch and come out through the opposite side of the wound and tie the suture. This method secures the tube in place, and when it is time to remove the tube the two ends of the suture marked *C* and *D* can be cut and tied with an instrument tie using hemostats to grasp the short suture ends. The incision is then closed similar to a horizontal mattress closure, the exception being that there is a knot on both ends of the suture (Fig. 4.26D inset).

Aftercare

1. The physician must check for any leaks in the system. Leaks are indicated by persistent bubbling or failure to reexpand the lung. When a leak is found, this indicates one of the following causes:
   a. Leakage of air through a connection in the tubing. One must check the connecting sites and make sure there is no leak. In addition, check for a hole in the tubing.
   b. One of the holes in the chest tube is not in the chest itself but in the subcutaneous tissue, thus, air is leaking out of the chest tube.
   c. Air is continuing to leak through a bronchiole with a bronchopleural fistula formed. If this continues, one should suspect a ruptured bronchus. When an air leak is massive and neither *a* nor *b* above are the cause, then a rupture of the main stem bronchus or other larger bronchi should be suspected. Occasionally a small bronchopleural fistula may be "overpowered" and reduced by the insertion of two or three chest tubes.
   d. Rupture of the esophagus, although rare, is another possible cause of continuing air leak in the chest tube. With a ruptured esophagus, air dissects into the mediastinum and pleural spaces and is drained by the chest tube, causing a persistent air leak.
2. Close the remainder of the incision with simple interrupted vertical mattress sutures.
3. Apply antibacterial ointment to the incision site, followed by a Xeroform[R] dressing over the wound. Following this, apply two sterile 4 × 4 dressings with a slit cut ½ across the center of the 4 × 4 and advance the

pads around the chest tube via the slit so that two 4 × 4 dressings encircle the chest tube.

4. Secure the dressing in place with adhesive tape, followed by an Elastoplast® dressing. It is the authors' preference to attach adhesive tape between the dressing and the chest tube and spiral additional strips of 1 inch adhesive tape around the chest tube before application of the Elastoplast® dressing to provide additional security against pulling the tube out.

Anterior Chest Tube

In discussing the placement of an anterior chest tube, only those differences between the insertion of the anterior and the posterolateral chest tube will be discussed. Anterior chest tube is used only when dealing with a simple or tension pneumothorax in which there is no fluid to be drained. Remember then that when dealing with a tension pneumothorax a needle should be inserted before insertion of the anterior chest tube to relieve the tension pneumothorax.

1. The second or third intercostal space in the midclavicular line is the preferred site for placement of an anterior chest tube (29).
2. In passing the tube, it is aimed anteriorly toward the apex of the lung. The hole nearest the proximal portion of the tube should be located just behind the first rib, as this is where most air tends to accumulate in a pneumothorax (3).

Complications

1. Unilateral pulmonary edema. Unilateral pulmonary edema may occur from rapid reexpansion and excessive negative pressures. Rapid reexpansion causes a rapid increase in the pulmonary capillary pressure and blood flow, resulting in transudation of fluid across the capillary membrane which in turn results in pulmonary edema. When dealing with a large hemothorax, drainage should be interrupted by clamping the tube after 200 to 300 cc have been evacu-

Figure 4.26 The authors' preferred method of securing a chest tube in place. Pass 0 silk suture into the skin through the subcutaneous tissue at the point marked *A*. Come out through the opposite side. Wrap the suture around the tube several times and tie it securely in place as shown in 4.26 B, C, and D. Following this, pass the needle through the skin at the point marked *B* as if to complete the horizontal mattress stitch and come out through the opposite side of the wound, tying the suture. This method secures the tube in place while making removal easy. When it is time to remove the tube, the two ends of the suture marked *C* and *D* then can be cut and tied together. The incision then is closed similar to a horizontal mattress closure with the exception that there is a knot at both ends (4.26D inset).

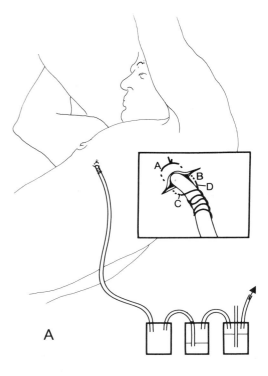

A

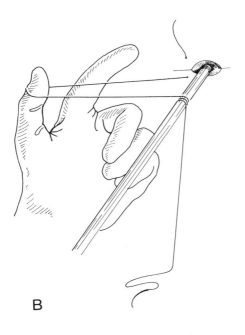

B

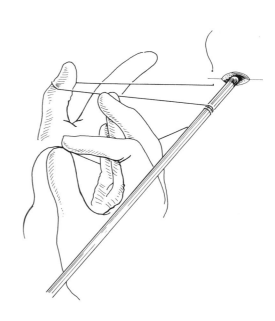

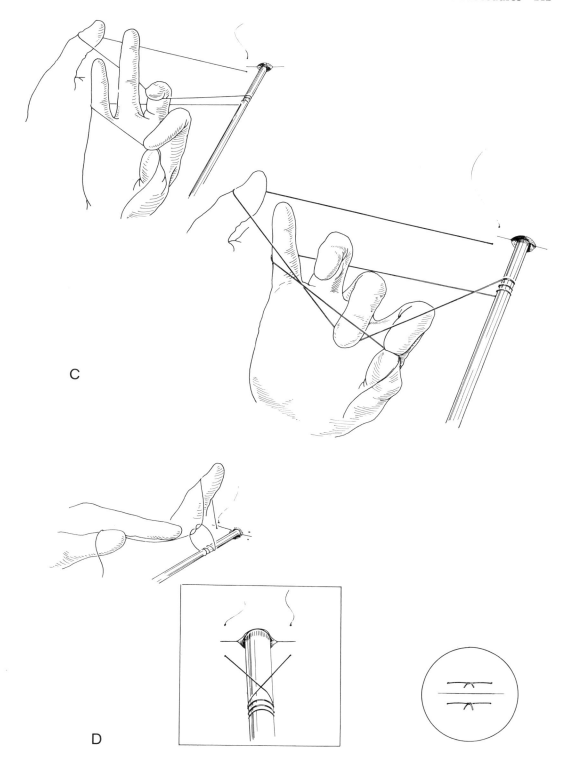

C

D

ated, followed by intermittent release so that reexpansion can be in a staged, slow fashion. Anoxia may have also damaged these capillary membranes, facilitating the development of pulmonary edema. This phenomenon occurs 2 to 3 hours post-thoracostomy (22, 46, 49, 58).

2. Injury to the lung. The thoracostomy can be placed into nonresilient lung fixed to the chest wall by pleural adhesions. This intrapulmonary insertion will cause a pneumothorax with persistent air leak and possibly hemoptysis (57). This complication is extremely common in neonates and has been reported as frequently as 25% in neonates with respiratory distress syndrome who require chest tubes (36). Laceration of the lung may result also from improper placement of the tube or the use of a trocar. This can be prevented by careful placement of the tube, using the technique outlined in this section.

3. Bleeding from the chest wall. This complication may result from laceration of an intercostal artery in placing a posterolateral chest tube or laceration of an internal mammary vessel in placing an anterior chest tube. This complication may be prevented by inserting the chest tube along the superior edge of the rib below the interspace being entered, to avoid the neurovascular bundle which courses under the ribs. With an anterior chest tube, one should not place the tube any more medial than the midclavicular line to avoid the internal mammary vessels.

4. Continuing air leak. This has been discussed above and one must check for holes in the tubing, loose connections, and chest tube holes being external to the pleural cavity. The problem of loose connections may be prevented by taping the connection of the tubing.

5. Occlusion of the chest tube. Occlusion of the chest tube may occur from a large clot or kinking of the chest tube. This can be prevented by inserting a sufficiently large chest tube when dealing with a hemothorax in the adult. Kinking of the tube may be prevented by inserting the chest tube at the midaxillary line rather than the posterior axillary line. In the latter position, the patient may kink the tube by lying on it.

6. Persistent pneumothorax. A persistent pneumothorax on repeat radiograph indicates that a large air leak is present, with failure of the lung to expand. The treatment of this is to increase suction and, if this does not provide relief of the pneumothorax, then consider placing a second chest tube (anteriorly or laterally). In patients with a large air leak and a persistent pneumothorax, the defect usually involves a large bronchus and surgical closure may be indicated.

7. Subcutaneous emphysema. This may result from continuing air leak into the subcutaneous space from a pneumothorax which is inadequately decompressed by the chest tube, resulting in leakage of air into the subcutaneous tissue. Another cause is that the skin may be too tightly sealed around the chest tube, resulting in air leakage into the subcutaneous tissue rather than through the skin incision. This is an unusual cause of this problem; however, when it occurs it can be treated by removing the suture closest to the chest tube at the incision site to permit venting of the subcutaneous tissue.

THORACENTESIS

Thoracentesis can be performed in the emergency center to drain a pleural effusion in a patient with respiratory compromise (51). In addition, a small pneumothorax may be drained by thoracentesis and observed for any recurrence.

Equipment

Iodinated skin prep with sterile sponges
Sterile towels
Local anesthetic
10 ml syringe
10 gauge 1½ inch needle

25 gauge ⅝ inch needle
Lidocaine 1% with epinephrine, 10 ml
22 gauge 2 inch needle
18 gauge 2 inch needle
3-way stopcock
Curved clamp
14 gauge Intracath
10 ml and 50 ml plastic syringe
Sterile intravenous tubing
Plasma vacuum bottle
Sterile dressings and 1 inch adhesive tape
Supplemental oxygen

Technique

Preparatory Steps

1. Position the patient. The position of the patient will vary, depending on whether one is performing thoracocentesis for the removal of air or fluid. For the removal of air the patient should be supine with the head elevated 30 degrees. For the removal of fluid, the patient should be sitting upright with the arms supported over a table next to the bedside.
2. Locate the effusion. Check the chest radiographs to ascertain the highest level of the effusion. In addition, percuss for dullness to find the level of the fluid.
3. Locate the site of insertion. When removing fluid by thoracentesis, one should aspirate at the angle of the rib posteriorly which is just lateral to the muscle mass of the erector spinal muscles. An alternate site is the posterior axillary line. The site of aspiration should be contingent on the location of the fluid level on the chest radiographs and confirmed by percussion. One should never perform thoracentesis lower than the eighth intercostal space without fluoroscopy. The ideal site for aspiration is the midscapular line at the sixth intercostal space (2). When thoracentesis is performed for the evacuation of air, the second interspace anteriorly in the midclavicular line should be used unless adhesions are present at this site (37).

4. Infiltrate a local anesthetic at the site selected using a 22 gauge, 2 inch needle. After this area is infiltrated, inject along the superior margin of the rub to avoid the intercostal neurovascular bundle. Pass the needle through the pleura and aspirate to confirm the presence of air or fluid. Mark the needle depth upon entering the pleura by attaching a curved clamp at the skin level and withdraw the needle.

Procedural Steps

1. Using a 14 gauge needle from a Bardic® Intracath with an 8 inch long catheter, one may begin the procedure. In children, a #15 Gelco® intravenous catheter may be used (56). Detach the needle from the catheter and connect a 3-way stopcock (not shown in the diagram) to the needle, followed by a 10 ml syringe. Using the clamped needle which was used for infiltrating the site of injection with anesthetic, measure the distance from the tip of the needle to the clamp and place the clamp on the needle of the 14 gauge Intracath at that same distance (Fig. 4.27). This marks the depth of the insertion of the needle and prevents insertion into lung tissue.
2. Insert the needle of the Intracath at the site anesthetized up to the level of the clamp as shown in Figure 4.27. Aspirate to confirm entrance into the pleural cavity and then introduce the 8 inch Intracath catheter through the needle, advancing it inferiorly toward the diaphragm (21).

CAUTION!

When removing the needle to insert the cannula, one must place a thumb over the hub of the needle to prevent a pneumothorax.

CAUTION!

Never move the catheter back through the needle. This may result in shearing of

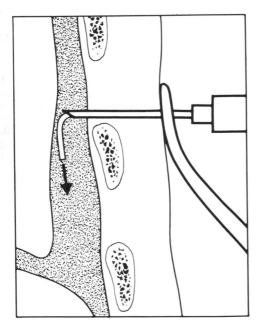

Figure 4.27. Thoracentesis. See text for discussion. Insert the needle of the Intercath® at the anesthetized site up to the level of the clamp. Once the pleural cavity is entered, introduce the 8 inch Intracath® directed inferiorly.

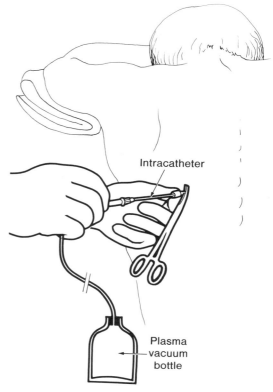

Intracatheter

Plasma vacuum bottle

Figure 4.28. Connect the intravenous tubing to the catheter and to a plasma vacuum bottle.

the catheter, and the catheter would have to be removed by a thoracotomy.

3. Connect the intravenous tubing to the catheter and to a plasma vacuum bottle as shown in Figure 4.28 (21). Alternately one may simply aspirate the fluid with a 50 ml syringe while covering the catheter orifice between aspirations.

Aftercare

1. Obtain a chest radiograph to ascertain the amount of fluid that has been evacuated. Send the fluid for specimens as desired. The fluid should be sent for cell count, Gram stain, culture, glucose, and cytology.
2. Remove the needle and the catheter as a *single unit*. Never remove the catheter separately through the needle as this may result in shearing off the catheter. Apply a sterile dressing over the site and obtain a chest radiograph to check for pneumothorax.

Complications

1. Pneumothorax (17, 27, 44, 54). This may result from laceration of the lung by the needle or from inadvertent entrance of air during removal of the syringe from the needle hub while advancing the cannula. This can be prevented by inserting the needle no farther than absolutely necessary as determined by the clamp technique noted earlier. When this complication does occur, if it is <20% pneumothorax, the patient may be observed; if it is >20%, drainage may be performed using the anterior thoracentesis procedure noted in this section or inserting a chest tube.
2. Laceration of an intercostal artery or vein. This may occur from insertion of the needle underneath the rib rather than just above the upper margin of the rib in the interspace se-

lected. When this complication occurs, a small hematoma may develop and can be treated symptomatically. If the injury results in a hemothorax greater than 300 ml, it should be drained with a closed thoracostomy.

3. Hypoxia. At 20 minutes and at 2 hours postthoracocentesis, hypoxia may be observed with an average decrease in PO_2 of 10 mm/Hg. The drop in PO_2 ranges from 10 to 16 mm of mercury (14). This hypoxemia is due to ventilation-perfusion abnormalities postthoracocentesis due to perfusion of atelectatic lung. The more fluid that is removed the worse the hypoxemia (14). All patients having thoracocentesis should have supplemental oxygen, particularly those with pulmonary compromise, such as patients with emphysema, chronic obstructive pulmonary disease (COPD), asthma, or carcinoma.

4. Pulmonary edema. Rapid removal of large volumes of fluid can result in pulmonary edema (14). Rapid reexpansion of the lung causes a rapid increase in the pulmonary capillary pressure and blood flow, resulting in transudation of fluid across the capillary membrane and leading to pulmonary edema.

5. Puncture of the liver or spleen. This results from placing the needle too deep (can be prevented by using the clamp technique as indicated above) or from placing the needle in an interspace below the eighth intercostal space posteriorly.

TRANSTHORACIC PACEMAKER INSERTION

A transthoracic pacemaker is indicated when a transvenous pacemaker cannot be inserted. This procedure is easy to perform and the incidence of successful capture is higher than when using transvenous pacemakers in the emergency setting without the guidance of fluoroscopy.

Indications

The indications are the same as for transvenous pacemakers.

Equipment

Elecath^R transthoracic pacemaker set. These sets are commercially available and contain all the equipment necessary to perform this procedure.
Prep solution
ECG machine
Local anesthetic
  1% Xylocaine® with epinephrine
10 ml syringe
18 gauge 1½ inch needle
22 gauge 2 inch needle.

Technique

Preparatory Steps

1. Prepare and drape the skin around the xyphoid process.
2. Keep the patient on an ECG monitor continuously throughout the procedure.
3. Infiltrate a local anesthetic to the left of the xyphoid process in the left costosternal angle.

Procedural Steps

1. Insert the 6 inch needle with the obturator in place in the left costosternal angle as indicated in Figure 4.29. After penetrating the skin, the needle should be directed toward the midclavicular line at an angle of 30 degrees to the skin. Alternately, the needle may be aimed at either the right or the left shoulders.
2. Remove the obturator from the needle to ascertain entrance into the cardiac chamber (Fig. 4.30). A brisk flow of

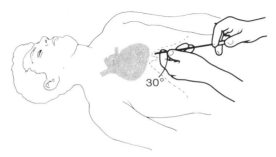

Figure 4.29. Passage of a transthoracic pacemaker. Insert the needle as shown above, directed toward the midclavicular line at an angle of 30 degrees to the skin.

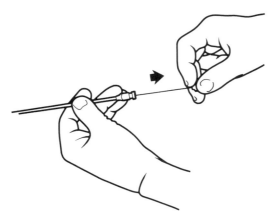

Figure 4.30. Remove the obturator from the needle to ascertain entrance into the cardiac chamber. A brisk flow of blood through the needle indicates the ventricle has been entered. When the procedure is being performed in a patient who has an asystole, aspiration intermittently performed during passage of the needle will indicate when the cardiac chamber has been entered.

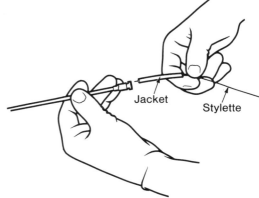

Figure 4.31. Pass a bipolar pacing stylette with a jacket around the J-shaped tip (to straighten the tip of the stylette to permit passage through the needle). The stylette should be passed through the needle until well within the cardiac chamber.

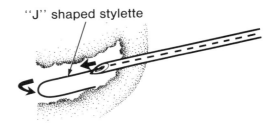

Figure 4.32. Pull the stylette back until its J-shaped tip enters the endocardial surface of the heart at which point a resistance is met to withdrawal of the stylette.

blood through the needle indicates the ventricle has been entered. When ventricular pressures are too low to produce this rapid flow, a syringe may be attached to the needle and aspiration of blood performed to ascertain entrance into the heart.

3. Pass a bipolar pacing stylette with a jacket around the J-shaped tip (to straighten the tip of the stylette to permit passage through the needle) (Fig. 4.31). The stylette should be passed through the needle until well within the cardiac chamber.

4. Withdraw the needle over the stylette.

5. Pull the stylette back until its J-shaped tip enters the endocardial surface of the heart, at which point resistence is met and prevents further withdrawal of the stylette (Fig. 4.32). The jacket shown in Figure 4.31 remains at the proximal end of the stylette and can be removed at this point.

6. Attach the stylette to the pacemaker unit via the connecting adaptor which is supplied in the set. The connecting adaptor has two leads extending from it, one marked *distal* which is secured to the *negative* pole and another marked *proximal* which is attached to the *positive* pole of the pacemaker generator.

7. Set the pacemaker at 1.5 to 2 ma and at a rate of 70 and check for capture. The level of the current may have to be elevated over 2 ma for capture to occur.

8. Once capture occurs, the stylette should be sutured to the chest wall and a sterile dressing applied.

Aftercare

1. The patient should be moved as little

as possible to prevent inadvertent removal of the stylette or perforation of the heart.

Complications

1. Injury to the coronary arteries. This complication is extremely common and can be prevented by using the fourth intercostal space as recommended by some authors. By using the technique described above and aiming the needle either at the midclavicular line or at the right shoulder, this problem generally can be avoided.
2. Pericardial hemorrhage and tamponade. This may result from puncture of a coronary vessel by the needle or from injury to the myocardium. There is very little, with the exception of exercising caution in performing the procedure, which one can do to prevent this complication.
3. Breakage of the stylette. This occurs from withdrawal of the stylette through the needle which should never be done, because it may shear this when placing an Intracath®. During CPR, external cardiac massage must be stopped or the stylette may break. One author (BB) has seen such a case in which the stylette was retrievable only by open thoracotomy.

References

1. Aslam, P.A., Insertion of apical chest tube. Surg., Gynecol. Obstet. 130:1097, 1970.
2. Baldwin, J.N., Fishman, N.H., A simplified method of thoracentesis. Surg. Gynecol. Obstet. 125:1321, 1967.
3. Batchelder, T.L., Morris, K.A., Critical factors in determining adequate pleural drainage in both the operated and non-operated chest. J. Trauma 8:176, 1972.
4. Beall, A.C., Bricker, A.L., Crawford, H.W., et al., Surgical management of penetrating thoracic trauma. Dis. Chest. 49:568, 1966.
5. Beall, A.C., Crawford, H.W., DeBakey, M.E., Considerations in the management of acute traumatic hemothorax. J. Thorac. Cardiovasc. Surg. 52:351, 1966.
6. Beall, A.C., Gasior, R.M., Bricker, D.L., Gunshot wounds of the heart: Changing patterns of surgical management. Ann. Thorac. Surg. 11:523, 1971.
7. Beall, A.C., Patrick, T.A., Okies, J.E., et al., Penetrating wounds of the heart: Changing patterns of surgical management. J. Trauma 12:468, 1972.
8. Beck, C.S., Further observations on stab wounds of the heart Ann. Surg. 115:698, 1942.
9. Bigger, I.A., Heart wounds. J. Thoracic Surg. 8:239, 1939.
10. Bishop, L.H., Estes, E.H., McIntosh, H.D., The electrocardiogram as a safeguard in pericardiocentesis. J.A.M.A. 162:264, 1956.
11. Bolanowski, P., Swaminathan, A.P., Neville, W., Aggressive surgical management of penetrating cardiac injuries. J. Thorac. Cardiovasc. Surg. 66:52, 1973.
12. Borja, A.R., Lansing, A., Randell, H., Immediate operative treatment for stab wounds of the heart. J. Thorac. Cardiovasc. Surg. 59:662, 1970.
13. Boyd, T.F., Strieder, J.W., Immediate surgery for traumatic heart disease. J. Thorac. Cardiovasc. Surg. 50:305, 1965.
14. Brandstetter, R.D., Cohen, R.P., Hypoxemia after thoracentesis: A predictable and treatable condition. J.A.M.A. 242:1060, 1979.
15. Breaux, E.P., Dupont, J.B., Albert, H.M., et al., Cardiac tamponade following penetrating mediastinal injuries: Improved survival with early pericardiocentesis. J. Trauma 19:461, 1979.
16. Callaham, M., Acute traumatic cardiac tamponade: Diagnosis and treatment. J.A.C.E.P. 7:306, 1978.
17. Cameron, G.R., Pulmonary edema. Br. Med. J. 1:965, 1948.
18. Carrasquilla, C., Wilson, R.F., Walt, A.J., et al., Gunshot wounds of the heart. Ann. Thorac. Surg. 13:208, 1972.
18a. Elerding, S., Aragon, G.E., Fatal hepatic hemorrhage after trauma. Am. J. Surg. 138:883, 1979.
19. Fry, W.A., Adams, W.E., Thoracic emergencies: Indications for closed tube drainage and early open thoracotomy. Arch. Surg. 94:532, 1966.
20. Griswold, R.A., Drye, J.C., Cardiac wounds. Ann. Surg. 139:783, 1954.
21. Griswold, R.A., Maquire, C.H., Penetrating wounds of the heart and pericardium. Surg. Gynecol. Obstet. 74:406, 1942.
22. Humphreys, R.L., Berne, A.S., Rapid reexpansion of pneumothorax: A cause of unilateral pulmonary edema. Radiology 96:509, 1970.
23. Isaacs, J.P., Sixty penetrating wounds of the heart: Clinical and experimental observations. Surgery 45:696, 1959.
24. Kerber, R.E., Ridges, J.D., Harrison, D.C., Electrocardiographic indications of atrial puncture during pericardiocentesis. N. Engl. J. Med. 282:1142, 1970.
25. Kilpatrick, Z.M., Chapman, C.B., On pericardiocentesis. Am. J. Cardiol. 16:722, 1965.
25a. Ledgerwood, A.M., Kazmers, M., The role of thoracic aortic occlusion for massive hemoperitoneum. J. Trauma 16:610, 1976.
25b. Levitsky, S., New insights in cardiac trauma. Surg. Clin. North Am. 55:43, 1975.
26. Lucido, J.L., Voorhees, R.J., Immediate thoracotomy for wounds of the heart. Am. J. Surg. 108:664, 1964.
27. Luisada, A.A., Cardi, L., Acute pulmonary edema: Pathology, physiology and clinical management. Circulation 13:113, 1956.

28. MacDonald, J.R., McDowell, R.M., Emergency department thoracotomies in a community hospital. J.A.C.E.P. 7:423, 1978.
29. Malonev, J.V., McDonald, L., Treatment of blunt trauma to the thorax. Am. J. Surg. 105:484, 1963.
30. Massumi, R.A., Rios, J.C., Ross, A.M., et al., Technique for insertion of an indwelling intrapericardial catheter. Br. Heart J. 30:333, 1968.
31. Mattox, K.L., Beall, A.C., Jordan, G.L., et al., Cardiorrhaphy in the emergency center. J. Thorac. Cardiovasc. Surg. 68:886, 1974.
32. Mattox, K.L., Espada, R., Beall, A.C., et al., Performing thoracotomy in the emergency center. J.A.C.E.P. 3:13, 1974.
33. Mattox, K.L., Von Koch, L., Beall, A.C., et al., Logistic and technical considerations in the treatment of the wounded heart. Circulation 51,52 (suppl. 1): 1, 1975.
34. Maynard, A.L., Avecilla, M.J., Naclerio, E.A., The management of wounds of the heart: A recent series of 43 cases with comment on pericardiocentesis in hemopericardium. Ann. Surg. 144:1018, 1956.
35. Maynard, A.L., Cordice, J.W.V., Naclerio, E.A., Penetrating wounds of the heart: A report of 81 cases. Surg., Gynecol. Obstet. 94:605, 1952.
36. Moessinger, A.C., Driscoll, J.M., Wigger, H.J., High incidence of lung perforation by chest tube in neonatal pneumothorax. J. Pediatr. 92:635, 1978.
37. Munnell, E.R., Thomas, E.K., Current concepts in thoracic drainage systems. Ann. Thorac. Surg. 19:261, 1975.
38. Neall, A.C., Bricker, D.L., Considerations in the management of penetrating thoracic trauma. J. Trauma 8:408, 1968.
39. Peddie, G.H., Creech, O., Halpert, B., Structural changes in the heart resulting from cardiac massage. Surgery 40:481, 1956.
40. Pomerantz, M., Hutchison, D., Traumatic wounds of the heart. J. Trauma 9:135, 1969.
41. Pories, W.J., Gaudiani, V.A., Cardiac tamponade. Surg. Clin. North Am. 55:573, 1975.
42. Ravitch, M.M., Blalock, A., Aspiration of blood from pericardium in treatment of acute cardiac tamponade after injury. Arch. Surg. 58:463, 1949.
43. Reul, G.J., Mattox, K.L., Beall, A.C., Jordan, G.L., Recent advances in the operative management of massive chest trauma. Ann. Thorac. Surg. 16:52, 1973.
44. Riesman, D., Albuminous expectoration following thoracentesis. Am. J. Med. Sci. 123:620, 1902.
45. Sankaran, S., Lucas, C., Walt, A.J., Thoracic aortic clamping for prophylaxis against sudden cardiac arrest during laparotomy for acute massive hemoperitoneum. J. Trauma 15:290, 1975.
46. Sautter, R.D., Dreher, W.H., MacIndoe, J.H., et al., Fatal pulmonary edema and pneumonitis after reexpansion of chronic pneumothorax. Chest 60:399, 1971.
47. Schaffer, A.I., Pericardiocentesis with the aid of a plastic catheter and ECG monitor. Am. J. Cardiol. 4:83, 1959.
48. Shoemaker, W.C., Algorithm for early recognition and management of cardiac tamponade. Crit. Care Med. 3:59, 1975.
49. Steckel, R.J., Unilateral pulmonary edema after pneumothorax. N. Engl. J. Med. 289:621, 1973.
50. Steichen, F.M., Dargan, E.L., A graded approach to the management of penetrating wounds of the heart. Arch. Surg. 103:574, 1971.
51. Stein, L., Shubin, H., Weil, M.H., Recognition and management of pericardial tamponade. J.A.M.A. 225:503, 1973.
52. Sugg, W.L., Rea, W.J., Ecker, R.R., et al., Penetrating wounds of the heart: An analysis of 459 cases. J. Thorac. Cardiovasc. Surg. 56:531, 1968.
53. Symbas, P.N., Harlaftis, N., Waldo, W.J., Penetrating cardiac wounds: A comparison of different therapeutic methods. Ann. Surg. 183:377, 1977.
54. Trapnell, D.H., Thurston, J.G.B., Unilateral pulmonary edema after pleural aspiration. Lancet 1:1367, 1970.
55. Trinkle, J.K., Marcas, J., Grover, F., et al., Management of the wounded heart. Ann. Thorac. Surg. 17:230, 1974.
56. van Heerden, J.A., Laufenberg, H.J., Simplified thoracentesis. Mayo Clin. Proc. 43:311, 1965.
57. Wilson, A.J., Kraus, H.F., Lung perforation during chest tube placement in the stiff lung syndrome. J. Pediatr. Surg. 9:213, 1974.
58. Ziskind, M.M., Weill, H., George, R.A., Acute pulmonary edema following the treatment of spontaneous pneumothorax with excessive negative intrapleural pressure. Am. Rev. Respir. Dis. 92:632, 1965.

Neurosurgical Procedures

5

BURR HOLES (12, 16, 21)

In a study involving 30,000 head injuries, conducted by Echlin et al. (12), it was found that the incidence of operable subdural hematoma was approximately 1% of all head injuries and about 5% of the severe cases. In addition, about 1% of the severely injured patients developed an epidural hemorrhage and another 1% developed an intracerebral blood clot (12).

Acute subdural hematoma may present with abnormal neurological signs. Although these signs are indicative of an organic lesion, they are frequently not of localizing value. In the series of 247 patients with subdural hematoma by Echlin et al. (12), 79 patients had the localizing signs correctly indicate the side of the hematoma; however, in 29 patients the signs were the result of lesions on the opposite side than predicted. In 139 patients in this series the neurological findings were inconclusive in determining the side of the lesion. Unilateral motor weakness was present in a large number of patients. Inequality in the size of the pupils was noted in 115 of the patients with subdural hematoma before operative intervention. The large pupil was on the side of the hematoma in 74 of these patients and on the opposite side in 41. In 30 patients there was a bilateral hematoma or a hematoma on one side and a laceration of the brain on the other side. Moreover, of 57 patients with a marked dilatation of one pupil, 36 demonstrated a hematoma on the same side, 9 had hematoma on the other side, and 12 had bilateral hematoma. These findings indicate that a fully dilated pupil is of some value in localization; however, a slight to moderate enlargement of one pupil is of no value.

An acute epidural hematoma is a true neurosurgical emergency. When a patient with the classical findings of an acute epidural hematoma presents to the community hospital emergency center, death often ensues rapidly when there is no emergency decompression (7). Craig states that the mortality rate due to epidural hematoma is 50%. This mortality rate has remained unchanged in spite of striking improvements in the mortality and morbidity rates of other cranial and cerebral injuries over the past several decades. Craig feels that the delay in treatment of an epidural hematoma is responsible for the continuing high mortality rate (7).

An epidural hematoma is formed between the dura and the skull. The source of the bleeding is usually the middle meningeal artery. After the artery courses through the foramen spinosum, it courses along the inner surface of the temporal bone. The main branch of this artery lies about 1 fingerbreadth anterior and superior to the external auditory meatus. This artery is usually torn by a linear fracture which passes through the temporal bone (Fig. 5.1). In many cases the fracture may not be seen on routine radiographs of the skull (7). Temporal muscle edema overlying the fracture is an almost constant clinical finding with middle meningeal artery bleeding. In some cases, although not all, a lucid interval is described and represents the period between recovery from concussion and lapse into coma due to increased

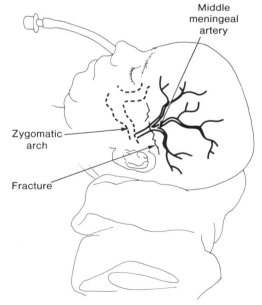

Figure 5.1. A fracture of the temporal bone and its relationship to the middle meningeal artery is shown. A burr hole placed in the temporal area just superior to the xygomatic arch will relieve the pressure of a hematoma.

intracranial pressure secondary to the acute epidural hematoma. The duration of the lucid interval depends on the rate of recovery from initial concussion and the rapidity of development of cerebral compression from the accumulating hematoma. At this time the patient may complain of severe headache on the side of the lesion. There also may be some nausea, vomiting, and lethargy. This is followed by a variable period after which there is rapid development of unconsciousness, dilatation of the ipsilateral pupil, and contralateral hemiplegia progressing to decerebrate rigidity (7). This development of unconsciousness is a terminal event, and unless immediate decompression is performed, changes in the brain will be irreversible and death will ensue. Such a patient should never be transported from a community hospital to a distant neurosurgical facility without first decompressing the extradural space.

Treatment of the Patient who has Severe Head Injury

A number of measures must be taken in the patient with severe head injury as described above. The stuporous patient should be kept on his side to prevent swallowing of the tongue and aspiration of secretions. The airway must be protected and oxygen should be administered. When necessary, endotracheal intubation should be performed (see Chapter 2: "Airway Procedures," for indication) or even tracheostomy. Shock is almost never secondary to the head injury until the terminal stage and should be presumed to be due to injury elsewhere in the body. Shock must be corrected to adequately treat the patient with severe head injury. The most important adjuncts to the treatment of the patient with a severe head injury are the correction of hypovolemia, maintenance of the airway, and adequate oxygenation. Also, every unconscious patient should be treated as if they had a fractured cervical spine until proven otherwise.

Patients who have sustained severe head injury and are suspected of having an intracranial hemorrhage may demonstrate signs of increased intracranial pressure. In addition to maintaining the airway and restricting fluids in these patients, a number of ancillary modalities which aid in decreasing intracranial pressure have been described. Hyperventilation has an effect on reducing PCO_2 which decreases cerebral blood flow markedly. A drop in PCO_2 from 40 to 30 mm of mercury decreases cerebral blood flow by one third. Hyperventilation has an onset of action almost immediately, making it the first choice in patients who are normotensive and who have increased intracranial pressure. Mannitol has been used to decrease intracranial pressure preoperatively in many patients. In some cases, mannitol may increase bleeding by decreasing brain size and releasing the tamponaded cerebral vessels (30). The onset of action of mannitol is 20 to 30 minutes and it reaches its peak effectiveness in 30 to 60 minutes. Steroids such as dexamethasone do not reach their peak effect in decreasing intracranial pressure for 12 to 24 hours. The use of steroids to decrease cerebral edema in head trauma is controversial (31). Table 5.1 compares the various agents used in decreasing intracranial pressure in patients with head injuries.

Indications

Unilateral neurological signs with deterioration despite usual therapy (hyperventilation, mannitol, and/or steroids).

Equipment

Smedberg hand drill
$7/64$ inch regular angle carbon bit or a chisel point bit
20 ml syringe
Anesthetic prep (usually not necessary)
1% Xylocaine^R with epinephrine, 1/100,000
10 ml syringe
25 gauge needle
18 gauge 1½ inch needle
Prep solution
Medicine cups
Iodinated prep
4 × 4 gauze
Single-edge recessed-blade shaver
#11 Bard-Parker blade
#16 or #18 cone ventricular needle

Table 5.1. Treatment of Increased Intracranial Pressure—Airway; Restrict Fluids*

Drug	Dose	Administration	Onset	Peak	Duration	Rebound	Effect on CBF	Mech. of Effect on CBF	Mech. of Red'n. on ICP
Mannitol (20%)	2–3 g/kg	Q4–6 hr IV	20–30 min	30–60 min	6 hr	+	incr	Vasodilation, decreased blood viscosity	Osmotic gradient
Urea (30%)	1–1.5 g/kg	Q4–6 hr IV	10 min	20–30 min	4–6 hr	++	incr	Vasodilation, decreased blood viscosity	Osmotic gradient
Decadron	0.2 mg/kg	Q6 hr IV	2–12 hr	12–24 hr		±	$\bar{0}$		Restore blood brain barrier (BBB)
Solumedrol	1 mg/kg	Q6 hr IV							
Glycerol	0.5–1.5 gr/kg	Q4–6 hr PO or IV	15–60 min			$\bar{0}$	decr		Osmotic gradient
Hyperventilation	Reduce PCO_2 from: a. 40 to 30 mm → ↓CBF by 1/3 b. 40 to 20 mm → ↓CBF by 1/2	Short periods				$\bar{0}$		Vasoconstriction, increased venous drainage	
Hypothermia	32°C or 90°F						decr	Vasoconstriction, increased blood viscosity	CBF effects
Other									

* CBF, cerebral blood flow; ICP, intracranial pressure.

4 curved hemostats
Drapes, mask, and gown
Frazier suction catheter
Self-retaining retractors

Technique

NOTE

It should be noted that a twist drill is good for the evacuation of a chronic (i.e., watery) subdural hematoma; however, it may be useless for evacuation of solid or semisolid clotted blood. This is true whether the hematoma is a subdural or a epidural hematoma. Such clots are too viscous for removal from such a small hole.

Preparatory Steps

Several types of drills are available for performing trephination within the emergency center. A burr hole may be placed in the underlying skull using either a standard drill or a drill bit with a chisel head (Fig. 5.2). Recently a new twist drill has been introduced for placing burr holes (Fig. 5.2).

1. The patient is placed in a supine position with the head of the bed elevated to 15 to 20 degrees.
2. The scalp then is shaved throughout, including the temporal areas.
3. The scalp is prepped with an iodinated solution.

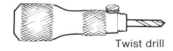

Twist drill

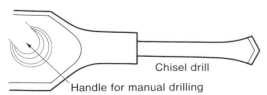

Chisel drill

Handle for manual drilling

Figure 5.2.   The twist drill and the chisel drill are shown. See text for discussion.

NOTE

The patient should be endotracheally intubated before the procedure is performed both to protect the airway should vomiting occur and for purposes of hyperventilating the patient. In addition, it is advisable that a nasogastric tube be inserted for decompression of the stomach and removal of gastric contents.

4. Drape the head of the patient with sterile towels and wear a mask and gown when performing this procedure.
5. Locate the sites of trephination. In cases of trauma in which an epidural hematoma is highly suspected, a temporal burr hole is generally placed. If this is unsuccessful in localizing a hematoma and in relieving elevated intracranial pressures, then an anterior and a posterior burr hole are placed on both sides of the midline as shown in Figure 5.3.

Temporal Burr Hole. A 3 cm vertical scalp incision is made and carried through the temporalis muscle to the bone. The most common site for placing a burr hole to drain an epidural hematoma is just above the root of the zygoma and one

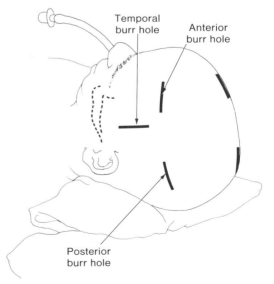

Temporal
burr hole   Anterior
burr hole

Posterior
burr hole

Figure 5.3.   The sites of incision and burr hole placement are noted. See text for discussion.

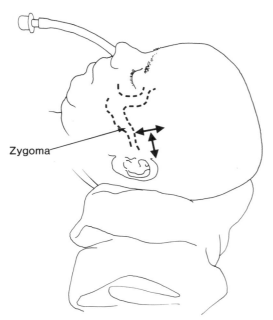

Figure 5.4. The temporal burr hole is placed just above the mid-point of the zygomatic arch and one fingerbreadth anterior to the external auditory canal.

fingerbreadth anterior to the external auditory canal (Fig. 5.4). When this successfully reduces intracranial pressure, the anterior and posterior holes are not necessary.

Anterior Burr Hole. The anterior burr hole is placed just in front of the coronal suture and 4 to 5 cm from the midline (Figure 5.3).

Posterior Burr Hole. The posterior or parietal burr hole is placed over the parietal boss approximately 7 to 8 cm from the midline (Fig. 5.3) (5, 6, 7, 27).

Procedural Steps

1. Using a #11 Bard-Parker blade, a small stab wound is made through the scalp and periosteum when using the twist drill. When using the standard drill, a linear incision is made as indicated in Figure 5.3. When a scalp bleeder is encountered, it can be treated by infiltrating anesthesia with epinephrine or by applying pressure. After the scalp incision has been made, a self-retaining retractor should be placed in the wound.

2. Twist drill. A ⁷⁄₆₄ inch regular angle carbon bit driven by a Smedberg hand-drill is used to perforate the skull. It is inserted through the scalp incision perpendicular to the skull. When beginning the drill hole, one must be careful not to permit the drill point to "walk" by applying the drill firmly to the skull and drilling slowly. The dura is generally found to be tightly adherent to the inner table. The handle design of the twist drill provides for maximum amount of control and force to be applied by alternately pronating and supinating the hand while the wrist is held in a neutral position. When the drill bit has penetrated the diploic space, the drill can be turned in a clockwise motion which will permit the bit to emerge through the inner table of the skull. This is usually felt as a definite endpoint by the physician.

Standard hand-held drill. The drill bit is introduced perpendicular to the skull through the site of incision (Fig. 5.5). The outer table is penetrated and the drill often catches in the diploë

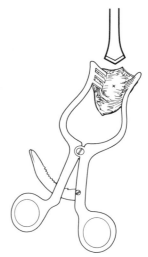

Figure 5.5. The standard hand-held drill introduced through an incision is shown. The drill is centered along the periosteal surface of the outer table.

between the inner and outer tables. The inner table is then penetrated.

3. Twist drill. After carefully passing through the inner table, but no further, the drill is removed and the bone dust is irrigated from the area. The dura is palpated then with a #16 or #18 cone ventricular needle. Following placement of the burr hole the physician has access to the epidural and subdural spaces. If a hematoma is obvious and the dura is not visible and one is certain that perforation of the dura has not taken place, then one is generally dealing with an epidural hematoma. Aspiration can be attempted; however, the hematoma usually is clotted, making aspiration difficult. In such a case the hole must be enlarged in the operating room with a rongeur to 4 cm and suction applied to remove the hematoma.

When dealing with a subdural hematoma, one can see the blue dura bulging through the burr hole. Ballot the hematoma with the cone needle, and, if fluctuant, incise the dura with a scalpel, #11 blade. Aspirate the hematoma with a suction catheter. When the pressure is relieved, the

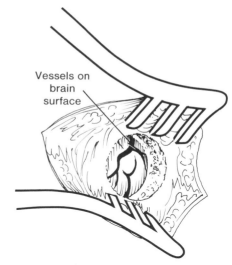

Figure 5.7. Once the pressure is relieved, swelling of the brain will cause the convolutions of the underlying cortex as well as overlying vessels to be visualized.

convolutions of the underlying brain may be visualized (Fig. 5.7). Aspiration of a chronic subdural hematoma which presents acutely to the emergency center is performed easily through a simple burr hole, and the hematoma can be removed by needle aspiration through either a twist drill hole or a standard drill burr hole. However, when an acute or subacute subdural hematoma is encountered, further surgical intervention may be warranted.

Standard hand-held drill. Once the epidural space is entered, a hematoma may be noted and should be suctioned (Fig. 5.6). After the clot is evacuated a bleeding point is searched for and, if found, is ligated or coagulated. When this is not possible the epidural space may be loosely packed, permitting some bleeding to the outside to continue decompression. In some cases in which the hematoma cannot be evacuated by this procedure, the hole may be enlarged with a rongeur in the operating room in a radial fashion to a diameter of approximately 4 cm, thus permitting evacuation.

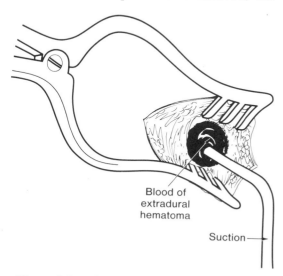

Figure 5.6. Once the extradural space is entered, a hematoma may be noted. The hematoma may be partially clotted or gelled or may be in liquid form. This should be suctioned.

4. A loose dressing is applied over the area and the patient then may be transported to a neurosurgical center.

NOTE

Brain decompression, while this is ideally performed in the operating room by a neurosurgeon, may have to be performed in the emergency center in a rapidly deteriorating patient. Where time is of the essence, burr or twist-drill holes offer access to the intracranial cavity and permit decompression by the removal of fluid contents as a prelude to formal surgery. Immediate decompression in these situations may prevent further irreversible neurological deterioration and may be lifesaving (5).

Complications

1. Penetration of the sagittal sinus. This complication has been reported to occur in use of the twist drill (27). One must be certain to stay several centimeters from the midline, as indicated above.
2. Broken twist drill point in the skull. This complication can be avoided by keeping the drill perpendicular to the skull and avoiding angulating the drill, which may cause breaking of the bit.
3. Subdural empyema. This complication can be avoided by maintaining sterile conditions. The physician should wear a mask and gown as with any major surgical procedure.
4. Superficial intracerebral hematoma mistaken for a subdural hematoma. This complication has been reported to occur in 3 cases in a large series (27).
5. False positive or false negative taps, A false positive or negative tap has been reported to occur with use of the twist-drill (5, 27). When one considers the total number of complications with use of this instrument, false negatives account for one third of all the complications seen in the series by Rand et al.
6. Laceration of an afferent middle me-

ningeal artery. One must be very careful to avoid penetration beyond the inner table. The authors recommend looking at the lateral radiograph of the skull and determining the location of the meningeal vessel by looking for the grooves in the skull x-ray. One should note the position of these grooves in relation to the external auditory meatus and avoid these grooves in performing the temporal burr hole.

LUMBAR PUNCTURE

Lumbar puncture is one of the most frequently performed procedures in the emergency center. The usual information obtained from examination of the spinal fluid is pressure reading, glucose, protein cell count and differential, Gram stain and culture. This information is important in establishing a diagnosis of meningitis and other inflammatory conditions affecting the brain and spinal canal. In addition, when performing a microscopic examination on the fluid, one should not only determine the number of lymphocytes, polymorphonuclear cells, and red blood cells, but a search should be made for abnormal cells such as fat-laden histiocytes indicative of acute brain damage, tumor cells, and leukemic cells. γ-Globulins and VDRL may be measured directly in the cerebral spinal fluid (CSF). Individual antibodies such as CSF measles titer also can be ascertained. Immunofluorescent techniques now are available and aid in the identification of cells coated by antigen in *Herpes simplex* encephalitis and in *Hemophilus influenzae* meningoencephalitis. Antigens to bacteria in CSF can be demonstrated rapidly by counterimmunoelectrophoresis diagnosing partially treated bacterial meningitis.

When a spontaneous subarachnoid hemorrhage is suspected, a lumbar puncture may be performed to confirm the diagnosis. In this situation the most experienced physician available should do the lumbar puncture. A number of situations have occurred in which many questions could have been avoided if it were not for a traumatic lumbar puncture.

Indications

1. Diagnostic lumbar puncture is performed in patients with suspected meningitis or encephalitis, such as fever and acutely altered mental status.
2. Inflammatory conditions involving the brain and leptomeninges such as abscesses.
3. Diagnosis of metastatic carcinoma, leukemia, or demyelinating conditions affecting the brain or leptomeninges.
4. Diagnosis of subarachnoid hemorrhage.
5. Relief of intracranial hypertension, e.g., pseudotumor cerebri.

Contraindications

1. Signs of increased intracranial pressure. With the advent of computerized axial tomography (CAT) the indications for lumbar puncture in patients with suspected intracranial mass lesions has decreased markedly. When the suspicion is high, a CAT scan should be obtained before performing lumbar puncture. With intracranial mass lesions, it is rare that a lumbar puncture will give enough information to justify the risk (25).

   There is a significant amount of controversy surrounding the issue of lumbar puncture in patients with intracranial mass lesions. In one series reported by Lubic and Marotta (20) of 401 patients with histologically verified brain tumors in whom lumbar puncture was performed, it was found that only 1 patient showed evidence indicating an untoward effect of the lumbar puncture. Papilledema and increased CSF pressure were present in 32% of the patients. Mass lesions were located in the temporal lobe in 14% of the patients and in the posterior fossa in 18.5%. Even with this extraordinarily low complication rate, Lubic and Marotta emphasized that the procedure should not be performed routinely on such patients (20). In a study involving 30 patients with raised intracranial pressure, Duffy (11) showed that their condition worsened after lumbar puncture was performed. In half the cases, deterioration occurred immediately and was dramatic; in the other half, it occurred within 12 hours following lumbar puncture. The overall mortality rate in Duffy's series was 40%.

   A history of progressively increasing headache associated with mental status changes *and* the development of localizing neurological signs is highly suggestive of increased intracranial pressure due to a mass lesion (11).

   In a study by Korein et al. (17) involving 129 patients with increased cerebrospinal fluid pressure in which 70 of the patients had papilledema while 59 did not, it was found that the incidence of complications following lumbar puncture was significantly higher in the group without papilledema. From their extensive review of the literature, they state that the actual complication rate of lumbar puncture in the presence of papilledema is less than 1.2%. They further state that careful lumbar puncture in the diagnosis and management of patients with papilledema is of definite value and may prevent unnecessary surgical intervention. This is no longer relevant in the days of CAT scanning.

   The authors feel that when the following are present, a lumbar puncture should not be performed before evaluation for signs of increased intracranial pressure which may include a CAT scan:

   a. History of progressively increasing headache.
   b. Presence of localizing neurological signs or symptoms.
   c. History of progressive deterioration in mental status.
   d. Presence of papilledema.
   e. History or physical examination suggesting frontal sinusitis or otitis media.

2. In patients with coagulation defects or with anticoagulant therapy, lumbar puncture is generally contraindicated. While careful lumbar puncture

seldom induces complications in these patients, Edelson et al. (13) have described 8 patients with thrombocytopenia (25) in whom a lumbar subdural hematoma developed following lumbar puncture. When lumbar puncture is indicated in such patients, it must be done with extreme care with a small gauge needle and by an experienced physician. All reported patients with spinal epidural hematomas (a rare complication of lumbar puncture) were receiving anticoagulant therapy before performance of the procedure (18). Thus, patients with thrombocytopenia, leukemia, hemophilia, or advanced liver disease and those receiving anticoagulant therapy pose a significant danger with regard to intraspinal bleeding with this procedure (23).

3. Cutaneous infection at the site of puncture.

Equipment

Standard lumbar puncture kits are available for performing lumbar puncture in both children and adults. These kits contain all of the material needed.

Local anesthetic
25 gauge ⅝ inch, 22 gauge 1½ inch needles
3 ml syringe
1% lidocaine with epinephrine 1/100,000, 10 ml
Skin prep
Iodinated solution
4 × 4 sponges
Sterile towels and barrier
Spinal needles with stylette

NOTE

While a number of authors have used 18 and 20 gauge spinal needles in performing this procedure, we advocate the use of the smallest needle possible. In the adult the commonly used needle is a 20 or 22 gauge 3 inch spinal needle with a stylette. The authors advocate the use of a 25 gauge 2½ inch needle for performing this procedure. This needle has been found to reduce

greatly the incidence of headache following lumbar puncture (35). A common fallacy is that a 25 gauge needle is more prone to breakage than is a 20 or 22 gauge needle. In a study by Dessloch (10) it was found that the breakage rate of a 20 or 22 gauge needle was higher than that of a 24 or 25 gauge needle. The advantages of a 25 gauge needle are as follows (35):

1. Loss of spinal fluid is negligible.
2. There is a small puncture hole in the dura and skin, providing for a smaller portal of entry.
3. Headache following lumbar puncture is decreased markedly.
4. Needle breakage is less than with a larger size needle.
5. Needle insertion is both rapid and relatively painless to the patient. In the child, a 25 gauge needle also is used.

3-way stopcock
Manometer
4 specimen collection tubes
Band-Aid[R]
Sterile sponges

Technique
Preparatory Steps

1. Position the patient. Place the patient in a lateral decubitus position with the back flexed maximally. Unless the lumbar spinous processes are "separated" by spinal flexion and the patient's back is positioned perpendicular to the examining table, the chances of painfully snagging the periosteum or a nerve root as well as an unsuccessful attempt are increased (25). The following position should be used (Fig. 5.8):
   a. The back should be at the edge of the table with the knees and hips flexed maximally.
   b. Place a small pillow under the head of the patient.
   c. Check the shoulders and the pelvis to be certain they are *perpendicular* to the examining table.
Alternate position. In patients who have scoliosis or ankylosing spondylitis or those who are very obese, the

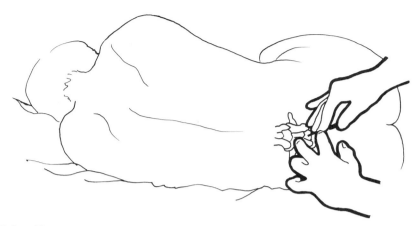

Figure 5.8. The position in which to place a patient for performing a lumbar puncture. The back should be at the edge of the table with the knees, hips, and neck flexed maximally. Place a small pillow under the head of the patient. The shoulders and the pelvis should be perpendicular to the examining table. The needle then is introduced in the midline with the bevel directed in the horizontal plane.

midline may be difficult to localize in the position indicated above. In these patients the midline is more accurately found by placing the patient in the sitting position at the edge of the table with his head and arms leaning over a pillow on a bedside stand. Once the midline of the spinal column is localized, the patient should be changed to the position indicated above.

2. Localize the site for needle insertion. The site for needle puncture is in the L4-L5 or L5-S1 interspace. Palpate the posterior aspect of the iliac crest bilaterally and draw an imaginary line connecting the two. The spinous process of L4 is at the level of the iliac crest and such a line traverses this point. The optimal site of needle puncture is in the midline in the L4-L5 interspace. Alternately, the L5-S1 interspace or the L3-L4 interspace can be used.

3. Prep the patient's back, beginning at the site of needle puncture and working outward in the routine fashion, with iodinated solution and drape the area at the puncture site.

4. Locally infiltrate 1% Xylocaine^R with epinephrine into the skin and subcutaneous tissue with a 25 gauge needle.

A 22 gauge needle can be used to infiltrate the interspinous region which is between the spinous process of the areas selected.

Procedural Steps

1. Insert the needle in the midline with the bevel directed in the horizontal plane (parallel to the axis of the spine). Accurate puncture requires keeping the needle point in the midline during advancement. Patients often can aid in this procedure by reporting whether or not the needle is going to the left or to the right as this can be felt by the patient (25). Hold the needle as shown in Figure 5.8 and advance it through the interspinous ligament, directing it at an angle of approximately 10 degrees cephalad and toward the umbilicus. A "pop" may be noted as the needle passes through the ligamentum flavum.

Once the subarachnoid space is approached, there is a real danger that one will advance the needle too far rather than not deep enough. The sharp needles contained in disposable lumbar puncture sets reduce the dural "pop" markedly. Thus, as the physician advances the needle beyond this point the stylette must be removed every 1 to 2 mm to avoid going through the subarachnoid space and penetrating the ventral epidural space, which is richly endowed by a venous plexus and is responsible for most traumatic lumbar puncture (25). A second "pop" may be felt as the needle advances through the dura mater and into the subarachnoid space. If this second "pop" is felt, remove the stylette and check for CSF immediately as one is almost certain to be in the subarachnoid space at this point.

NOTE

Once the spinal needle is engaged in the interspinous ligament, a technique described by Livingston (19) aids in determining when the subarachnoid space has been entered. The stylette is removed and a drop of fluid is placed in the adaptor of the needle once the needle is in the interspinous ligament. As the tip of the needle is advanced it displaces the dura, thus creating a negative pressure in the extradural space which "sucks" the drop inward. This is a maneuver which is often used by anesthesiologists in guiding them with placement of epidural anesthesia in the proper space. Since overpenetration can be a significant problem in lumbar punctures and has a risk of nerve root impingement and pain as well as inducing a traumatic tap, this procedure is indicated whenever one is involved with a case which may be difficult.

Traumatic Tap vs. Intracranial Bleed. It may be difficult to interpret the meaning of a bloody tap in some patients. One must distinguish between intrinsic bleeding and that caused by trauma of the lumbar puncture. If bloody fluid is obtained, the examiner should note closely if it clears as more fluid is withdrawn. In addition, cell counts should be obtained in the first and the last tubes of fluid to aid in determining and quantifying this value. In addition, the supernatant of the centrifuged sample of fluid should be examined. The supernatant should be crystal clear when red cells are

present for less than 2 hours, and the red cell count should be decreased from the first to the last tube if the lumbar puncture is traumatic. One must remember when looking at the supernatant that nonhemorrhagic fluid can be mildly to moderately xanthrochromic when the patient is deeply jaundiced or if the CSF protein is greater than 150 mg/100 ml (34). Tourtellotte et al. (32) observed that if a traumatic tap contains more than 12,000 red cells/cc, the oxyhemoglobin will stain the fluid within half an hour after puncture. In most patients the absence of xanthochromia and a declining cell count are the two most reliable criteria for determining if a lumbar puncture is traumatic.

When bone is encountered during advancement of the needle, it should be withdrawn to the subcutaneous tissue and the angle changed. Puncturing bone is usually due to directing the needle away from the midline during advancement.

2. Once the subarachnoid sac is punctured, a manometer is applied to the needle after the stylette is removed, and the patient is asked to straighten his legs and neck and relax to decrease intraabdominal pressure (19, 25).

NOTE

Forced deep breathing is contraindicated as this results in hypocapnea and induces a falsely low CSF pressure reading due to cerebral vasoconstriction. Lundberg (8) has found that increased cerebral intraventricular pressure may drop to normal within 1 minute after introduction of a spinal needle before withdrawal of fluid. Thus, one should not wait more than a minute before checking the pressure of the fluid in the canal.

3. Attach the manometer and 3-way stopcock to the needle after CSF is noted at the hub (Fig. 5.9). The zero point in measuring the CSF pressure is the needle itself. The normal range of CSF pressure is 70 to 180 mm of water.

4. Collect 4 samples of CSF (Fig. 5.10).

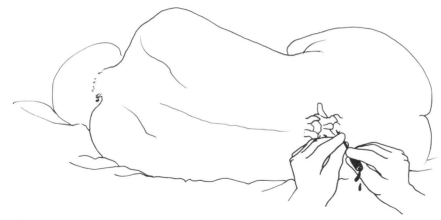

Figure 5.9. Once cerebrospinal fluid is noted at the hub of the needle, a manometer and 3-way stopcock are attached.

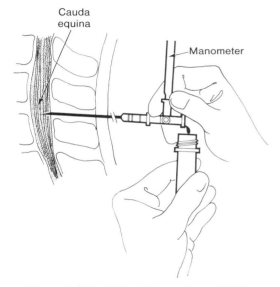

Cauda equina

Manometer

Figure 5.10. Collect 4 samples of CSF.

In the first tube, place 1 to 2 ml which is used for Gram stain and culture and sensitivity. In the second tube, collect 0.5 to 1 ml of fluid which is used for glucose and protein determination. A third tube is sent for antibodies, antigens, or cytology as indicated. In the fourth tube, 1 ml of fluid is collected which is used for cell count.

NOTE

If the flow rate decreases while collecting samples, rotate the needle 180 degrees as this decrease may be due to a nerve root which is impinging on the orifice of the needle.

5. Remove the needle after reinserting the stylette. The stylette should be reinserted before withdrawal of the needle as this will protect the patient from nerve root herniation (33). Rapid withdrawal of a spinal needle may initiate enough suction to herniate a spinal nerve root and adjacent arachnoid and fix them into the epidural space (33).

Aftercare

1. Apply a Band-Aid^R over the puncture site.
2. The patient should be instructed to lie in the *prone* position for several hours. In a large study by Brocker (2) 894 patients were placed on their abdomens for 3 hours before ambulation after lumbar puncture was performed in the routine position. Only 4 patients developed post-lumbar puncture headache, or an incidence of less than 0.5%. In a control group of 200 patients in whom lumbar puncture was performed using the same

size needle in the decubitus position but who were placed in the supine position for a period of 3 hours, the incidence of post-lumbar-puncture headache was 36.5%. It is believed that the dural, arachnoid, and ligamentum flavum holes are "staggered" during extension of the spine while in the prone position, thereby decreasing cerebrospinal fluid leak and decreasing post-lumbar-puncture headache (2).

Complications

1. Post-lumbar-puncture headache. Spinal headaches cause significant discomfort to the patient. The incidence of lumbar puncture headaches in the literature is approximately 41% (2). The size of the tear left in the dura is the most important factor in the production of these headaches, and one should be careful to produce only one hole and to use the smallest possible needle (2, 25, 35). Post-spinodural arachnoid *rents* can occasionally persist for months, with accompanying leakage of CSF and persisting headaches (3). Two key points with regard to preventing lumbar puncture headaches deserve reemphasis here:
   a. A small 25 gauge needle should be used (35).
   b. The patient should be placed in the prone position for a period of *3 hours* following the procedure.
2. Intraspinal epidermoid tumors (1). Intraspinal epidermoid tumors may be induced by lumbar punctures performed with needles without a stylette or with an ill-fitting stylette. This results from the implantation of epidermal fragments into the spinal canal. The most common symptoms are pain in the back or lower extremities, which may appear months later in these patients. Myelography should be considered in every patient who has pain in the lower extremities or back and who has had a previous lumbar puncture (1).

3. Spinal subdural hematoma (13). This complication has been reported in patients with thrombocytopenia in whom lumbar puncture was performed. The symptoms of a spinal subdural hematoma in some patients are weakness and sensory loss in the lower extremities. Some patients may have bladder dysfunction. Removal of large volumes of CSF in an elderly patient also may cause a subdural hematoma, due to avulsion of a perforating vein. One can prevent this problem by avoiding the procedure in patients with thrombocytopenia and in those who are on anticoagulants or who have coagulopathies. When performing the procedure in the elderly, remove the fluid slowly and in small volumes.
4. Spinal epidural hematoma. This is a rare complication of lumbar puncture (9, 29). All reported patients were receiving anticoagulant therapy or had severe hepatic dysfunction. The complication is usually due to laceration of the ventral epidural venous plexus. Such bleeding may result in paraplegia (23). Needle aspiration of the clot or laminectomy may or may not be beneficial in these patients. One can avoid this complication by avoiding deep penetration of the needle during lumbar puncture and maintaining the needle in the midline during advancement, as lateral displacement also will cause injury to the venous plexus anteriorly. When performing lumbar puncture on a patient who has a blood dyscrasia or who is on anticoagulants, one should place a drop of sterile saline at the hub of the needle after penetrating the interspinous ligament to aid in determining when the extradural space is penetrated, as indicated above in the section on technique. This procedure will aid in avoiding deep penetration in such patients.
5. Herniation of the spinal cord. This complication is due to the removal of CSF from below the foramen

magnum in patients in whom there is a site of neural impaction and increased CSF pressure proximally, resulting in a pressure gradient and herniation. Lumbar puncture distal to an intraspinal mass should not be performed.

6. Exacerbation of peripheral neurological symptoms secondary to an intraspinal tumor. Following removal of CSF distal to a complete intraspinal block (usually due to a tumor), the patient may experience exacerbation of symptoms secondary to a tumor or to herniation of the spinal cord. Small volumes of CSF should be removed slowly.

7. Dry tap. This is most commonly due to lateral displacement of the tip of the needle. One should keep the needle in the midline during advancement, as indicated above, to avoid this problem.

8. Transient sixth nerve palsy. This is due to the removal of large volumes of CSF, resulting in traction on the sixth cranial nerve. Cerebrospinal fluid should be removed slowly and in only those quantities which are needed.

9. Injury to the annulus fibrosus or rupture of the nucleus pulposus. This is due to excessively deep penetration of the spinal needle, resulting in injury to the intervertebral disc. One should avoid further advancement of the needle when it is obvious that it has gone beyond the subarachnoid space.

10. Infection. Epidural or subdural empyema has occurred following lumbar puncture. Meningitis also has been reported. Introduction of organisms into the epidural, subdural, or subarachnoid space from a contaminated needle is the cause. This may be due to inadequate skin prep or to puncture placed in the presence of focal skin infection. One must avoid puncturing skin which is infected, macerated or involved in any skin disease. In addition, strict aseptic technique must be followed.

11. Subarachnoid hematoma. Hematomas can occur in the epidural, subdural, or subarachnoid spaces or within the spinal cord following lumbar puncture. Bleeding within the spinal subarachnoid space usually produces a clinical syndrome characterized by the sudden onset of intense back pain followed by neck stiffness and headache (26). A subarachnoid hematoma following a lumbar puncture can cause compression of the cauda equina, resulting in neurological deficits to the legs, urinary bladder and anus. When such a deficit is encountered, particularly in a patient who was previously on anticoagulants, one should suspect this complication. This is a rare complication (28).

12. Stylette injury syndrome. A stylette must be inserted before withdrawing a spinal puncture needle to avoid aspiration of the lumbar nerve root and adjacent arachnoid tissue, thus fixing the nerve in the epidural space. This syndrome is characterized by pain which requires laminectomy and replacement of the nerve root within the subarachnoid space (33).

Lumbar Puncture in the Neonate

The performance of a lumbar puncture in the young infant and neonate is often difficult. Greensher and Mofensen (15) have introduced a simplified technique for performing lumbar punctures in the neonate. The puncture is performed using a butterfly needle—21 gauge produced by Abbott Laboratories. This needle has a 20 gauge bore, is thin-walled and has a plastic tubing which is approximately 30 cm long attached to its end. The dead space volume of the tubing is 0.25 ml. One of the problems routinely encountered in performing punctures on neonates is that fluid is lost and the pressure is difficult to obtain because the infant is squirming and difficult to handle. The needle is inserted in the third, fourth, or fifth lumbar interspace and is advanced into the spinal canal in the routine manner. When spinal fluid flows into the plastic tubing, the tube is elevated and a pressure measurement is taken, as shown in Figure 5.11. Following this, the plastic tubing is lowered and samples are collected in collecting tubes. The advantages of this technique are that it is simple and the spinal fluid is easily visualized through the tube. If the tap becomes traumatic, then the needle can be removed before contamination of previously collected specimens. In a study by Naidoo (24) involving 136 newborn infants, no complications were found in using this type of needle without a stylette. The discomfort of lumbar puncture should not be minimized as the stimulation may cause tonic fits in the asphyxiated newborn or even vagal cardiac arrest in children with cardiopulmonary disease (4). The child should be held firmly but not tightly flexed as this can embarrass respiration and cause restriction in venous return from the head.

SKELETAL TRACTION FOR CERVICAL SPINE DISLOCATIONS AND FRACTURES

Immediate treatment in the emergency center may be indicated for patients who present with severe dislocations of the cervical spine without evidence of spinal cord compression. The need for treatment depends largely on the degree of displacement. Fractures and dislocations of the cervical spine requiring tongs within the emergency center are those which are accompanied by neurological compromise on initial evaluation or those in which minimal motion of the cervical spine produces paresthesias. Those fractures and dislocations which are so unstable as to make movement of the patient dangerous also should be placed in tongs before moving the patient. Collars and braces are often of no value in treating these patients as immobilization of the cervical spine is not achieved (8). Crutchfield first introduced the Crutchfield tongs which were inserted into the calvarium and provided traction for patients with cervical spine fractures and dislocations (8). Since then a number of devices have been introduced

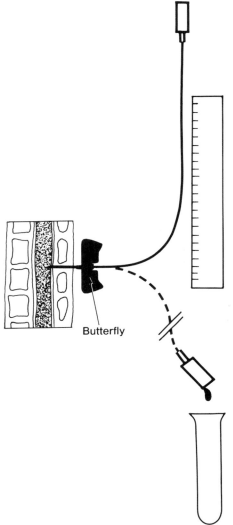

Butterfly

Figure 5.11.   Lumbar puncture in the neonate. The needle is inserted in the third, fourth, or fifth lumbar interspace. A 21 gauge butterfly is excellent for performing this procedure in the neonate. The butterfly is introduced into the spinal canal and once fluid is noted to be advancing into the catheter tubing of the butterfly, the catheter is lifted vertically and the pressure is measured with a standard centimeter ruler. After the pressure is measured, the samples are then taken.

on the market including the Gardner tongs, the Heifetz tongs, Vinke tongs, and Blackburn tongs. Two of these devices (which, in the authors' opinions, represent the best ones on the market) are described here. Both devices can be applied in the emergency center with very little difficulty.

Gardner Tong (14)

This tong consists of a rigid member which follows the coronal contour of the calvarium. A threaded hole which accommodates a screw for the advancement of the cone-shaped points is retractable by an enclosed spring which is calibrated to indicate when a squeeze pressure of 30 pounds is reached. The instrument is designed for emergency bedside application under antiseptic rather than aseptic conditions. This makes its utility in the emergency center excellent, and it is the tong most commonly applied in the emergency center at UCLA Hospital.

Technique of Application

Hair should be shaved around the site where the tong is to be applied. This will decrease the chance of osteomyelitis of the skull. The scalp is then prepped with an antiseptic solution. One percent Xylo-caine[R] is injected at the sites where the points of the tongs will be applied. The points of the tong are inserted above the ears and below the "equator" (Fig. 5.12). Flexion and extension of the head is obtained by adjusting the height of the pulley. The tapered points are advanced into the skin. Since the points are directed upward, as they advance, the skin is stretched increasingly snugly about them. This seals the point of entry and prevents bleeding. When bone is encountered, the stiff spring yields until the posterior end of the spring-loaded point just protrudes out of the casing. This indicates that the spring is fully compressed and is exerting 30 pounds of squeeze between the points. The tong then is tilted back and forth to insure proper seating, after which it is retightened if the posterior end of the spring-loaded point has recessed. The total excursion of the spring is approximately 5 mm, thus avoiding the possibility of penetrating too deeply and resultant pressure atrophy. The points of the tong, when applied properly, rarely pull out because of their

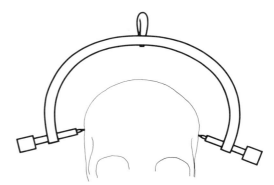

Figure 5.12. The Gardner tong. This tong consists of a rigid member and two cone-shaped points. See text for discussion.

angle. The points should be just below the temporal ridges. The tong will tolerate easily a traction of 65 pounds, if necessary. In the first 24 hours, the points will have to be tightened. With the patient supine, rotation of the head is prevented by placing a sandbag under each projecting end of the points. This is especially important when dealing with fractures of the odontoid.

Heifetz Tong

The Heifetz tong has the advantage of being able to maintain constant position of the patient's head and neck in flexion or extension when dealing with fractures or dislocations of the cervical spine. The Gardner tongs and other tongs available will permit flexion, extension or "swivel" of the skull within the tongs. The Heifetz tongs can be applied without the use of drills or incisions. The device consists of a rigid stainless steel arc with 3 self-drilling bolt drills providing for skull fixation (Fig. 5.13). The three-pronged principle avoids the tendency of swivel which occurs in other tongs. The traction device literally becomes an integral part of the patient's head. The physician is able to drill into the skull with simple hand rotation of the bolt drill, similar to the technique used with the Gardner tongs. The depth of penetration of the bolt is easily determined because there are 2 mm increment markings on the side of the bolt drill.

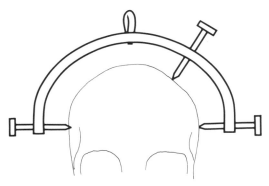

Figure 5.13.   The Heifetz tong. This tong consists of a rigid stainless steel arc with 3 self-drilling bolt drills providing firm fixation of the skull. See text for discussion.

Technique of Application

The site of penetration is along the lateral aspect of the calvarium. The optimal angle of insertion is perpendicular to the plane of traction desired. The area of insertion along the scalp is cleansed and prepped and a local anesthetic is injected. The arc containing the three bolt drills is then placed in position along the parietal fossa. The bitemporal bolt drills are then advanced into the scalp until they firmly impinge upon the skull. At this point the millimeter markings on the bolts are noted. The temporal bolt drills then are advanced into the skull alternately using the following technique: One bolt drill is advanced by turning it clockwise three complete revolutions. This bolt drill then is retreated by unscrewing it two complete revolutions. The opposite bolt drill then is advanced three turns and is retreated two turns. Using this maneuver of alternately advancing and then retracting the temporal bolt drills, one continues until each drill has penetrated the outer table by 2 to 3 mm as determined by notches on the drill. When insertion is complete, the bolt is rotated so that the flat edge of the bolt is facing the patient's feet. The locked bolt at the end of the arc then is tightened (Fig. 5.13) to maintain the temporal bolts in their position. The parietal bolt is then tightened and traction is applied.

SUBDURAL ASPIRATION

Subdural aspiration may be necessary in the infant for diagnostic purposes. The procedure is indicated when a subdural hematoma is suspected in an infant. The procedure is safe as long as the physician remains away from the midline, thus avoiding the sagittal sinus. The procedure should be performed bilaterally even when one side is positive, as a bilateral subdural hematoma is often present in these patients. The physician must remember that a negative subdural tap does not rule out the presence of a subdural hematoma.

Technique (Fig. 5.14)

1. Restrain the child and have an assistant immobilize the head. The child's head should be placed at the edge of the examining table.
2. Shave the top of the scalp over the region of the fontanelle.
3. Prep the scalp with an iodinated solution and drape the area of the fontanelle.
4. Locate the point of puncture. The point of puncture is in the anterior fontanelle at the junction of the coronal suture with the fontanelle. This point must be 3 cm lateral to the midline to avoid the sagittal sinus.
5. Anesthetize the area of puncture with a 25 gauge needle and 1% Xylocaine[R] with epinephrine.
6. Insert a 20 gauge spinal needle at the point selected. Direct the needle laterally after it has penetrated the skin.

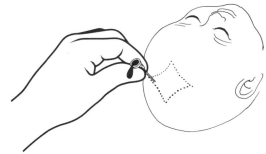

Figure 5.14.   Subdural aspiration in the infant. See text for discussion.

A "pop" will be felt as the subdural space is entered. In addition there is a decrease in resistance to advancement of the needle when the space is entered.

7. The stylette should then be removed from the spinal needle and fluid permitted to drip from the needle on its own. A syringe never should be attached and the fluid aspirated. If a subdural hematoma is present, it will appear usually as a brown or pale yellow color.

8. Remove the needle and apply pressure at the puncture site. Apply a sterile dressing to the scalp.

References

1. Batnitzky, S., Keucher, T.R., Mealey, J., et al., Iatrogenic intraspinal epidermoid tumors. J.A.M.A. 237:148, 1977.
2. Brocker, R.J., Technique to avoid spinal tap headache. J.A.M.A. 168:261, 1958.
3. Brown, B.A., Jones, O.W., Jr., Prolonged headache following spinal puncture: Response to surgical treatment. J. Neurosurg. 19:349, 1962.
4. Brown, J.K., Lumbar puncture and its hazards. Dev. Med. Child Neurol. 18:803, 1976.
5. Burton, C., Blacker, H.M., A compact hand drill for emergency brain decompression. J. Trauma 5:643, 1965.
6. Caldwell, R.B., Epidural hematoma: A true emergency. J.A.C.E.P. 4:49, 1975.
7. Craig, T.V., Hunt, W.E., Emergency care of extradural hematoma. J.A.M.A. 171:405, 1959.
8. Crutchfield, W.G., Skeletal traction for dislocation of the cervical spine. South. Surg. 2:156, 1933.
9. DeAngelis, J., Hazards of subdural and epidural anesthesia during anticoagulant therapy: A case report and review. Anesth. Analg. 51:676, 1972.
10. Dessloch, J.C., Problem of broken needles in spinal anesthesia: A survey. Anesth. Analg. 18:353, 1939.
11. Duffy, G.P., Lumbar puncture in the presence of a raised intracranial pressure. Br. Med. J. 1:407, 1969.
12. Echlin, F.A., Sordillo, S.V.R., Garvey, T.Q., Jr. Acute, subacute and chronic subdural hematoma. J.A.M.A. 161:1345, 1956.
13. Edelson, R.N., Chernik, N.L., Posner, J.B., Spinal subdural hematoma complicating lumbar puncture. Arch. Neurol. 31:134, 1974.
14. Gardner, W.J., The principle of spring-loaded points for cervical traction: Technical note. J. Neurosurg. 39:543, 1973.
15. Greensher, J., Mofensen, H.C., Lumbar puncture in the neonate: A simplified technique. J. Pediatr. 78:1034, 1971.
16. Horrax, G., Poppen, J.L., The frequency, recognition and treatment of chronic subdural hematomas. N. Engl. J. Med. 216:381, 1937.
17. Korein, J., Cravioto, H., Leicach, M., Reevaluation of lumbar puncture: A study of 129 patients with papilledema or intracranial hypertension. Neurology 9:290, 1959.
18. Laglia, A.G., Eisenberg, R.L., Weinstein, P.R., et al., Spinal epidural hematoma after lumbar puncture in liver disease. Ann. Intern. Med. 88:515, 1978.
19. Livingston, K.E., Technic of lumbar puncture (letter). N. Engl. J. Med. 287:724, 1974.
20. Lubic, L.G., Marotta, J.T., Brain tumor and lumbar puncture. Arch. Neurol. Psychiatry 72:568, 1954.
21. McKenzie, K.G., A surgical and clinical study of nine cases of chronic subdural hematoma. Can. Med. Assoc. J. 26:534, 1932.
22. McKissock, W., Richardson, A., Bloom, W.H., Subdural hematoma: A review of 389 cases. Lancet 1:1365, 1960.
23. Messer, H.D., Forshan, V.R., Brust, J.C.M., et al., Transient paraplegia from hematoma after lumbar puncture: A consequence of anticoagulant therapy. J.A.M.A. 235:529, 1976.
24. Naidoo, B.T., The cerebrospinal fluid in the healthy newborn infant. S. Afr. Med. J. 42:933, 1968.
25. Petito, F., Plum, F., The lumbar puncture (letter). N. Engl. J. Med. 290:225, 1974.
26. Prieto, A., Jr., Cantu, R.C., Spinal subarachnoid hemorrhage and associated neurofibroma of the cauda equina. J. Neurosurg. 27:63, 1968.
27. Rand, B.O., Ward, A.A., White, L.E., Jr., The use of the twist drill to evaluate head trauma. J. Neurosurg. 25:410, 1966.
28. Rengachary, S.S., Murphy, D., Subarachnoid hematoma following lumbar puncture causing compression of the cauda equina: Case report. J. Neurosurg. 41:252, 1974.
29. Senelick, R.C., Norwood, C.W., Cohen, G.H., "Painless" spinal epidural hematoma during anticoagulant therapy. Neurology 26:213, 1976.
30. Shenkin, H.A., Bouzarth, W.F., Clinical methods of reducing intracranial pressure: Role of the cerebral circulation. N. Engl. J. Med. 282:1465, 1970.
31. Tornheim, P.A., McLaurin, R.L. The effect of dexamethasone on cerebral edema from cranial impaction in the cat. J. Neurosurg. 48:220, 1978.
32. Tourtellotte, W.W., Somers, J.F., Parker, J.A. et al., A study on traumatic lumbar punctures. Neurology 8:129, 1958.
33. Trupp, M., Stylet injury syndrome. J.A.M.A. 237:2424, 1977.
34. Vastola, E.F., Non-hemorrhagic xanthochromia of cerebrospinal fluid. J. Neuropathol. Exp. Neurol. 19:292, 1960.
35. Wetchler, B.V., Brace, D.E., A technique to minimize the occurrence of headache after lumbar puncture by use of small bore spinal needles. Anesthesiology 16:270, 1955.

Obstetrics and Gynecology

6

NORMAL DELIVERY OF THE INFANT

Infrequently the emergency physician is called upon to deliver an infant when the obstetrician is not available or when the mother is brought in with the cervix completely dilated and the delivery is imminent. He must be capable of performing a normal delivery and a breech extraction. The occiput or vertex presentation occurs in approximately 95% of all labors. The fetus may enter the pelvis in either an occiput anterior position or an occiput posterior position, the former being by far the most common. A detailed discussion of the various steps and stages of labor is beyond the scope of this chapter. The reader is referred to any one of a number of excellent obstetrical texts available (5).

Examination

Inquiry must be made as to the frequency and intensity of the uterine contractions. The heart rate, presentation, and the size of the fetus may be evaluated abdominally. The fetal heart rate should be checked at the end of a contraction and immediately thereafter to identify any pathologic bradycardia which may foretell danger to the fetus. Always ask the patient whether there has been rupture of the membranes with a leaking of fluid vaginally and whether there has been any significant vaginal bleeding in excess of a bloody show. To minimize bacterial contamination if there is a question of rupture of the membranes, a *sterile* speculum is carefully inserted, and the physician looks for fluid in the posterior vaginal fornix. The fluid is observed for vernix, meconium, and frank blood. Three tests are commonly used to document rupture of membranes. In the Nitrazine test, Nitrazine paper is placed in the fluid and one looks for an alkaline pH. If the paper turns blue, this documents rupture of membranes. Fluid can be placed on a microscope slide and permitted to dry. If the fluid crystallizes as it dries this is a positive "ferning" test. Finally, the accumulation of fluid in the posterior vagina is known as pooling, and this also is indicative of rupture of the membranes. No speculum examination is done if the patient is bleeding more than a bloody show.

A diagnosis of ruptured membrane is not always easy to make unless amniotic fluid is seen escaping from the cervical os by the examiner. Although a Nitrazine test is commonly performed to ascertain rupture of the membranes, it is not completely reliable. The basis of the test is that normally the pH of the vagina ranges from 4.5 to 5.5 and if aminotic fluid has leaked into the vagina the pH of the amniotic fluid is usually 7.0 to 7.5. Nitrazine-impregnated paper is inserted into the vagina, and the color of the reaction is interpreted by comparison with a standard color chart. Intact membranes generally result in a color ranging from yellow to olive green. When ruptured membranes have occurred, the color of the paper changes from blue-green to deep blue depending on the pH.

The cervix then is palpated for softness and effacement as well as for dilatation. The degree of effacement of the cervix is expressed in terms of the length of the cervical canal compared to that of an uneffaced cervix. When its length is only 1 cm, the cervix is usually said to be 50% effaced since normal uneffaced cervix averages approximately 2 cm in length. At the point when the cervix becomes essentially a thin ring of tissue flush to the vaginal fornix, it is termed "completely effaced" or 100% effaced. The amount of dilatation of the cervix is ascertained by estimating the average diameter of the cervical opening. The examiner places his finger within the margins of the cervix and the diameter traversed is expressed in centimeters. When the diameter of the opening measures 10 cm the presenting part can usually pass through the cervix without difficulty, and this is termed "fully dilated."

The onset of the second stage of labor is indicated by full dilatation of the cervix. The duration of the second stage of labor from complete dilatation of the cervix to delivery of the fetus is highly variable between patients; however, on the average, in the nulliparous woman it is 50 minutes and in the multiparous woman it is approximately 20 minutes. It is imperative that the status of the fetus be monitored closely during this critical period since the force of contraction during labor may significantly reduce the placental blood flow. The presenting part should be positively determined and its position identified.

STATION

It is important to identify the level of the presenting part within the birth canal. The ischial spines are approximately halfway between the pelvic inlet and the pelvic outlet. When the lowermost portion of the presenting part is at the level of the ischial spines, it is designated as being at zero station. The birth canal above the ischial spines is arbitrarily divided into thirds. If the presenting part is at the level of the pelvic inlet, it is at −3 station. If it has descended one third the distance from the pelvic inlet to the ischial spines, it is termed a −2 station. Finally, two thirds of the distance from the inlet to the spines is termed a −1 station. Similarly, the birth canal is divided into thirds below the ischial spines. When the presenting part is two thirds of the distance between the ischial spines and the pelvic outlet, this is termed a +2 station. When the presenting part reaches the perineum, delivery may be imminent and the station is termed +3. A few of the preparatory steps taken in normal delivery are bypassed in the emergency center when delivery is imminent; this is the only time that the emergency physician performs delivery within the emergency center.

FETAL DISTRESS

It is important to ascertain the fetal heart rate with either a Delee-Hillis fetoscope or a Doppler ultrasonic device. Fetal distress is suggested if the fetal heart rate immediately following a contraction decreases below 120 or increases above 160 per minute. The diagnosis is definite if the fetal distress is anticipated, the fetus is at high risk and the obstetrician should be contacted immediately.

Preparation For Delivery In The Emergency Center

The mother's temperature should be checked initially and blood pressure should be checked periodically. An 18 to 19 gauge intravenous line should be placed and blood drawn for hemoglobin, hematocrit, and typing. If the patient is high-risk, include a blood sample for cross matching. If the membranes have been ruptured previously, many hours before arrival at the emergency center, the pregnancy is considered at high risk. All oral intake should be withheld during labor and delivery since gastric emptying time is prolonged once labor is established. The bladder should be emptied either spontaneously with the mother voiding in a bed-pan or, if this is not possible, by catheterization of the bladder.

The vulva, perineum, and adjacent areas should be scrubbed with Betadine[R] or soap and sterile drapes applied in preparation for delivery. An obstetrical kit containing the necessary items for delivery is then opened. The physician should scrub his hands and wear sterile rubber gloves.

A transvaginal pudendal nerve block should be employed in the emergency center as discussed in Chapter 3: "Anesthesia and Regional Blocks." As the head descends through the vaginal canal, the perineum begins to bulge. The scalp of the fetus may be seen through a slitlike vulvar opening at this time.

Spontaneous Delivery

As the head descends with each contraction, the perineum bulges and the vulvar opening becomes more and more dilated. Its shape changes from an oval to an almost circular opening. With the cessation of each contraction, the head recedes and the opening becomes smaller. As labor progresses, the vulva is stretched further and ultimately encircles the baby's head, known as "crowning."

An *episiotomy* can be performed at but not before crowning. The technique of performing an episiotomy is discussed later in the chapter. The perineum now may be extremely thin and in danger of rupture with subsequent contractions. In multiparous females, an episiotomy may not be necessary. The anus becomes greatly stretched and protuberant, and, if an episiotomy is not performed, perineal and rectal lacerations may occur during passage of the head. This may lead to permanent relaxation of the pelvic floor and the possibility of cystocele and uterine prolapse. An episiotomy is formed by making a midline incision with a sharp scissors to relax the tense perineum as shown in Figure 6.1A. As the head appears through the perineum, a towel should be draped over the physician's hand to protect the fetus from the anus and fecal excretions and to exert forward pressure against the forehead of the fetus (Fig. 6.1B). This procedure is called modified Ritgen maneuver and permits the physician to control the delivery of the head. The head should be delivered slowly with the base of the occiput rotating around the lower margin of the symphysis pubis. Upon delivery of the head the physician should pass his finger along the neck of the fetus to ascertain if there are any encircling coils of umbilical cord. While these commonly are noted and usually cause no harm, they may occasionally be so tight as to constrict the cord vessels and result in hypoxia. If the coil is

loose, it can be slipped over the infant's head; however, if it is too tightly applied to the neck and the probability of constriction is present, the cord should be clamped and cut immediately between the two clamps, and the infant then delivered.

After the head is delivered, it generally rotates laterally to the right occipitanterior (ROA) or left occipittransverse (LOT) (Fig. 6.1C). Usually the shoulders appear in the vulva in A-P position. The sides of the head are grasped with both hands of the physician, and gentle downward traction is applied until the anterior shoulder is delivered under the pubic symphysis. Completion of delivery of the anterior shoulder can be performed before delivery of the posterior shoulder (Fig. 6.1D). Following this, apply an upward movement to deliver the posterior shoulder (Fig. 6.1E–F).

The remainder of the body almost always follows the delivery of the shoulders without difficulty.

DELIVERY OF THE PLACENTA

Two clamps are applied to the cord, and the cord is cut between the clamps. The cord should be cut approximately 2 cm from the abdomen of the fetus. A sample of cord blood should be taken for VDRL and Coombs' test. Following delivery of the infant, the consistency and height of the uterus should be ascertained. As long as there is minimal bleeding the placenta never should be manually pulled to accomplish delivery, but rather patient waiting is advised. When the placenta is to be delivered, the uterus becomes globular and firm. This is the earliest sign of placental delivery. The umbilical cord protrudes farther out of the vagina, indicating that the placenta has descended; this is often preceded by a sudden gush of blood. The above signs generally appear within 5 to 15 minutes after delivery of the infant (maximally 30 minutes unless bleeding is profuse).

Following delivery of the placenta, one enters a critical period with regard to postpartum hemorrhage. Postpartum hemorrhage due to uterine relaxation is most likely to occur at this time. It is mandatory that the patient be observed constantly

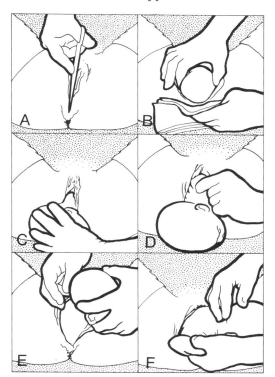

Figure 6.1.   The normal vaginal delivery of an infant. See text for discussion.

throughout this period. Oxytocin is often placed in the intravenous solution and infused at this point; 20 units of oxytocin should be placed in a liter of intravenous fluid and administered at a rate of 10 ml/minute over a few minutes until the uterus remains firmly contracted and the bleeding is controlled. Following this, the infusion rate is reduced to 1 to 2 ml/minute. Bimanual uterine massage may also decrease bleeding due to postpartum uterine atony. One must examine for cervical and vaginal wall lacerations at this point and be sure that all sponges which have been used are removed.

Repair of Episiotomy Incision

While a medial lateral episiotomy has been described, the midline episiotomy is more commonly used. The more common practice is to begin the episiotomy in the midline and to direct it downward toward the rectum. Episiotomies are performed to prevent tears of the perineum which may extend into the rectum. The episiotomy also serves to shorten the second stage of labor. In addition, the episiotomy serves to protect the fetal head, to prevent jagged or irregular perineal lacerations which may extend, and to prevent excessive stretch of the pelvic diaphragm (3).

When an episiotomy is performed too early, bleeding from the wound may be significant. It is common practice to perform an episiotomy when the head of the fetus is visible for a diameter of 3 to 4 cm with a contraction. The episiotomy is generally not repaired until after the placenta has been delivered.

Technique

Repair of the episiotomy should be performed with 2-0 chromic catgut. The vaginal epithelium is first closed with a continuous interlocking suture. Following this, 3 or 4 interrupted sutures of 2-0 catgut are placed in the fascia and muscle layer of the perineum with care to avoid the underlying rectum (Fig. 6.2A). The continuous suture is then used to close the subcutaneous tissue. A subcuticular stitch can be used to close the skin, or several interrupted sutures of chromic 3-0 catgut can

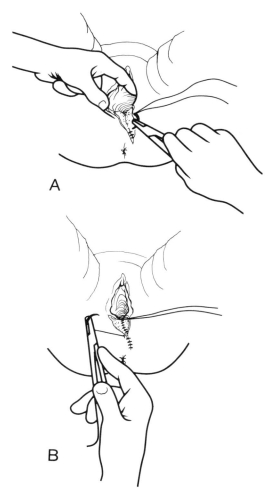

Figure 6.2. Repair of an episiotomy incision. The vaginal mucosa is first closed with a continuous suture. Following this, 3 or 4 interrupted sutures of 2-0 catgut are placed in the fascia and muscle layers of the perineum (*A*). The episiotomy should be repaired from posterior to anterior. A continuous suture is used to repair the skin and subcutaneous fascia (*B*).

be placed through the skin to loosely close the skin and subcutaneous tissue (Fig. 6.2B).

BREECH EXTRACTION

Three types of breech deliveries are described: a spontaneous breech delivery in which the entire infant is expelled without manipulation; partial breech extraction in which the infant is delivered spontaneously as far as the umbilicus and the remainder of the body needs to be extracted manually; and total breech extraction in which the entire body of the infant is extracted by the physician. Fortunately, breech extraction is an uncommon procedure for the emergency physician to be required to perform. It is best for a breech fetus to be allowed to deliver spontaneously to the umbilicus and then to be extracted. However, if fetal distress develops a decision must be made as to whether to perform a total breech extraction or a cesarean section. For breech extraction to be performed vaginally, the birth canal must be sufficiently large to permit passage of the fetus without trauma and the cervix must be effaced and fully dilated. If these conditions are not present, cesarean section is often necessary.

A breech delivery should be done by the emergency physician when vaginal delivery is likely before the obstetrician arrives and when acute fetal distress occurs and breech extraction is possible and cesarean section is impossible (i.e., due to prolapsed cord, etc.). The ideal anesthesia for breech extraction is epidural spinal anesthesia, with the ability to use general anesthesia with halothane after delivery to the umbilicus. This is usually not available to the emergency physician.

Technique

Prepare for extraction when the buttocks or the feet of the fetus appear at the vulva. The physician's hand should be introduced into the vagina and both feet of the fetus grasped. The ankles of the fetus should be held with the second finger of the physician lying between them. The feet are then brought down by gentle traction until they appear at the vulva (Fig. 6.3). A midline episiotomy is best performed at this time, before delivery of any larger parts. Once the feet are drawn through the vulva, they should be wrapped in a sterile towel to obtain a firmer grasp since vernix caseosa makes them slippery and difficult to hold. Continuous downward traction is applied and the legs and

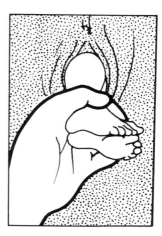

Figure 6.3. Breech extraction. The feet are brought down by gentle traction until they appear at the vulva.

then the thighs are grasped. When the buttocks appears at the vulva, gentle traction is applied until the hips are delivered. The physician's thumbs are then placed over the posterior iliac spines and sacroiliac area as shown in Figure 6.4. With the fingers of the examiner encircling the hips, downward traction is continued until the rib cage is visible. Further downward traction produces the scapulas. Once the buttocks is delivered, the back of the child generally faces upward; however, as further traction is exerted it tends to rotate spontaneously. If rotation does not occur during traction, slight rotation should be added while traction is maintained to bring the bisacromial diameter of the child into an anterior posterior position with the outlet and the back of the fetus facing laterally. One should not attempt to deliver the shoulders and arms until one axilla becomes visible during downward traction. Once one of the axillae appears through the vulva, the shoulder may be delivered. There are two methods of delivering the shoulders:

1. The infant's trunk is rotated in such a way that the anterior shoulder and arm appear at the vulva and can easily be released and delivered first. This can be accomplished by rotating the trunk of the infant in a clockwise

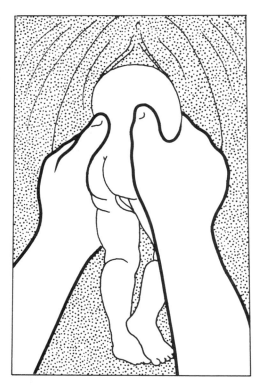

direction to deliver the anterior shoulder and arm. The body of the infant then is rotated in the reverse direction to deliver the other shoulder and arm. One must generally extract the arm by sweeping it across the chest.

2. If this method of trunk rotation is not successful, the posterior shoulder should be delivered first since the posterior and lateral portions of the normal pelvis are wider. The feet are grasped in one hand and drawn upward. In this way, leverage is exerted upon the posterior shoulder, which slips out over the perineal margin and is followed by the arm and hand (Fig. 6.5). Following this the body of the infant is depressed and the anterior shoulder is delivered beneath the pu-

Figure 6.4. The physician's thumbs are then placed over the posterior iliac spines and sacroiliac area, and his hands are placed around the infant's pelvis anteriorly. Downward traction is applied until the rib cage is visualized.

Figure 6.5. The posterior shoulder should be delivered first. Leverage superiorly is exerted such that the shoulder slips out over the perineal margin followed by the arm and the hand.

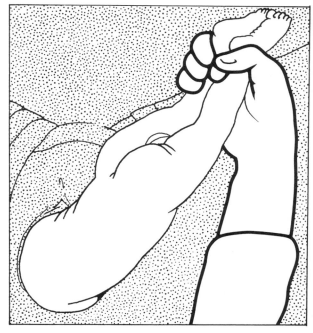

bic arch followed by the arm (Fig. 6.6). Following this the back generally rotates spontaneously and faces the pubic symphysis of the mother. If rotation does not occur, it is effected by manual rotation of the body.

Once the shoulders are delivered, the head rotates in the pelvis so that the chin is directed posteriorly and the head may be extracted by the Mauriceau maneuver.

Mauriceau Maneuver. The index finger of one hand is introduced into the mouth of the child while the body rests upon the palm and forearm of the hand as shown in Figure 6.7. The index and long fingers of the other hand are then placed around the neck posteriorly grasping the shoulders,

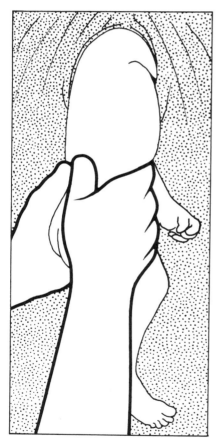

Figure 6.6. The body of the infant then is depressed as shown and the anterior shoulder is delivered beneath the pubic arch.

and downward traction is applied until the suboccipital region appears under the symphysis. An assistant applies downward suprapubic pressure at this point. The body of the infant is now elevated toward the mother's abdomen, and the mouth, nose, brow, and occiput emerge successively over the perineum. Downward traction during this procedure should be exerted only by the fingers over the shoulders and not by the fingers placed in the infant's mouth.

When the physician is dealing with a prolapsed cord, the treatment must be total breech extraction or cesarean section. When the head is not deliverable by routine methods, suprapubic pressure as well as a piper forceps should be used as shown in Figure 6.7B.

CESAREAN SECTION

The emergency physician is rarely called upon to perform a cesarean section in the emergency center. The indications are described; however, most obstetricians would feel that this sort of C-section should be done for *maternal* indications only. The risk of saving the fetus may impose incredible maternal risk. Four indications for performing a cesarean section within the emergency center are:

1. A postmortem (maternal) cesarean section. An example of this would be when a mother has been involved in an automobile accident and is severely injured, with impending death.
2. Severe traumatic abruptio placentae or bleeding from placenta praevia. When blood loss is greater than the ability to transfuse the patient.
3. Suspected uterine rupture.
4. Questionable fetal indications are continuous bradycardia and acute cord prolapse.

An emergency cesarean section should be performed in the operating room by the obstetrician or general surgeon whenever possible; however, in the situations indicated above, it may become necessary for the emergency physician to perform this procedure. While there is continuing con-

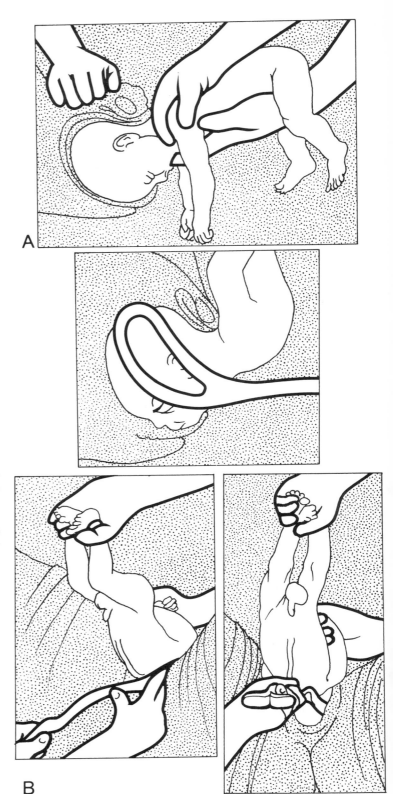

Figure 6.7. Mauriceau maneuver. *A.* The index finger of the left hand is introduced into the mouth of the child to open the mouth. The remainder of the infant's body rests on the palm and forearm of the left hand as shown. The index and long fingers of the right hand then are placed around the neck posteriorly grasping the shoulders, and downward traction is applied until the suboccipital region appears under the symphysis. *B.* The piper forceps may be used for extracting a breech pregnancy. When inserting the forceps, one must do so gently, placing the forceps as shown above. Gentle traction permits the head to be more easily extracted.

troversy over this issue, the authors believe that the procedure should at least be known to the emergency physician should a case arise in which the mother's life is in jeopardy, and the fetus is viable.

Equipment

12 Kellys	on 2
20 hemostats	ring
8 towel clips	forceps
6 Allis clamps	
4 Babcocks	
12 Penningtons	
6 straight Kochers	on 2
1 bandage scissors	ring
1 Mentzenbaum	forceps
2 Suture scissors	
1 Curved Mayo scissors	
3 needle holders, 8 inch	
1 needle holder, 6 inch	

2 knife holders
2 Adson forceps
1 dressing forceps, 10 inch
1 dressing forceps, 5½ inch
2 Russian forceps, 5½ inch
1 Debakey forceps, 8 inch
1 bladder retractor
2 Goulet retractors
1 Richardson retractor, large
1 Richardson retractor, medium
2 tonsil suction tips
2 clip applicators
2 sets skin clips
2 cord clamps
2 red top tubes
1 sterile strip
1 # 10 scalpel and blade
drapes
gloves
1% lidocaine anesthesia with epinephrine

wrap separate	1 baby de Lee forceps
	1 Bovie tip
	1 Bovie cord
	1 bulb syringe
	3 suction tubing sets

Technique

NOTE

In performing an emergency cesarean section within the emergency department,

one may have to eliminate a number of the steps detailed below. The authors feel that to perform a procedure such as this as an emergency, one must be aware of the steps to follow in performing the procedure somewhat more electively. It then becomes obvious which steps can be excluded. In performing the emergency cesarean section, those steps which are preceded by an asterisk are regarded as the essential steps in performing the procedure in the emergency center.

Preparatory Steps

1. Anesthesia. Anesthesia for this procedure should be provided by epidural or spinal anesthesia. If this is not possible, local infiltration nerve block anesthesia will suffice as described in Chapter 3: "Anesthesia and Regional Blocks."

2. The hair is shaved from the abdominal wall, from the mons pubis to above the umbilicus in the midline and laterally to the length of the abdomen.

3. Prep the area with iodinated solution.

*4. Empty the bladder through an indwelling catheter, which should remain in place during the entire procedure.

5. Apply sterile drapes to the area bounded by the mons pubis below and 4 to 6 cm above the umbilicus and 2 to 3 cm to each side of the midline. The physician should use a mask and gown as for any major operative procedure.

Procedural Steps

*1. Make an infraumbilical vertical incision, as this is the quickest technique for entering the abdomen. The incision should extend from just above the upper margin of the pubic symphysis to just below the umbilicus.

2. Dissect the subcutaneous fat away from the anterior rectus sheath to expose a strip of fascia in the midline approximately 2 cm wide.

*3. Make a small opening in the rectus sheath with a #11 scalpel and then insert a scissors and incise the fascia in the midline vertically to expose the uterus. Do not incise the rectus sheath with a scalpel or without being able to visualize it adequately, or one risks inadvertently entering the bowel which might be lying beneath the peritoneum. Separate the rectus muscles in the midline and expose the underlying transversalis fascia and the peritoneum.

4. Any bleeding which is encountered along the abdominal incision is treated by clamping with hemostats rather than by ligation. Ligation usually is performed later, unless the hemostat is in the way.

5. The transversalis fascia and the properitoneal fat are dissected carefully to reach the underlying peritoneum.

*6. At the upper end of the incision, the peritoneum is picked up by two hemostats placed approximately 2 cm apart in the midline. The fold of peritoneum between the clamps is palpated to rule out inclusion of bowel, bladder, or mesentery. An incision is made between the hemostats and is carried superiorly to the upper pole of the abdominal incision and inferiorly to just above the peritoneal reflection over the bladder.

*7. A retractor is placed firmly against the pubic symphysis, as shown in Figure 6.8.

*8. The bladder is identified and the serosa overlying the upper margin of it and extending along the anterior aspect of the lower uterine segment is grasped in the midline with forceps, as shown in Figure 6.8. Scissors are inserted between the edge of the serosa of the bladder and the myometrium over the lower uterine segment, and a 2 cm wide strip of serosa is separated from the uterus by blunt dissection with the scissors. The dissection is extended laterally along both sides of the bladder-uterus interface. The

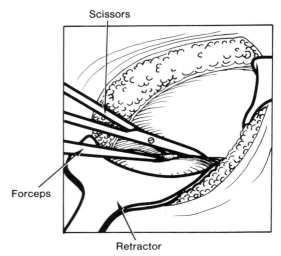

Figure 6.8. Cesarean section. The bladder is identified and separated from the lower uterine segment and retracted inferiorly. See text for discussion.

area dissected then is incised with the scissors and the bladder is separated gently by blunt dissection from the underlying uterus. The bladder should not be separated more than 5 cm from the uterus.

*9. The bladder then is retracted inferiorly beneath the pubic symphysis with a bladder retractor.

10. The uterus is palpated quickly to identify the size of the presenting part of the fetus.

NOTE

The uterus is usually rotated to the right so that the left round ligament is more anterior and closer to the midline than is the right.

*11. A transverse uterine incision then is made with the #10 scalpel into the exposed lower uterine segment midway between the lateral margins of the uterus (Fig. 6.9). As the initial incision is made into the uterus, a spurt of amniotic fluid will be noted as the uterine cavity is entered. This aids in determining

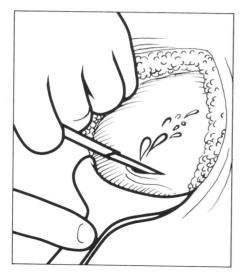

Figure 6.9. A small, 2 cm transverse incision is made over the exposed lower uterine segment. One will note amniotic fluid spurt out of the wound, once the uterine cavity is entered. This guides the physician as to the depth of the incision to avoid injury to the fetus.

the depth of the incision. The incision should be approximately 2 cm long. The transverse incision must be performed carefully so as not to cut completely through the uterine wall and injure the underlying fetus. Suction is very important during this procedure and should be carried out by an assistant. Once the uterus is opened, the incision is then extended by either placing the index fingers into the wound and applying lateral pressure as shown in Figure 6.10 or, preferably, by using either a bandage scissors or blunt-pointed scissors to extend the incision laterally. The uterine incision must be made large enough to allow delivery of the head and trunk of the fetus without tearing the uterus and cutting the uterine arteries which course along the lateral margins of the uterus. When this is a possibility, the uterine incision should be curved upward bilaterally rather than extending it farther laterally.

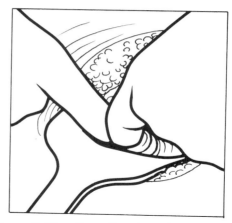

Figure 6.10. Once the uterus is opened, the incision is extended by placing the index fingers into the wound and applying lateral pressure. A bandage scissors or blunt-point scissors can be used alternately to extend the incision laterally.

CAUTION!

Uterine arteries and veins, both of which are quite large, course along the lateral margins of the uterus. When extending the transverse uterine incision, care must be taken to avoid these veins and arteries.

NOTE

The uterus can be opened by either a vertical or a transverse incision; however, the vertical incision which extends into the uterine fundus is not very commonly used in cesarean sections. The transverse incision over the lower uterine segment has the advantage of requiring very little dissection of the bladder as compared with the vertical incision. The vertical incision has the advantage that it avoids the laterally placed uterine vessels. Another disadvantage of the vertical incision is that if it extends too far inferiorly it may tear through the cervix and vagina.

NOTE

A Richardson retractor can be placed into the wound to retract the abdominal wall laterally when performing the uterine incision.

*12. The membranes should be incised at this time, and if the placenta is encountered during the incision it should be detached. If the placenta is incised, fetal hemorrhage may be severe. In this situation, the umbilical cord should be clamped as soon as possible.

*13. The hand then is placed into the uterus between the symphysis pubis and the head of the fetus. The fetal head then is gently elevated and lifted out of the uterus (Fig. 6.11). The nares and mouth are aspirated with a bulb syringe to minimize aspiration of amniotic fluid before delivery of the thorax of the infant. The shoulders then should be delivered using gentle traction plus fundal pressure (Fig. 6.12). Once the shoulders are delivered, the remainder of the body follows without any problem.

14. An intravenous infusion containing approximately 20 units of oxytocin per liter is then begun at the rate of approximately 10 ml/min until the

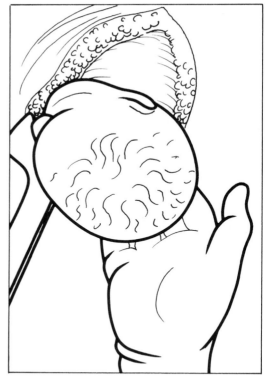

Figure 6.12. The shoulders should be delivered using gentle traction plus fundal pressure.

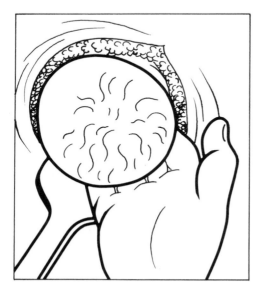

Figure 6.11. The hand is placed into the uterus after the membranes have been incised, and the head of the fetus is withdrawn.

uterus contracts satisfactorily, at which time the rate can be reduced to 2 to 4 ml/min. This infusion should be begun after the shoulders are delivered.

*15. The cord then is clamped and the infant is placed into an incubator; an attendant continues suctioning and any resuscitative maneuvers necessary. A sample of cord blood should be obtained at this time.

*16. As the uterus contracts, the placenta will bulge through the uterine incision and will be delivered.

Repair of the Uterus

1. The uterine incision must be searched at this time for any major bleeding points, which then are clamped and ligated. The placenta is examined to be certain that there are no retained fragments within the uterus. If this is

suspected, a gauze pack should be used to wipe out the uterine cavity.

2. The uterine incision then is closed with a continuous chromic suture. The technique used is a running lock suture begun just beyond the end of the uterine incision. Each stitch must be placed in the full thickness of the myometrium. The sutures should be passed through the myometrium carefully, and the running lock suture then is continued just beyond the opposite angle of the incision. Either a 1 layer or a 2 layer closure can be used (Fig. 6.13). The 1 layer closure generally is preferred when dealing with the very thin-walled lower uterine segment. Search for bleeding sites before closing the abdominal wall; when encountered, they should be ligated.

2. The serosa overlying the bladder is then approximated to its original location using 2-0 chromic catgut suture. The abdominal wound is closed in a layer-by-layer fashion.

CULDOCENTESIS

Culdocentesis is used to identify blood or pus within the peritoneal cavity (1, 2, 4, 7). Its most common application is in the diagnosis of a ruptured ectopic pregnancy or ruptured ovarian cyst. Some authors state that culdocentesis is more reliable in the adult female than is peritoneal lavage

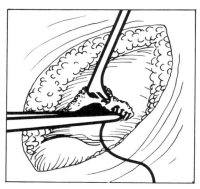

Figure 6.13. A 2 layer closure of the uterus is shown. A 1 layer closure will suffice in which a continuous running locked suture is used.

in determining if there is intra-abdominal bleeding following blunt abdominal trauma (6). Gravity places small amounts of intra-abdominal fluid or blood within the pouch of Douglas where it can be aspirated with a single needle puncture. In addition, the pouch of Douglas normally contains a small amount of clear peritoneal fluid which, upon aspiration, is very valuable in ascertaining a negative lavage.

Indications

1. To identify the presence of peritoneal fluid, blood, or pus within the peritoneal cavity. This is most useful in the diagnosis of ectopic pregnancy.

Contraindications

1. Mass in the cul-de-sac (especially if there is a possibility of a tubo-ovarian abscess or ovarian neoplasm).
2. Cases in which the introduction of intraperitoneal air may confuse the radiological diagnosis.

Equipment

Grave's bivalve vaginal speculum
Tenaculum
18 gauge spinal needle
10 ml glass syringe
Iodinated prep
5 ml syringe, 1% Xylocaine[R] with epinephrine, and a 25 gauge spinal needle

Technique

Preparatory Steps

1. The patient should be placed in the lithotomy position.

Procedural Steps (Fig. 6.14)

1. Grave's bivalve vaginal speculum is inserted and the cervix is identified.
2. The posterior lip of the cervix is grasped with the tenaculum.
3. The posterior vaginal fornix is cleansed with an antiseptic solution.
4. Anesthetic solution is deposited at the point of puncture, although this is usually unnecessary.
5. The cul-de-sac is then punctured with an 18 gauge spinal needle attached to

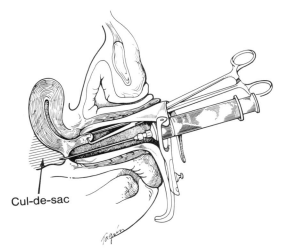

Cul-de-sac

Figure 6.14. Culdocentesis. See text for discussion.

a 10 ml syringe. This puncture should be made in the midline of the posterior fornix, 1 to 1.5 cm posterior to the cervix. The needle is inserted, but not more than 2 cm, while gentle suction is applied. Have an assistant sit the patient up slightly at this point. This will permit the pooling of blood in the cul-de-sac.

The aspiration of nonclotted blood indicates a positive tap. If no aspiration of blood is noted, then there is no diagnostic value to the procedure. When a serosanguinous aspirate is obtained, the rupture of an ovarian cyst should be considered. If purulent material is obtained, this often indicates a ruptured tubo-ovarian abscess or ruptured appendix.

Thus, a *positive* tap is when nonclotting blood is obtained. This indicates either a ruptured ectopic, a ruptured ovarian cyst, or a ruptured spleen. A *negative* tap is indicated when pus is withdrawn into the syringe or a clear straw-colored peritoneal or cystic fluid is withdrawn. A *nondiagnostic* tap is indicated when there is no return of blood or when clotting blood is obtained. If the clotting blood is less than 1 to 2 ml, this usually comes from the vaginal epithelium or small vessels. Greater than 2 ml indicates that one could be dealing with an intraperitoneal bleed.

BARTHOLIN'S ABSCESS

Bartholin's gland and duct may become obstructed, resulting in a Bartholin's cyst or abscess. This obstruction may be secondary to infections and abscess formation may occur primarily with the cyst.

Technique Of Drainage And Marsupialization

Incision and drainage of a Bartholin's abscess, while providing immediate relief of symptoms, is occasionally followed by a recurrence of a cyst or abscess. When an abscess occurs, it is best drained after local anesthesia by vertical incision of the mucocutaneous junction of the labia minora, followed by culture, lysis of loculations, and then packing or insertion of a wound catheter (Fig. 6.15). Definitive treatment then can be delayed, and the patient referred for follow-up. When a painless Bartholin's cyst is the presenting complaint, refer the patient. Marsupialization involves opening the Bartholin's abscess and emptying its contents, and then the edges of the abscess are stitched to the edges of the external incision. This keeps the cavity open while the interior of the cyst suppurates and closes by granulation.

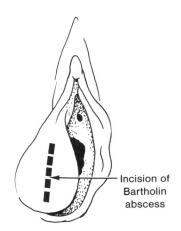

Incision of Bartholin abscess

Figure 6.15. Incision and drainage of a Bartholin's cyst or abscess. Marsupialization of the gland involves suturing the inner layer of the cyst to the outside to keep the cavity open, which promotes granulation and healing from within outward.

For treatment of a Bartholin's abscess, infiltrate a small amount of 1% lidocaine vertically along the mucocutaneous junction at the incision site. An incision then is made and extended vertically as shown in Figure 6.15. The contents of the cyst are drained, and the cavity is irrigated with saline. For marsupialization, the lining of the cyst is everted and sutured to the skin with interrupted 3-0 chromic catgut.

While it is not the procedure recommended by the authors, the Bartholin's abscess may be marsupialized initially rather than awaiting a delayed procedure. In either case the patient should be advised to use sitz baths twice daily; if a packing is placed for a Bartholin's abscess, this should be removed in 24 to 48 hours.

In summary, when cellulitis is present, a sitz bath three or four times a day and antibiotics are indicated. One should be certain not to incise an area of cellulitis, which can be prevented by the insertion of a needle to ascertain whether pus is present. These patients should always be given antibiotics when cellulitis is present. Most obstetricians incise and drain an abscess and then insert a wound catheter or marsupialize. One should refer a painless cyst to a gynecologist.

References

1. Clarke, J.M., Culdocentesis in the evaluation of blunt abdominal trauma. Surg. Gynecol. Obstet. 129:809, 1969.
2. Generelly, P., Moore, T. A. 3rd, LeMay, J.T., Delayed splenic rupture. J.A.C.E.P. 6:369, 1977.
3. Harris, R.E., An evaluation of the median episiotomy. Am. J. Obstet. Gynecol. 106:660, 1970.
4. Lucas, C., Hassim, A.M., Place of culdocentesis in the diagnosis of ectopic pregnancy. Br. Med. J. 1:200, 1970.
5. Pritchard, J., MacDonald, P.C., Williams Obstetrics. Appleton-Century-Crofts, New York, 1976.
6. Rothenberg, D., Quattlebaum, F.W., Blunt maternal trauma: A review of 103 cases. J. Trauma 18:173, 1978.
7. Webb, M.J., Culdocentesis. J.A.C.E.P. 7:451, 1978.

Orthopedic Procedures 7

NOTE

This chapter on orthopedic procedures for the emergency physician is divided into five sections:

Arthrocentesis

Fracture Principles, Casting Techniques and Common Splints

The Reduction of Selected Common Fractures

The Reduction of Selected Common Dislocations

The Injection and Aspiration of Selected Soft Tissue Disorders

This chapter is not intended to be a detailed presentation of each of the disorders discussed, as this is beyond the scope of this text. A number of excellent orthopedic texts are available for a detailed discussion of the mechanism of injury, clinical findings, and complications of each of the disorders. Some of the key features which are pertinent to the procedure being discussed are, however, presented briefly. In the sections on reductions of selected fractures and dislocations, only those procedures which should be performed by the emergency physician are discussed. It should be noted that a number of those procedures discussed are not routinely performed by the emergency physician; nevertheless, the emergency physician must be familiar with the procedure so that when an urgent indication for the procedure arises he can be prepared.

ARTHROCENTESIS (14, 17)

The optimal site for arthrocentesis is usually over the extensor surface of the joint, where the synovial pouch is close to the skin and is as removed as possible from major nerves, arteries, and veins (22, 39, 40, 54). The flexor surfaces of the joints generally have a high concentration of periarticular nerves, vascular structures, and tendons, making aspiration of the flexor side more difficult (39, 54).

Techniques of aspiration based on absolute measurements are unreliable since there is a striking variation between individuals and races (39). In this section, few measurements are offered; instead, the size and position of each anatomic structure are used to aid in the localization of the injection site. Bony prominences are more readily palpable, constant, and closely related to each articulation. Palpable bony landmarks are usually available in the immediate vicinity of the injection site (39, 40). When the landmarks are not easily palpable when the joint is placed in the best position for aspiration, these landmarks may become more readily palpable by changing the position of the joint and subsequently moving it to a more optimal position for aspiration (40). Two points are critical in performing arthrocentesis in any joint, *positioning and traction on the joint.* Proper positioning enlarges the target area of a joint which is to be aspirated. This almost always involves placing the joint in 20 to 30 degrees of flexion. Since arthrocentesis is usually performed on the *extensor surface* of a joint, flexion enlarges the joint space. The application of traction along the long axis of the bone distal to the joint opens the joint space and is especially important in small joints. Traction of the metacarpophalangeal joint is applied by pulling on the digit, which opens the metacarpophalangeal joint space. These techniques stretch the capsule and any supporting ligaments which might be penetrated by the needle (40). To enlarge the target area, the technique of traction can be used most effectively in the wrist and metacarpal phalangeal and interphalangeal articulations where the joint capsules are sufficiently loose to permit this technique (39, 40). The technique of positioning also may be used to enlarge the target area and is especially helpful in aspirations of the knee, due to the shape of the femoral condyles in which the vertical extent of the joint cavity is largest when the knee is flexed. Proper positioning, as will be discussed, also aids in enlarging the target area for aspiration of the first carpometacarpal articulation. Medial rotation of the thigh facilitates palpation of the greater trochanter of the femur by moving it out from under the gluteus maximus thus aiding in hip arthrocentesis. When a joint is aspirated the direction at which the needle enters should be such as to minimize the damage to the articular cartilage from scoring with the needle tip since hyaline cartilage regenerates poorly (39, 40). In the discussion below, the angle to pass the needle will not be discussed since it varies and is easily forgotten. By knowing the space to enter and the osseous anatomy, the angle to pass the needle is obvious.

If the site of aspiration is properly prepped, the incidence of infection is reduced to 1:15,000 (58). After preparation, in some patients with a markedly distended joint capsule, there is no need to raise a wheal with Xylocaine® and only a brief spray with ethyl chloride solution gives sufficient anesthesia to perform the procedure (22). When the synovial lining is entered, the folds of synovium or cellular debris may act as a flap valve on the end of the needle, preventing easy withdrawal of fluid (22). When this is suspected, the needle should be moved about gently and a little fluid already withdrawn reinjected to push the tissue or clot away from the tip of the needle. When aspiration must be performed in joints with little fluid, e.g., for the detection of septic arthritis, aspiration may be facilitated by wrapping the joint, except for the site of aspiration, with an elastic bandage to compress the free fluid into that portion of the sac being punctured (22). In general, always aspirate all readily accessible fluid at the time of aspiration.

In summary three points should be stressed
1. Arthrocentesis is usually performed on the extensor surface of a joint.
2. The joint usually is placed in 20 to 30 degrees of flexion.
3. Traction is important to open the joint space.

Synovial Analysis

Synovial fluid is an ultradialysate of plasma. Joints may be swollen in disorders such as protein-losing syndrome, nephrotic syndrome, and congestive heart failure, but these are usually not very painful or inflamed and pose little problem in differentiation.

One of the major concerns relating to an unnecessary arthrocentesis is the introduction of infection. In properly prepared patients, the incidence of infection is extremely low and occurs in less than 1/15,000 procedures (58).

Joint fluid varies in composition depending on the cellular responses, which can be classified into three groups: minimal inflammatory reactions such as would occur in mild trauma; mild inflammatory reactions such as occur in rheumatic fever, systemic lupus erythematosus, and viral arthritides; and severe inflammatory reactions such as occur in septic arthritis, acute gout and acute rheumatoid arthritis. Normally, joint fluid is straw colored; as an inflammatory reaction occurs, it changes to a lemon-yellow or a greenish hue. In some conditions, such as osteoarthritis and osteochondritis dissecans presenting with a joint effusion, the color remains normal. Hemorrhagic fluid suggests trauma to the joint; however, one must remember that there are four causes of a hemorrhagic effusion: trauma, coagulation defects, hemangiomas of the synovium, and villonodular synovitis. In the normal knee, the most common site for a joint effusion, there is 0.5 to 2 ml of fluid (59). The total protein content is 1.8 gm % and glucose is normally 10 mg % less than it is in the serum. A very low joint fluid glucose suggests septic arthritis. Noninflammatory arthritides usually have less than 2.5 gm % protein, while inflammatory fluids show a protein concentration of 6 to 8 mg %.

Viscosity is a function of the concentration and quality of hyaluronic acid in the fluid. The *mucin clot test* can be performed on all joint aspirates by adding glacial acetic acid drop by drop to a small amount of joint fluid in a test tube. In the normal synovial aspirate, the fluid will form a white clot. A clot which breaks up easily on agitation is indicative of an inflammatory or an infected fluid. Mucin clots of noninflammatory fluids do not break when agitated. An alternative method of checking for the viscosity is by placing a drop of joint fluid between the thumb and index finger and separating the fingers. In normally viscous fluid, "stringing" of the fluid between the fingers occurs and reflects a noninflammatory condition. In inflammatory conditions, the synovial fluid will not "stretch" between the fingers.

The turbidity of the fluid is proportional to the number of cells present and is influenced by the presence of crystals and cartilage debris in the effusion (59). Normally the synovial fluid contains 10 to 200 cells/ml. A high white cell count can occur with acute gout; in which case, uric acid crystals can be seen under a polarizing light within white cells or even free in the synovial fluid. Infectious arthritis usually contains leukocyte counts in excess of 50,000 cells/ml, accompanied by a variable blood sugar that is less than half the serum sugar and a high protein count. Other forms of arthritis which are accompanied by high cell count include acute pseudogout, acute gout, and rheumatic fever. In patients with rheumatoid arthritis, mononuclear cells predominate in the first 6 weeks. Later, with acute exacerbations, the fluid may contain 65 to 85% neutrophils, many of which appear degenerated.

Joint aspiration is done either for therapy of an acutely swollen joint or for diagnostic purposes within the emergency center. Relief of joint pain is achieved rapidly, whether the joint aspirate is due to a traumatic arthritis, gouty arthritis, infectious arthritis, or rheumatoid arthritis. The only time one should attempt to aspirate a joint which does not contain an effusion is when there is a suspicion of septic arthritis (54). This relief varies directly with the rapidity with which the fluid has accumulated. Table 7.1 indicates the findings in different joint effusions. The tests which should be performed on aspirated joint fluid include a leukocyte count with differential, a search under a polarizing light for crystals, a mucin clot test or "string test," a Gram stain in patients suspected of having septic arthritis, and a synovial fluid glucose and protein.

Equipment

Prep solution—Betadine®
Anesthetic prep
18 gauge, 1.5 inch needle
23 gauge, ⅜ inch needle
3 cc syringe
1% lidocaine with epinephrine
Assortment of needles (Specific needle sizes and lengths are indicated in the description of the specific procedure especially when longer needles are required.)
18 gauge, 1.5 inch
22 gauge, 1.5 inch
23 gauge, 1.5 inch
10 cc syringe
20 cc syringe
Sterile gloves and towels
4 × 4 gauze
Sample tubes for specimens

Surgical Preparation of a Joint Surface

Arthrocentesis should be performed under sterile conditions. When a joint surface is prepared properly, the incidence of infection is extremely low. The site of aspiration should be scrubbed with Betadine® for a 5 minute preparation. The area should be draped with sterile towels, and the procedure should be performed under sterile conditions. When performing arthrocentesis over the sites indicated for

Table 7.1. Characteristics of Synovial Fluid Effusions

	Color	Clarity	Viscosity	Leukocytes/ml	Protein
Normal	Clear	Transparent	High	200	3.5
Noninflammatory Degenerative joint disease, osteochondritis dessicans	Yellow	Transparent	High	200–2000	3.5
Inflammatory Acute gout, pseudogout, rheumatic fever, rheumatoid arthritis, Reiter's syndrome*	Yellow-green	Opaque	Low	2000–50,000	3.5
Septic Bacterial infections	Yellow-green	Opaque	Low	50,000–200,000	3.5

* Synovial fluid complement is high in Reiter's syndrome but is low in other acute inflammatory arthritides.

the various joints, one avoids vessels and nerves.

Metacarpophalangeal And Interphalangeal Joint Aspiration

The metacarpophalangeal and interphalangeal joints of the hand have a wide range of motion which makes traction an effective means of increasing the target area, especially when aspirating the joints of the thumb and little finger. This technique is least effective in cases involving the third and fourth fingers. The volar surface of the joint contains the volar plate, nerves, and vessels all of which contraindicate aspiration on the volar surface. Therefore, the optimal site for aspiration is over the dorsal surface on either side of the extensor tendons (39). The best landmark for aspiration of the metacarpophalangeal joints is at the head of the metacarpal with the fingers flexed. If the first metacarpophalangeal joint is passively flexed and traction is applied, there is a separation noted between the metacarpal and the proximal phalanx which is accentuated by this technique, making penetration easier. The interphalangeal joints have a smaller space and tighter capsules; therefore, traction is of limited value here. The landmark in second to fourth metacarpophalangeal joint aspiration is the head of the metacarpal, immediately medial or lateral to the extensor tendon with the joint held in flexion (22, 39) (Fig. 7.1).

Carpometacarpal Aspiration Of The Thumb

This is a small joint which is a common site of arthridities which may require aspiration for diagnostic purposes. The best site from which to enter this joint is the dorsal aspect over the radial side of the hand (Fig. 7.2) (22). Traction of the thumb and flexion of the wrist and thumb with the hand held in slight ulnar deviation will aid in increasing the target area.

Radiocarpal Arthrocentesis (Wrist Arthrocentesis)

The joint line of the radiocarpal joint runs between the radial and ulnar styloid

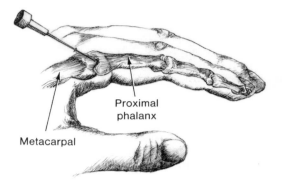

Figure 7.1. Metacarpophalangeal joint aspiration. One should enter the joint immediately medial or lateral to the extensor tendon where a small depression or "pit" often is seen when traction is applied. Traction is critical in aspiration of this joint. The joint should be flexed in the position shown and opened by traction performed by an assistant.

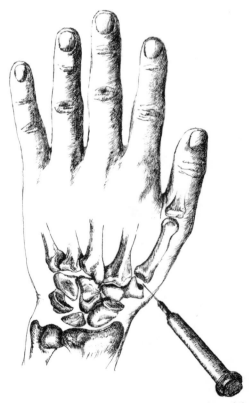

Figure 7.2. Carpometacarpal aspiration of the thumb. See text for details.

processes. The best site for aspirating the radiocarpal joint is dorsally, as the volar aspect contains numerous tendons, vessels, and nerves. While it might appear at first glance that the radial side of the dorsum of the wrist would be the optimal site for aspiration, this area should be avoided. From lateral to medial, the following structures crisscross that region: the abductor pollicis longus tendon; the extensor pollicis brevis tendon (which forms the radial side of the anatomic snuffbox) the radial artery, which in the snuffbox branches into a dorsocarpal branch and a first dorsometacarpal branch; the extensor pollicis longus tendon, forming the ulnar border of the snuffbox; and the extensor carpi radialis brevis tendon (Fig. 7.3). Thus, although one can enter the joint through the anatomic snuffbox, better sites can be selected. Between the ulnar border of the anatomic snuffbox and the common extensor tendons is a space containing no large vessels, nerves, or tendons. This space is just ulnar and distal to a bony landmark on the dorsal aspect of the ra-

dius called the tubercle of Lister (Fig. 7.3). Extending the thumb makes the extensor pollicis longus tendon stand out and defines the ulnar border of the anatomic snuffbox. It will be noted that the extensor pollicis longus tendon courses around Lister's tubercle. *Relax* the wrist in a flexed position and palpate Lister's tubercle with the index finger. Now, extend the wrist slightly and one can feel the extensor carpi radialis brevis tendon stand out as it courses just distal to the tubercle and almost obliterating it as the wrist is extended. With the wrist relaxed, a slight depression will be noted just ulnar to the extensor carpi radialis brevis tendon at a point just distal to the dorsal rim of the radius. This depression marks the site of choice for arthrocentesis of the radiocarpal joint. It should be noted that this depression lies between the extensor carpi radialis tendon and the common extensor tendon. With the index finger in the depression it always will point directly at the third metacarpal. This depression can be easily palpated in most patients, and the needle should be inserted at that site (Fig. 7.4). Flexion and ulnar deviation opens the joint cavity dorsally and stretches the capsule and the extensor retinaculum. Traction on the hand may further increase the radiocarpal joint space (22, 39, 54). A needle is inserted just distal to the rim of the radius in the depression. The needle should be directed between the radius and

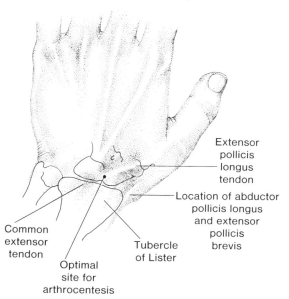

Extensor pollicis longus tendon

Location of abductor pollicis longus and extensor pollicis brevis

Common extensor tendon

Tubercle of Lister

Optimal site for arthrocentesis

Figure 7.3. Radiocarpal arthrocentesis. The optimal site for arthrocentesis is shown and is discussed in the text. A depression can be palpated just ulnar to the course of the extensor pollicis longus tendon distal and ulnar to Lister's tubercle. This is the site of aspiration.

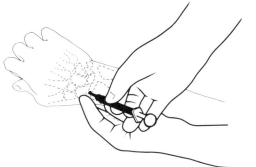

Figure 7.4. Radiocarpal arthrocentesis. Palpate Lister's tubercle and enter the joint with the wrist in 15 to 20 degrees of flexion over the fossa shown in Figure 7.3.

the lunate (the bone which lies at the floor of the depression).

A technique has been described for arthrocentesis of the wrist (ulnocarpal) joint, when there is marked bulging noted over the ulnar surface of that joint. The ulnar surface of this joint may be entered by insertion of the needle just distal to the ulnar styloid process and dorsal to the pisiform bone (Fig. 7.5) (22). This is not the optimal site for routine aspiration of this joint since there are tendons coursing through this area through which the needle must pass. The authors prefer the radiocarpal approach.

Since the joint cavities of the *intercarpal* joints usually communicate freely through a common synovial space, a single site for either aspiration or injection is usually adequate (39). In performing intercarpal arthrocentesis, palpate Lister's tubercle with the patient clenching his fist. Place the examining finger just distal and ulnar to the tubercle between the tendons of the extensor carpi radialis brevis and the extensor digitorum communis. As the patient flexes his wrist the dorsum of the lunate bone becomes palpable and just distal to it is a depression between the lunate and the capitate. This is the optimal site for intercarpal aspiration (39). Thus radiocarpal arthrocentesis is performed in the depression proximal to the lunate (beween it and the distal radius) and intercarpal arthrocentesis is performed distal to the lunate with the wrist more acutely flexed.

Elbow Arthrocentesis

Aspiration of the elbow joint is one of the easiest procedures to perform in the emergency center. Arthrocentesis of the elbow joint medial to the olecranon is not recommended (22, 39, 54). While a number of techniques have been described (22, 39, 54) for arthrocentesis over the lateral aspect of this joint, the optimal site is through the anconeus muscle. With the elbow extended, three bony landmarks are readily palpable on the lateral side of this joint: the lateral epicondyle, the head of the radius, and the tip of the olecranon process. The radial head can be identified by supinating and pronating the forearm. The elbow is extended to approximately 135 degrees with the forearm held midway between pronation and supination after identifying the three bony landmarks (54). The needle should then be inserted in the middle of a triangle formed by connecting these three points. The needle should enter the joint from posteriorly at a 90 degree angle to the humerus and traverse the skin and anconeus muscle and enter the joint space between the olecranon and lateral epicondyle (39). There are no major nerves or vessels traversing this area of the joint (Fig. 7.6).

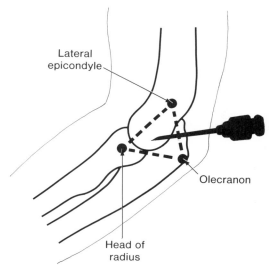

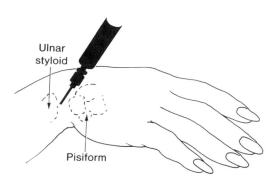

Figure 7.5. The ulnocarpal joint arthrocentesis.

Figure 7.6. Elbow joint arthrocentesis. See text for details.

Shoulder Aspiration

Anterior Approach

Aspiration of the shoulder joint (gleno-humeral) through the anterior approach is the most common approach for aspirating the shoulder. The bony landmarks are readily palpable and include the coracoid process and the head of the humerus, which is palpable just medial to the lesser tuberosity. The arm is abducted 15 to 20 degrees and the capsule is relaxed (54). Further opening of the joint space is obtained by an assistant applying gentle downward traction on the arm. The patient may be either sitting or supine; however, the procedure is more easily performed with the patient in the sitting position. The needle is then inserted just medial to the head of the humerus between it and the tip of the coracoid process (22) (Fig. 7.7).

Posterior Approach

The posterior approach is the technique preferred by the authors. One advantage of the posterior approach over the anterior approach is that to reach the synovial cavity by the anterior approach the needle must pass through the tendons of the coracobrachialis and the subscapularis, whereas with the posterior approach the needle passes through the posterior fibers of the deltoid only. In addition, the anterior portion of the capsule is strengthened by the glenohumeral ligaments which must be pierced by the needle in the anterior approach to enter the joint cavity. In addition, the patient sees the needle with the anterior approach. To perform the procedure by the posterior approach, the angle of the acromion forms the bony landmark for injection since it overlies posteriorly the contact surfaces between the humeral head and the glenoid fossa. The needle is inserted horizontally one fingerbreadth below the angle of the acromion and passes between the head of the humerus and the lip of the glenoid fossa (Fig. 7.8). A concavity can be palpated and even seen in some patients at this site. In performing this procedure, internal rotation of the humerus is recommended to tighten the posterior fibers of the joint capsule (39).

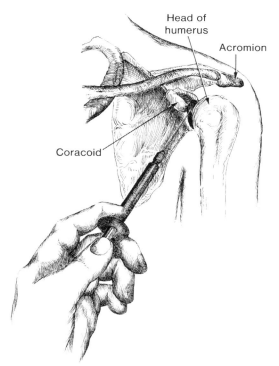

Head of humerus

Acromion

Coracoid

Figure 7.7.   The anterior approach for shoulder arthrocentesis. See text for discussion.

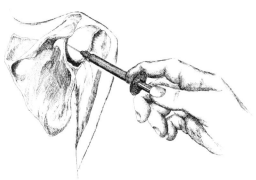

Figure 7.8.   The posterior approach for shoulder arthrocentesis. The needle is inserted one fingerbreadth below the angle of the acromion, which is easily palpable posteriorly at the junction of the spine of the scapula and acromion process. The patient should be placed so that the humerus is internally rotated to tighten the posterior capsule.

Aspiration Of The Sternoclavicular Joint

This joint is the most common site for septic arthritis and osteoarthritis in patients who abuse intravenous drugs (24, 45). The sternoclavicular joint is difficult to enter from directly anterior due to the fibrocartilaginous articular disc which lies within the joint (22). It is a rather difficult joint to aspirate or inject unless it is distended. For this procedure the patient should be placed in a supine position with the arm on the side to be aspirated abducted to 90 degrees and dropped backward over the edge of the table. This brings the clavicle forward and permits insertion of the needle from medially (adjacent to the suprasternal notch) and avoids the articular disc. Insert the needle into the joint just adjacent to the suprasternal notch, aiming the needle posteriorly. The joint should be entered after a few millimeters (Fig. 7.9).

Hip Arthrocentesis

The hip joint is the most difficult to aspirate or inject due to the large amount of soft tissue around this joint (22). In patients with osteoarthritis, it may be impossible to enter the joint space with certainty even with fluoroscopic guidance. In the best of hands, there is a more than 50% failure rate reported with hip arthrocentesis (20, 21, 23, 40). The anterior approach is the most frequently used for performing this procedure (43, 50), although some authors prefer to use the lateral approach (33, 35, 53). The anterior approach is the preferred method by the authors and the one that is primarily discussed here.

Anterior Approach

The head of the femur lies halfway between the anterior superior iliac spine and the lateral tubercle of the pubis and approximately 1 to 1½ inches distal to the inguinal ligament (Fig. 7.10). One should use a 19 or 20 gauge needle which is approximately 2½ to 4 inches long, depending on the size of the individual patient (22, 54). The site at which one should enter the joint is approximately 2 to 3 cm below the anterior superior iliac spine and 2 to 3 cm lateral to the femoral pulse, depending on the size of the patient (Fig. 7.10). One can localize this point by palpating the femoral pulse and going approximately 2 cm lateral to it, entering the skin 1 to 1½ inch distal to the inguinal ligament or measuring out the distances as indicated above. Insert the needle at a 60 degree angle with the skin, aiming it posteromedially through the capsular ligaments until the bone is reached (22). The tip is then slightly withdrawn and one should aspirate to check the po-

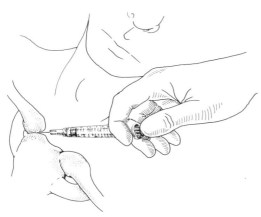

Figure 7.9. Sternoclavicular joint arthrocentesis. The needle is inserted adjacent to the suprasternal notch and is aimed posteriorly.·

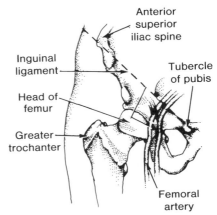

Figure 7.10. Hip arthrocentesis—anterior approach. The point of entrance is approximately 2 to 3 cm below the anterior superior iliac spine and 2 to 3 cm lateral to the femoral pulse, depending on the size of the patient.

sition and be certain the needle is not in a vein or artery. One may not aspirate anything even though the joint has been entered. One may have to rely on fluoroscopic guidance to ascertain entrance into the joint. In this procedure, it is easiest to enter the joint with the hip in maximal extension and internally rotated, which brings the greater trochanter out from under the gluteus maximus and brings the neck of the femur in a plane parallel to the table (40).

Lateral Approach

The landmark to localize in using this approach is the greater trochanter. The patient should be placed in the supine position, and the thigh should be rotated medially (internally) to bring the greater trochanter out from under the gluteus maximus muscle and to bring the neck of the femur into a plane parallel to the table. The thumb and index finger are placed on the greater trochanter and a 4 inch 20 gauge needle is inserted superior to the middle of the upper margin of the trochanter, parallel to the table, and at right angles to the femur (40). The needle will pass through the gluteus medius and will contact bone at a nonarticular surface. Injections here will be intrasynovial, as the capsule extends laterally if the needle is passed slightly superior over the head of the femur. This procedure should be performed under fluoroscopic control and has the advantage that there are no large vessels or nerves in the vicinity. The largest vessels in the area are the inferior branches of the superior gluteal artery and vein.

Knee Aspiration

The knee contains the largest synovial cavity in the body and is the largest weight-bearing structure. It is also one of the most common sites of synovial inflammation and the most commonly aspirated joint in the emergency center for various pathological processes. Due to the size of this joint and its relatively superficial nature, it is the easiest joint to aspirate, particularly when it is tightly distended with an effusion (22). Suprapatellar, infrapatel-

lar, and parapatellar approaches have been advocated by various authors (20–22, 40, 53, 54). The suprapatellar approach is a good method if large volumes of fluid are present in the suprapatellar bursa; however, this approach has the disadvantage that the suprapatellar bursa is not always continuous with the joint cavity. This problem is especially likely in patients with multilocular joint effusions, such as patients with chronic arthritis. If a small effusion or no effusion is present, the bursa may be little more than a potential space and is an irregular structure in patients with arthritis (40). The two approaches advocated here are the medial parapatellar approach by Hollander (22) and the infrapatellar approach (40). It should be noted that a tightly distended knee can be aspirated from almost any angle without difficulty; however, the techniques described below will allow ready entrance into the joint even if little fluid is present.

Parapatellar Approach (Medial or Lateral Approach)

The patient should lie in a supine position on the examining table with the knee fully extended. The medial surface of the knee should be adequately prepped using an iodinated solution. The site of puncture is on the medial border of the patella 1 to 2 cm proximal to the inferior pole. The needle should be inserted between the inferior surface of the patella and the patella groove of the femur (22, 54). The quadriceps muscle must be completely relaxed by placing the knee in 20 degrees flexion for the needle to advance readily and without difficulty (54) (Fig. 7.11). The needle tip may produce crepitance on the undersurface of the patella, demonstrating entrance into the joint space even with very little fluid (22). The advantages of this approach are that synovial membrane folds are seldom encountered. This is the preferred approach with a distended knee.

Infrapatellar Approach

The medial parapatellar approach advocated above has the disadvantage that the needle tip can easily contact the carti-

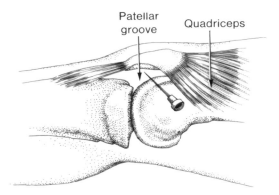

Figure 7.11. Medial view of the knee showing the parapatellar approach to knee arthrocentesis.

laginous surface, which some authors feel is a major disadvantage, since contacting the cartilage may result in damage (40). If the patella is ankylosed the optimal site for aspiration is in the infrapatellar region, coursing through the fat pad into the knee joint space between the condyles of the femur (22). In performing the aspiration, an 18 or 20 gauge needle on a 10 cc syringe should be used except when performing the procedure for purposes of aspirating a hemarthrosis; in which case, a 16 to 18 gauge needle on a 20 ml syringe is used. In addition, if the knee has a flexion deformity limit extension or has a small effusion in the knee, the medial approach may not be optimal. The infrapatellar approach has the advantage of a good landmark, the patellar tendon. In addition, there are no major vessels or nerves coursing through the area through which the needle may penetrate. Due to the shape of the femoral condyles, flexion in the intrapatellar approach greatly enlarges the vertical dimensions of the joint and stretches the patellar ligament, permitting easy entrance into the joint space without scoring the articular surface. In addition, there are very few pain fibers in the patellar ligament, making the procedure relatively painless; some authors regard it as the best approach of all (40).

In performing knee aspiration by the infrapatellar approach, the needle should be inserted immediately below the apex of the inferior pole of the patella, through the middle of the patellar ligament, and passing through the fat pad and into the intercondylar fossa. The knee is held at 90 degrees of flexion (the patient can be sitting with his legs hanging over the edge of the table) and the needle is directed perpendicular to the patellar tendon as shown in Figure 7.12 (40). Access to the joint can be readily demonstrated by aspiration.

Ankle Aspiration (Tibiotalar Joint Aspiration)

The ankle joint may be entered readily from either an anteromedial or an anterolateral approach. The anteromedial approach is preferred by most authors (22, 40, 54), as there is slightly more space for insertion of the needle between the joint surfaces when this approach is used.

Anteromedial Approach

As indicated above, this is the procedure of choice for ankle aspiration. Locate the

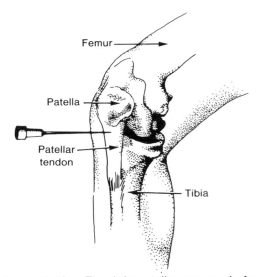

Figure 7.12. The infrapatellar approach for knee arthrocentesis. The anterior oblique view of the knee is shown with the needle inserted just inferior to the inferior pole of the patella, through the patellar tendon, and into the joint space after traversing the fat pad behind the patellar tendon. The knee should be flexed to 90 degrees with this approach, to avoid striking the articular surface.

medial malleolus and palpate the sulcus between the medial malleolus and the most distal articular surface of the tibia. With the foot plantar flexed, this sulcus can be palpated medial to the tendon of the tibialis anterior. Inversion of the foot aids in tensing the tibialis anterior and helps in localizing the point of entrance (40). A more easily noted landmark for performing the procedure is the extensor hallucis longus tendon which can be palpated and visualized by asking the patient to alternately flex and extend the great toe (22, 40, 54). This tendon is more laterally placed than is the tibialis anterior tendon; however, the extensor hallucis longus tendon is a more readily visible structure and allows easy entrance into the joint space (Fig. 7.13). Place the patient in a supine position with the ankle plantar flexed to permit a wider area for entrance into the joint. Insert the needle just medial to the extensor hallucis longus tendon, directing it perpendicularly to the floor (in the supine patient) and in line with the medial malleolus. The point of insertion should be just distal to the most distal edge of the tibia. The lateral side of the extensor hallucis longus tendon should definitely be avoided since the deep peroneal nerve and the dorsalis pedis artery and vein course on this side (Fig. 7.13). Alternately, the site of aspiration medial to the tibialis anterior tendon can be larger than the area medial to the extensor hallucis longus tendon (40). When the tibialis anterior tendon is easily palpable, it can be used as a reference point and landmark for insertion of the needle in the same fashion as the extensor hallucis longus tendon.

Anterolateral Approach

In performing ankle arthrocentesis with the anterolateral approach, the medial margin of the lateral malleolus should be palpated (Fig. 7.13). After asking the patient to extend his toes, palpate the extensor digitorum communis tendons. The point of entry is between the lateral margin of the extensor digitorum communis tendon and the medial margin of the fibular malleolus (Fig. 7.13) (54). The patient should be supine when this procedure is

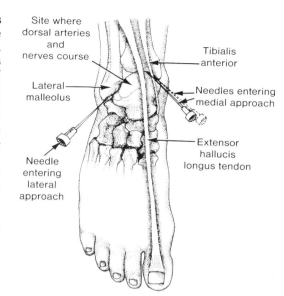

Figure 7.13. Arthrocentesis of the ankle. See text for discussion.

performed. The ankle should be plantar flexed after the point of entrance is identified. A depression can be palpated at the site of entrance, adjacent to the medial margin of the fibular malleolus. This approach is not the authors' preferred approach; however, in cases in which the medial approach is not feasible (cellulitis, rupture of the deltoid ligament) it may have to be used.

Subtalar Arthrocentesis

The subtalar joint is very difficult to enter and arthrocentesis of this joint is uncommonly performed in the emergency center. When an effusion is present within the subtalar joint, swelling will be noted below the lateral malleolus. This joint space, which lies between the talus and the calcaneus, may be widened as a result of an effusion. When an effusion is present and one needs to aspirate it for diagnostic purposes, the procedure should be performed while the patient is supine with the foot held perpendicular to the leg. The joint is entered by inserting a needle just below the lateral malleolus, perpendicular to the skin (54). The site of injection should be just proximal to the sinus tarsi (54) (Fig.

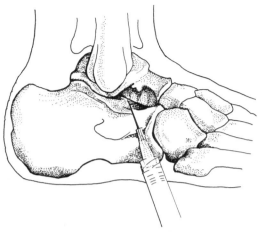

Figure 7.14. Subtalar arthrocentesis. The site of injection should be just proximal to the sinus tarsi.

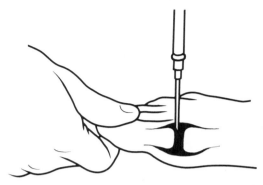

Figure 7.15. Metatarsophalangeal joint aspiration. The joint should be entered from the dorsal surface, just medial or lateral to the extensor hallucis longus tendon. Distraction is crucial in entering this joint.

7.14). The major indications for performing this procedure in the emergency center are suspected septic arthritis in this joint or suspected crystalline arthridites involving the joint.

Metatarsophalangeal Joint Aspirations

The first metatarsophalangeal joint is a frequent site of involvement in gouty arthritis. Aspiration is easily performed in the patient with a joint distended by an effusion. After linear traction is applied, insertion of the needle should be between the metatarsal head and the base of the first phalanx, and the needle should be inserted perpendicular to the toe from the dorsal surface of the foot (Fig. 7.15). Linear traction on the toe opens the space and facilitates entry into the joint (54). The point of entry into the dorsal surface should be just medial to the extensor hallucis longus tendon, as shown in Figure 7.16. The remainder of the metatarsophalangeal joints may be entered in a similar manner. A 22 gauge needle attached to a 5 cc syringe should be used in performing this procedure.

Interphalangeal Joint Aspiration

A 22 gauge needle should be used in performing interphalangeal joint aspira-

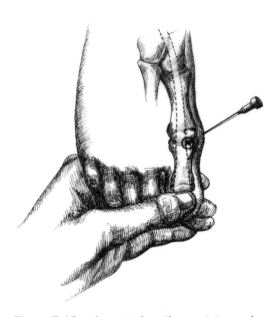

Figure 7.16. In entering the metatarsophalangeal joint, the needle should enter just medial to the extensor hallucis longus tendon over the point marked X.

tion of the toes (22). The needle should be inserted over the dorsal surface from either a medial or a lateral direction, slipping the needle beneath the extensor tendon between the cartilaginous surfaces forming the joint (22, 54). Traction of the toe may facilitate entry into the joint.

Temperomandibular Joint Aspiration (19)

Temperomandibular joint (TMJ) injections may be indicated in the emergency center in patients with rheumatoid arthritis involving this joint or in patients with TMJ syndrome; in which case, injections of anesthetic and a steroid are both diagnostic and therapeutic in selected cases (22). Anesthetic deposited in this joint is useful in reduction of TMJ dislocations. There is a fibrocartilaginous disc in the joint space, which makes it difficult to be certain that the needle is properly placed within the joint in some cases. A small needle should be used, preferably a 23 or 24 gauge. The point of insertion should be well anterior to the tragus of the ear to avoid damage to the facial nerve and the superficial temporal artery (Fig. 7.17). Insert the needle at a point just below the zygomatic arch, approximately 1.3 cm anterior to the tragus of the ear (22). Direct the needle slightly posteriorly and superiorly until it has penetrated to a depth of approximately 1.5 cm and one feels the

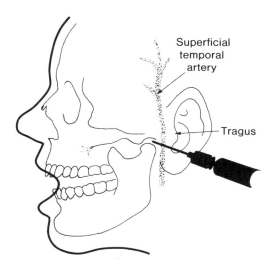

Figure 7.17. Temporomandibular joint aspiration. The joint should be entered just anterior to the tragus of the ear and anterior to the superficial temporal artery. The patient's mouth should be slightly open when this procedure is performed, to make entrance into the joint easier.

needle freely in the joint space. The joint can be localized by placing the finger over the site of insertion before performance of the procedure and asking the patient to open and close his mouth.

FRACTURE PRINCIPLES, CASTING TECHNIQUES AND COMMON SPLINTS

Initial Management

In the initial assessment of a fracture, a number of important questions must be answered. Is the fracture stable or unstable? If it is unstable, it must be stabilized by some form of external splinting or traction before any movement or transportation of the patient. There must be an assessment as to whether there is any associated injury involving the surrounding vessels, viscera, skin, or nerves. A well-documented neurovascular examination must be performed before any assessment is made of the patient with suspected or clinically obvious fracture. As a general rule, elevation is crucial when dealing with extremity injuries to promote adequate drainage and to permit healing without swelling. In the noncompliant patient, particularly in the pediatric age-group, one may apply a much larger dressing than is necessary in order that the involved extremity will be adequately immobilized, because the adult patient will be reluctant to remove and re-dress a large complicated dressing and the pediatric patient will forget about the existence of his injured part under a bulky dressing; both patient types will be less likely to unravel their dressing and move the injured extremity. Table 7.2 indicates the splints and casts which are commonly used and which are described in detail in this section.

EMERGENCY SPLINTING

The purposes of emergency splinting are threefold: to prevent further soft-tissue injury by the fracture fragments, for pain relief, and to decrease the incidence of clinical fat embolism. Perhaps the most commonly known splint is the Thomas splint, which is a half-ring splint used for femoral fractures. A modification of this

Table 7.2 Commonly Used Splints*

Splints	Indications	Comments
Dorsal distal phalanx splint	Avulsion fracture involving the extensor tendon of the distal phalanx	This must be maintained in position for 6 weeks. Splint must not interfere with motion at the PIP joint.
Hairpin splint	Comminuted fracture of the distal phalanx of a finger	This should remain in place until pain and swelling subside.
Volar and dorsal finger splints	Collateral ligament injuries of the PIP, DIP, or MP joint*	Place the MP joint in 50 to 90 degrees of flexion and the IP joint at 15 to 20 degrees of flexion.
Long arm posterior splint	Stable fractures of the forearm, fractures of the elbow, sprains and dislocations of the elbow	Apply a posterior slab with the elbow at 90 degrees and wrist in neutral position (unless contraindicated due to vascular compromise). Use sling after splint is applied.
Anterior-posterior splint of the forearm or arm	Fractures of the wrist and distal forearm in which more immobilization is necessary due to instability	With fractures of the forearm which are unstable, splints should extend above the elbow and thus be an anterior-posterior splint, immobilizing both the wrist and the elbow joint.
Sugar tong splint of the forearm	Fractures of the distal radius, wrist, and forearm	This splint permits immobilization in supination or pronation.
Sugar tong splint of the arm	Fractures of the humeral shaft	For stable fractures with no displacement, this splint along with a collar and cuff is all that is necessary. For unstable fractures, immobilize the fracture with this splint and refer the patient for definitive care.
Common sling	Used in numerous situations in which one desires immobilization of the upper extremity	
Collar and cuff	With a sugar tong splint of the arm for stable humeral fractures	
Stockinette valpeau	For immobilization of unstable fractures of the proximal humerus which have a tendency to displace due to the pull of the pectoralis major	This splint relaxes the pectoralis major which has a tendency to displace fractures of the proximal humerus.
Posterior splint of the ankle	Complex ankle sprains, initial treatment for immobilization of fractures of the ankles, initial management of foot fractures and distal tibial fractures	
Gutter splint	Stable phalangeal and metacarpal fractures	Splints should be applied so that the MP joint is at 50 to 90 degrees, depending on pain, and the IP joints are at 15 to 20 degrees.
Thumb spica	Scaphoid fractures	
Short arm cast	Simple fractures of the forearm, particularly incomplete fractures in children, stable distal forearm and metacarpal fractures	
Dynamic finger splint	Sprain of IP or MP joints of fingers or toes	

* PIP, proximal interphalangeal; DIP, distal interphalangeal; MP, metacarpophalangeal; IP, interphalangeal.

splint is the Hare traction splint, based on the same principle of applying continuous traction to the fracture to stabilize it and to prevent further soft-tissue injury (Fig. 7.18). These splints are practical and safe to use and provide good support for the patient in transport. Once a splint is applied, it should not be removed before x-ray evaluation. A new splint which is becoming popular is the Sager traction splint. This splint has many advantages over the Thomas splint, Hare traction splint, and other half-ring splints, including its relative ease of application and ability to provide stability of the femoral fracture without angulating the proximal femoral frac-

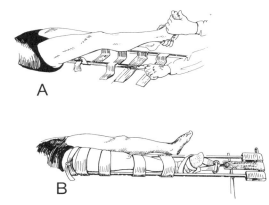

A

B

Figure 7.18. A half-ring fracture splint is shown. The two most commonly used are the Hare and the Thomas splints. *A.* Traction is applied to the patient's extremity in which there is a fractured femur, and the leg is lifted while an assistant places the half-ring splint beneath the involved leg as shown. *B.* With the splint in position, the ankle straps as well as straps along the thigh and leg are applied, and traction is applied through the ankle straps.

tured segment as occurs with use of the Thomas splint. The Sager traction splint is the authors' preference in emergency stabilization of all proximal femoral and shaft fractures of the femur in both the pediatric and the adult age-group. The splint is shown in Figure 7.19. It can be applied to the outer side or inner side of the leg, as shown and described in Figures 7.20 through 7.22. The splint does not have a half-ring posteriorly, which eliminates any pressure on the sciatic nerve and most importantly eliminates the angulation of the fracture site which occurs with half-ring splints. The advantages of this splint are listed in Table 7.3.

Inflatable splints, made of a double-walled polyvinyl jacket with a zipper fastener, placed around the injured limb are quite popular at the present time. While they afford the advantages of easy application and control of swelling, there are disadvantages to using them and these must be recognized. They are useful only

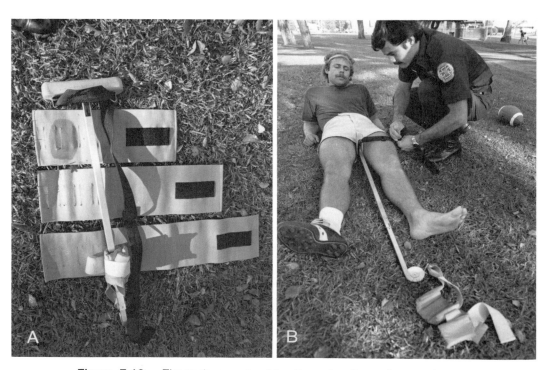

A

B

Figure 7.19. The various parts of the Sager traction splint are shown.

Table 7.3. Advantages of the Sager Traction Splint

1. No sciatic nerve compression as may occur with half-ring splint devices.
2. Flexion of the proximal femoral segment (as occurs with half-ring splint devices with midshaft and especially proximal one-third femoral fractures) is eliminated. This results in a more perfect bony alignment.
3. Overtraction, common with half-ring devices, resulting in knee edema and injury to epiphyseal growth centers in children is eliminated. The precise weight of traction, based on 10% of body weight of the patient and not to exceed 22 pounds, can be applied. The amount of traction applied is shown on the circular metered wheel.
4. The same splint can be used for pediatric and for adult patients.
5. This splint can be used with most trousers in place.
6. The splint can be used in patients with groin injuries by strapping it to the outer side of the leg.
7. The splint can be used in patients with severe pelvic fractures.
8. The ankle straps are so placed that one can monitor dorsalis pedis pulse with the splint in place.
9. The splint comes with a cross bar which permits splinting of bilateral femoral fractures with one splint between the legs.
10. Splints of the fracture are in a more anatomical position, so there is no rotation of the proximal fragment outward.

for fractures of the forearm, wrist, and ankle. All too often one sees patients with fractures in sites other than those indicated above who have been placed in an inflatable splint in the pre-hospital setting. This splint provides little or no support. When inflated at two pressures of 40 mm of mercury, they markedly reduce the blood flow to the limb and may even cause complete cessation of blood flow in some patients. Thus, circulatory embarrassment may occur at high pressures, and at lower pressures they may be ineffective in providing support. These splints should not be applied over clothing, as they may cause skin blisters. The application of these splints is shown in Figure 7.23. The pillow splint is an alternative type of splint which can be used in the pre-hospital setting and can be fashioned by wrapping an ordinary pillow tightly around a lower extremity fracture and securing it with safety pins as shown in Figure 7.24. A splint can be made from towels wrapped around a limb and supported on either side by wooden splints as demonstrated in Figure 7.25. This type of splint can be used for fractures of the forearm, as well as those of the lower extremity. The only additional support necessary when applying such a splint to the upper extremity is a sling. Patients who are seen in the pre-hospital setting with an open fracture can be splinted in a manner similar to those above. However, the site of skin puncture should be covered with a sterile dressing, and one should be careful not to reposition any exposed bony fragments through the skin back into the wound, as this will cause further contamination.

SELECTION OF DEFINITIVE TREATMENT

The selection of the definitive treatment of a fracture is a joint effort between the emergency physician and the referring doctor. Table 7.4 shows some of the common fractures, dislocations and sprains and gives general guidelines as to the initial splint or sling to use. Some fractures can be treated safely and followed by the emergency physician, while others need urgent consultation for operative intervention. These are discussed in the individual sections of the text. Closed treatment of fractures may include some form of manipulative reduction, which should be performed in the first 6 to 12 hours since swelling rapidly ensues and makes reduction more difficult. A displaced fracture usually leaves the periosteum intact on one side. Without this intact periosteal bridge, reduction would be difficult to maintain (Fig. 7.26). To reduce a fracture, one must apply traction in the long axis of the bone and reverse the mechanism that produced the fracture (Fig. 7.26B and C). One should align the fragment that can be manually maneuvered with the one which cannot. An intact periosteal bridge may help align the traction for reduction; however, soft-tissue interposition or a large hematoma may make reduction by closed means impossible. Once reduction is accomplished, immobilization with plaster, continuous traction or some form of splint is required to hold the position.

Traction is a good means for immobilization of some fractures. Skin traction should be used primarily, and usually temporarily, in children. When skin traction is used in adults, it should always be temporary and should never be applied with adhesive tape to the skin but rather with moleskin tape (Fig. 7.27). The limb is taped and traction is applied to the tape via a block of wood suspended from the end of the tape. One must be careful to protect all bony prominences with cotton wads. Skeletal traction applied through a pin placed through a bony prominence distal to the fracture site is a good form of immobilization, especially in comminuted fractures which cannot be held by plaster fixation. Skeletal traction is used most frequently in fractures of the femur and is also used in some humeral fractures.

Fractures through the metaphysis of a long bone have a good blood supply and heal well as a general rule, whereas diaphyseal fractures heal slower and need more attention due to the poor blood supply at this portion of the bone.

OPERATIVE TREATMENT OF FRACTURES

Indications

The emergency physician must be aware of the indications for operative intervention in fractures; while these are discussed in the individual sections, some general guidelines can be stated here. Operative intervention is indicated in the following circumstances:

In displaced intra-articular fractures
When there is associated arterial injury with the fracture
When experience shows that open treatment yields better results
When closed methods fail to heal
When the fracture is through a meta-

static lesion, open treatment is usually indicated.
In patients in whom continued confinement in bed would be undesirable, open reduction and internal fixation may be indicated.

Casting

One should not equate the presence of a fracture with the need for casting. Casts are used for three reasons: to immobilize a fracture to permit healing, to relieve pain by rest, and to stabilize an unstable fracture.

The plaster rolls or slabs used in casting are rolls of muslin stiffened by dextrose or starch and impregnated with a hemihydrate of calcium sulfate. When water is added, the calcium sulfate takes up the water and a reaction occurs which liberates heat; this heat is noted by both the patient and the physician applying the cast. Accelerator substances are added to the bandages which allow them to set at differing rates. Common table salt can be used to retard the setting of the plaster if this is desired, by simply adding the salt to the water. Acceleration of the setting occurs by increasing the temperature of the water or by adding alum to the water. The colder the water temperature, the longer the plaster takes to set. There are several methods to apply plaster.

Skin tight casts applied directly over the skin, although advocated by some in the past, are no longer used due to the complications of pressure sores and the circulatory embarrassment that may ensue. Most commonly today we use a stockinette applied at the ends of the cast (Fig. 7.28A), followed by a sheet of cotton padding (Webril®); the padding should be applied from the distal to the proximal end of the limb (Fig. 7.28B). Too much padding reduces the efficacy of the cast and permits excessive motion. Generally the more padding used, the more plaster is needed. The cotton padding interposed between the skin and the plaster provides elastic pressure and enhances the fixation of the limb by compensating for slight shrinkage in the tissues after the application of the cast.

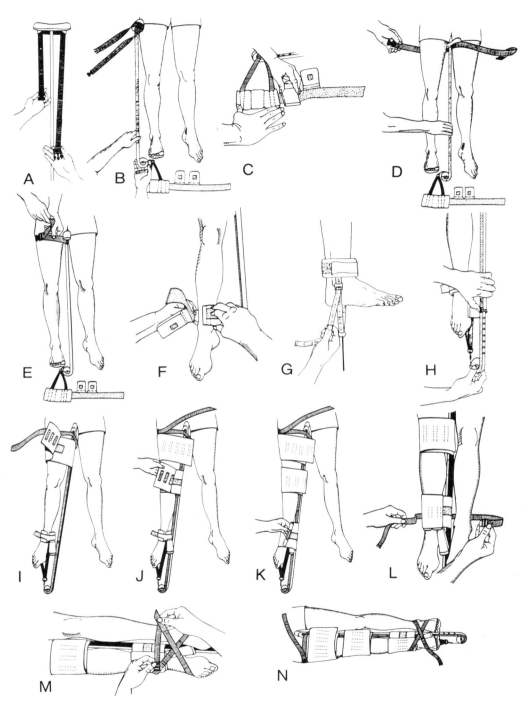

Figure 7.20. Standard application of the Sager emergency traction splint. *A.* Before applying the splint to the leg, slide the Kydex plastic buckle so that when it is closed it will be located on the anterior (top) surface of the thigh. *B.* Before application of the splint, obtain a rough measure of

Next the plaster is applied. The plaster bandage should be rolled in the same direction as the padding and each turn should overlap the preceding layer of plaster by half the width. Always lay the plaster on the limb transversely, keeping the roll of plaster in contact with the surface of the limb almost continuously. Instead of being lightly guided around the limb, the roll should be shaped and smoothed

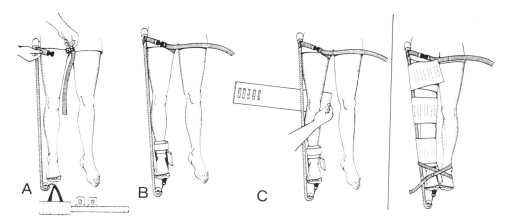

Figure 7.21.   Application of the Sager splint on the outside of the leg. *A.* Application of Sager splint on the outside of thigh is appropriate if perineal injuries or pelvic fractures are encountered. Carry out steps *A* through *C* shown in Figure 7.20, then apply the splint on the outside of the leg. *B.* Leave the Kydex buckle thigh strap loose so that it makes a sling around the upper thigh and forms an angle of about 55 degrees with the shaft of the splint. Pad the strap as needed. *C.* Apply the thigh straps in sequence, adding figure-eight strap as last step before securing the patient on the spine board.

---

length of splint needed. Extend the splint so that the wheel is at the heel. NOTE: Patients wearing tight jeans or tight underclothing, especially males, will find the splint uncomfortable to wear unless clothing is removed or cut open, which, of course, should be done as part of the secondary evaluation before application of the splint. *C.* Roughly estimate the size of the ankle and fold a number of gauze pads needed to provide padding all around the leg. *D.* Grasp the Kydex buckle and slide the thigh strap up under the leg so that the perineal cushion is snug against the perineum and ischial tuberosity. *E.* Tighten the Kydex buckle thigh strap, drawing the perineal-ischial pad to the lateral portion of the crotch. *F.* Apply the ankle harness tightly around the ankle, above the medial and lateral maleoli of the ankle. Check posterior tibial and dorsalis pedis pulses before hitch application and after traction is established. *G.* Shorten the loop of the harness connected to the cable ring by pulling on the strap threaded through the square "D" buckle. *H.* Extend the inner shaft of the splint by opening the shaft lock and pulling the inner shaft out until the desired amount of traction is noted on the calibrated wheel. Rough guide to determine amount of traction needed: apply traction equal to 10% of body weight to a maximum of 22 to 25 pounds (10 to 12 kilograms) of traction. *I.* Apply the longest 6 inch wide thigh strap as high up the thigh as possible. *J.* Apply the second longest thigh strap around the knee. Use padding if needed. *K.* Apply the shortest 6 inch wide strap over the ankle harness and lower leg. *L.* Apply figure-eight strap around both ankles by slipping the strap under the ankles. *M.* Cross strap over the feet as noted. Secure buckle snuggly. *N.* Patient's leg is now secured, traction is controlled, medial and lateral shift of distal fragment and internal and external rotation are prevented. Patient is ready for strapping to spine board for transport.

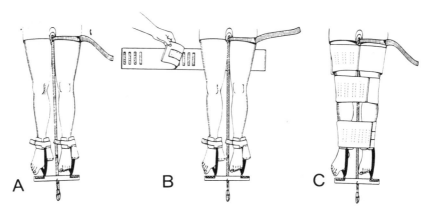

Figure 7.22. Application of the bilateral Sager splint. *A.* Application of double splint is accomplished in the same manner as with the single splint. Modify step *B* of Figure 7.20 by lengthening splint so that the harness bar is adjacent to the patient's heels. *B.* Apply the 6 inch wide thigh straps, hooking together more than one thigh strap to give you a proper length for wrapping strap around both thighs. *C.* Apply all three sections of leg strapping to secure the legs together. A figure-eight strap may be used around both ankles and feet, if needed.

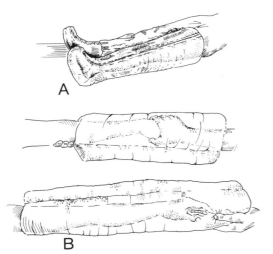

Figure 7.23. Inflatable splints are commonly used in field emergency care. *A.* An inflatable splint is shown applied over the leg and thigh in a patient with a fractured ankle. *B.* The deflated splint is applied by applying traction to the injured extremity and then applying the splint over the physician's hand and forearm onto the injured extremity. While traction is maintained the splint is inflated.

with pressure applied by the thenar eminence. This thenar pressure should be applied to the middle of the plaster roll, which permits no excessive pressure to

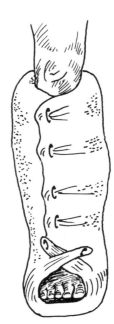

Figure 7.24. A pillow splint.

fall on either edge of the bandage so that no sharp ridges occur. Each turn should be smoothed with the thenar eminence of the left hand as the right hand guides the roll around the limb. As the limb tapers, the bandage is made to lie evenly by small tucks made with the index finger and

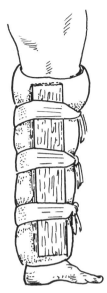

Figure 7.25. A splint fashioned from towels and wooden splints is shown. Towels are wrapped to protect the involved extremity, and wooden slabs are applied to both sides of the extremity; the entire device is secured with rags or pieces of towel as noted.

thumb of the left hand before each turn is smoothed into position (Fig. 7.28C). As the cast is applied, it is smoothed by the palms and the thenar eminences of both hands (Fig. 7.28D). Remember that the durability and strength of the cast depend on the welding together of each individual turn by these smoothing movements of the left hand and the final smoothing out with both hands (Fig. 7.28E). One should concentrate on making the two ends of the cast of adequate thickness; it is easy to make the center too thick, which provides no additional support at the fracture site (Fig. 7.29). A common problem is to use too many narrow bandages, which gives the cast a more lumpy appearance. Four, six and eight inch bandages should be the most commonly used bandages for most casting. Another common mistake in bandaging is not applying the plaster tightly enough, especially over the proximal fleshy portion of the limb, where greater tension is needed than at the distal bony parts, resulting in a loose cast.

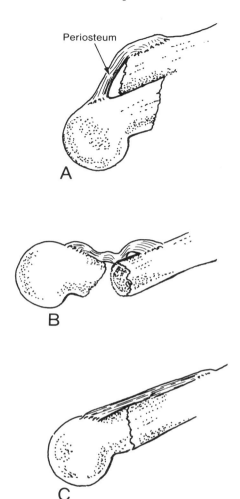

Figure 7.26. *A.* The intact periosteal bridge is shown. This aids in reducing a displaced fracture. *B.* To reduce a fracture, traction is applied in the long axis of the bone and the fracture is reduced by reversing the mechanism which produced it. *C.* The reduction is maintained by the intact periosteal sleeve as shown.

If one needs to reinforce the cast, as in an obese patient with a walking cast, this should be done by adding a fin to the front (Fig. 7.30) not by adding posterior splints to the back, as this adds no extra strength but only adds weight to the cast. Posterior slabs are used when one wants to add strength to the "sole of the foot" to prevent breakage there. Plaster boots are available and are preferred to walking heels by some

Table 7.4. Common Fractures, Dislocations and Sprains and Their Treatment

Fracture, Dislocation or Sprain	Treatment	Page
Comminuted fracture of distal phalanx—hand	Hairpin splint	
Mallet fracture of distal phalanx—hand	Dorsal distal phalanx splint	
Fracture of middle or proximal phalanx	Ulnar or radial gutter splint	
Fracture of metacarpals	Ulnar or radial gutter splint	
Suspected fracture of scaphoid	Sugar tong splint to forearm	
Suspected fracture of dorsal chip of carpal	Thumb spica cast, volar splint	
Stable fracture of distal radius	Sugar tong splint to forearm	
Unstable distal radius fracture	Anterior-posterior splint (short arm) or long arm	
Fracture of radius and ulna	Long arm anterior and posterior splint	
Fracture distal humerus	Long arm anterior and posterior splint	
Fracture of humerus shaft	Sugar tong splint of arm	
Fracture proximal humerus	Sugar tong splint of arm, sling and swathe, sling and valpeau	
Fracture of femur	Sager traction splint	
Fracture of ankle	Posterior splint ankle	
Fracture of phalanges—foot	Dynamic "toe" splint	
Collateral ligament		
Sprain of I.P. or M.P. joints (1° or mild 2°)	Dynamic finger splint	
Severe 2°	Dorsal or volar finger splint	
Complete rupture 3°	Gutter splint	
Elbow sprain	Posterior splint elbow	
Elbow dislocation	Posterior splint elbow	
Shoulder dislocation	Sling and swathe	
Collateral ligament sprain knee		
Mild or swelling	Jones compression swelling	
Moderate or severe	Posterior splint knee	
Patella dislocation	Posterior splint knee	
Knee dislocation	Posterior splint knee	
Ankle sprain	Posterior splint ankle	
Tibiotalar dislocation	Posterior splint ankle	
Sprain I.P. joints of foot	Dynamic "toe" splint	

patients, although currently in the emergency center a walking heel remains the most commonly applied device for ambulation (Fig. 7.31).

The application of a walking heel should be under the center of the foot (Fig. 7.32).

When applying a cast to the upper extremity, one should leave the hand free by stopping the cast at the metacarpal heads dorsally and the proximal flexor crease of the palm to permit normal finger motion (Fig. 7.33).

A window may be placed in a cast when a fracture is accompanied by a laceration or any skin lesions which need care while treating the fracture. Windows are best made as shown in Figure 7.34 by covering the wound with a bulky piece of sterile gauze and then applying the cast over the dressing in the normal manner (Fig. 7.34B). At the end, the window is cut out in the cast over the "bulge" created by the gauze dressing (Fig. 7.34C). The defect always should be covered with a dressing and, over the dressing, a piece of sponge rubber or felt held snugly in place with an Ace® bandage so that herniation of the soft tissue and subsequent swelling around the window and ulceration of the skin from pressure at the sides of the defect do not occur.

There are many types of casts such as

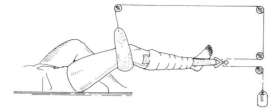

Figure 7.27. Skin traction applied to the leg. This type of traction is often provided in dealing with fractures of the distal femur and some distal humeral fractures.

spica casts, patellar tendon bearing casts and, more recently, cast braces; however, these are not used by the emergency physician and are not discussed here.

Recently, fiberglass casts which are made of light-weight plastic have been introduced. These casts are durable and radiolucent and have the advantage of not being softened or damaged when they become wet. These have limited application to fresh fractures since they are more difficult to apply and a snug fit is more difficult to achieve, but they are commonly used as a second or subsequent cast. They are especially useful for open fractures since the patient can use a whirlpool or other forms of "wet" therapy while in the cast.

Plaster sores are complications of plaster casts which can occur due to excessive pressure. Patients complain of a burning pain or discomfort. These can be avoided by eliminating sharp ends in the cast and by avoiding indented spots in the cast. Felt pads placed between the layers of padding in the cast tend to migrate and pressure sores may result.

Splints also are commonly used to immobilize injuries. The most common splints used are the posterior splints to the lower extremity for ankle and foot injuries, and similar splints are used in the upper extremity (Fig. 7.35). Splints offer the advantage of permitting soft-tissue swelling to occur without compromising the circulation. Ice packs can be applied to the site of injury along with elevation of the limb, since the splint will permit penetration of the cold to maximize its effect. These reasons, along with its ease of application,

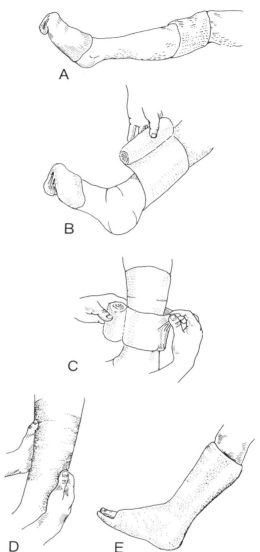

Figure 7.28. *A.* Stockinette is applied to the ends of the cast. *B.* Cotton padding or Webril® should be applied from the distal end of the limb proceeding proximally. See text for discussion. A plaster bandage should be rolled in the same direction as the padding, and each turn should overlap the preceding layer of plaster by half the width. *C.* As the limb tapers, the bandages are made to lie evenly by small tucks made with the index finger and thumb of the left hand as shown. *D.* This then is smoothed down by the palms of the hands and the thenar eminences as shown. *E.* The final outcome is a well-molded, smooth, and strong cast.

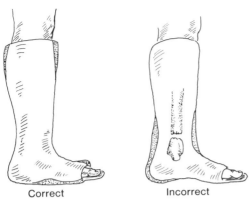

Figure 7.29. One of the most common mistakes is layering the plaster more thickly than is necessary around the fracture site by the physician who thinks this will increase the strength. One should concentrate on making the two ends of the cast of adequate thickness as this provides for the most durable cast.

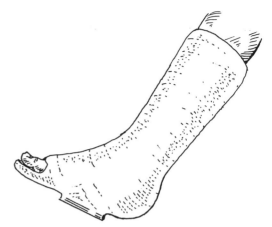

Figure 7.31. A walking heel is shown in the center of the foot. The cast may be extended distally from the sole to provide support for the toes; however, this is not necessary with more proximal injuries.

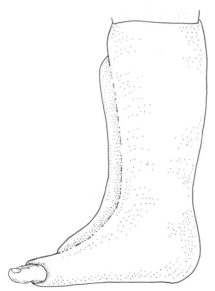

Figure 7.30. A fin applied to the front of the cast adds strength to the cast at the ankle to prevent breakage there and prevents breaking at the ankle. The fin is made of 2 or 3 strips of 2 inch plaster slab applied over the anterior aspect of the cast. This is covered by a final roll of plaster with the result being an anterior "fin".

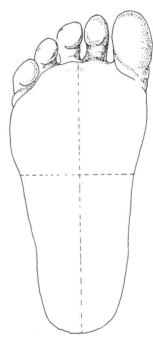

Figure 7.32. Walking heels should be applied under the center of the foot.

make splinting of upper and lower extremity fractures a commonly used method of immobilization in the emergency management; later a more definitive cast is applied. The disadvantages of splinting are that they permit excessive motion and provide little stability for a fracture which has been reduced and needs to be maintained in a certain position.

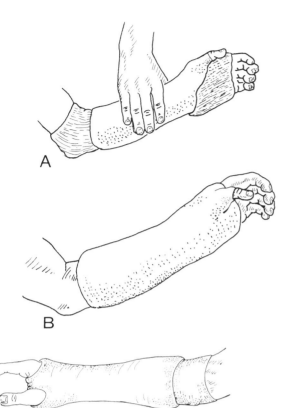

Figure 7.33. The fingers and the thumb should be free to move when a cast is applied to the forearm for fractures of the distal forearm.

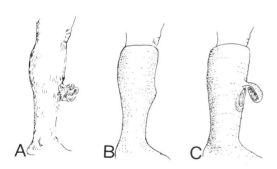

Figure 7.34. When a wound is present over the leg and the limb requires casting, a window can be cut out of the cast. *A.* A wad of gauze is applied over the wound after it is adequately dressed and/or sutured. *B.* A cast is then applied over the wad of gauze. This creates a lump in the cast as shown. *C.* The "lump" then is cut out, which permits a window through which the wound may be managed.

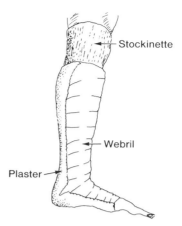

Figure 7.35. A posterior splint to the ankle. These splints offer the advantage of permitting soft tissue swelling without compromising circulation. Added support may be obtained by extending the splint over the medial and lateral sides to strengthen it. When Webril® is applied under the plaster, it should be incised longitudinally to permit swelling to occur.

CHECKING CASTS

Any circumferential cast applied should be accompanied by written instructions to the patient or family members instructing them about signs of the cast being too tight. *Increasing pain,* swelling, coolness, or change in skin color of the distal portions of the extremity are signs of a cast being too tight. Paresthesias, poor capillary refill, pain on passive extension of the phalanges distal to the cast are important signs and symptoms of ischemia from a too tight circumferential cast. The patient should be checked immediately and he must be made aware of the dangers of ignoring such problems. As a general rule, we recommend that any circumferential cast be checked the following day for signs of circulatory compromise. The patient must be instructed to elevate the limb for 24 hours after the application of a cast to avoid problems.

If the cast is too tight, one must remember to split not only the plaster casting but also the inner padding to reduce the pressure significantly. This was well demonstrated in a recent study which showed that there was no significant reduction in pressure when only the plaster was opened and that there was significant reduction when the padding also was incised (46).

ANESTHESIA FOR FRACTURES

There are many forms of anesthesia which can be used in fracture reduction. Many fractures require general anesthesia, particularly those in small children. One must weigh the risk of general anesthesia against the advantages of regional blocks, which can be satisfactorily used in most of the common reductions performed in the emergency center. Injection of anesthetic into the fracture hematoma is commonly done but may not achieve adequate pain control.

Bier Block

A Bier block is an excellent form of anesthesia for leg, foot, forearm, and hand fractures. This type of anesthesia is discussed in detail in Chapter 3: "Anesthesia and Regional Blocks"; the reader is referred to that chapter for contraindications, complications, technique, etc.

Regional Block

This is another good form of anesthesia for upper extremity reductions. See the chapter on anesthesia for complete information.

Special Considerations For Fracture Management

OPEN FRACTURES

Open fractures provide a significant challenge to the physician. One must check the skin around the wound and note what contaminants may be in the wound. There should be no attempt to digitally explore the wound in the emergency center, as little information will be provided, and an increased risk of infection will result. Local debridement is indicated in all cases. When a small wound is noted on the skin which overlies a fracture, and a question arises as to whether or not it communicates with the fracture, one can safely check the wound with a sterile blunt probe to see if bone is touched. If the question still remains, then prudent man-

agement mandates treatment as if it were an open fracture with debridement of the wound in the operating room. The wound should be dressed with a sterile dressing and the extremity should be splinted. There are some open fractures which do not require meticulous debridement and which have a good prognosis, including open fracture of the distal phalanx of the digits; this is the open fracture most commonly seen in the emergency center. The usual prudent therapy advocated for open fractures elsewhere is not necessary here, as the blood supply to the distal phalanx is excellent and fractures clinically heal without osteomyelitis in this area. The treatment of open fractures of the distal phalanx includes cleansing the area, treating the fracture and any open laceration as one would routinely and following the patient.

Gutter Splints

Gutter splints are used for the treatment of stable phalangeal and metacarpal fractures. The fractures which are most commonly treated by gutter splints are those which are simple with no rotational abnormality or significant displacement. In fractures involving the ring and little finger, the digit is immobilized in a gutter splint as shown in Figure 7.36A. The splint is formed by using plaster slabs cut to the proper size and then applied and molded into a U-shaped splint over the ring and little fingers, while the fingers are held in the position shown. The splint should extend from the fingertips to just below the elbow, permitting flexion and extension at the elbow joint. Approximately 6 to 8 sheets of plaster provide an adequate thickness to give good support. The plaster should be applied directly to the skin, as shown, with the fingers held at approximately 50 degrees of flexion at the metacarpophalangeal joint and 15 to 20 degrees of flexion at the interphalangeal joints. With fractures involving the index and long fingers a similar splint is used, as shown in Figure 7.36C. This splint has a piece cut out for the thumb. The splints are held in place with an elastic bandage, as shown in Figure 7.36B and D. Due to the light weight of these splints, the patients generally do not require a sling or support; however, the patient must be advised to elevate the hand continuously for the first 24 hours to prevent swelling, which is a common complication in fractures involving the hand and can lead to a significant loss of function.

Thumb Spica Or Wrist Gauntlet Cast

The thumb spica is the most commonly used cast for management of scaphoid fractures of the wrist in the emergency center. It is made by applying a stockinette dressing to the arm and extending the stockinette from the hand to the midarm, or more proximally when a long arm spica cast is desirable. The decision as to whether to use a short arm or a long arm cast must be individualized to the patient and is in part contingent upon the philosophy of the treating physician. This is fol-

lowed by the application of a cotton bandage (Webril)® which is then followed by the application of plaster rolls (Fig. 7.37). The method for applying plaster rolls has been discussed earlier in the chapter and is not repeated here. Before the application of the final roll, the stockinette should be folded back over the cast and the final plaster roll applied, as shown in Figure 7.38B where the distal end of the stockinette has been folded back. The position of the thumb must be maintained when applying this cast as shown. The optimal position in which the thumb should be held is provided by asking the patient to imagine he is holding a glass in his hand. Although the interphalangeal joint may be incorporated in the cast we have described, it should be mentioned that this is controversial regarding the need to immobilize this joint in treating scaphoid fractures. The fingers are left free so that there is full motion at the metacarpophalangeal joints. The position of the forearm shown here is the neutral position, midway between supination and pronation. In using this cast for scaphoid fractures some authors advocate extending it above the elbow joint, thus making it a long arm cast with the elbow flexed to 90 degrees; however, as mentioned above, there is controversy. It is the authors' preference to use a short arm cast in treating these fractures.

Short and Long Arm Cast

A short arm cast is used in the emergency center for immobilization of a number of simple fractures involving the distal forearm and metacarpals. The cast is made by applying the stockinette from the fingers to above the elbow as shown in Figure

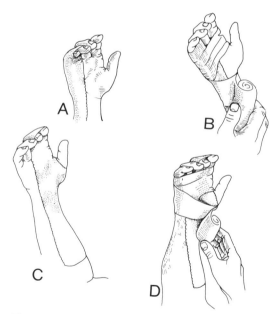

Figure 7.36. Ulnar (*A* and *B*) and radial (*C* and *D*) gutter splints are shown. These splints are used in management of proximal and middle phalanx fractures and metacarpal fractures. The U-shaped gutter splint is fashioned from strips of plaster and is applied to the ulnar or radial border of the hand as shown.

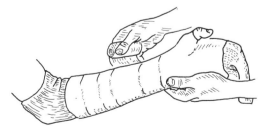

Figure 7.37. A thumb spica cast. See text for details.

7.38A. Following this a cotton bandage (Webril)® is applied over the stockinette with the thumb remaining free at the metacarpophalangeal joint and the fingers free at the same level. Two to three plaster rolls are then applied, while the hand is maintained in the position shown in Figure 7.38B. The stockinette then is folded over this cast, and a final roll of plaster bandages is applied (Fig. 7.38B and C). The patient should be able to use his fingers and thumb freely, without any impingement on normal motion after the cast is applied. A long arm cast is produced in a similar fashion with the exception that it is extended above the elbow to approximately the midarm position, with the elbow flexed at 90 degrees. The long arm cast is used in treating most fractures involving the forearm.

Dorsal Distal Phalanx Splint

Avulsion fractures involving the extensor tendon attachment to the distal phalanx can be treated in the emergency center with a dorsal extension splint applied over the dorsal surface of the distal inter-

phalangeal joint (Fig. 7.39B). Either a dorsal or a volar splint is useful in treating avulsion fractures of the distal phalanx; however, the authors prefer the dorsal splint because it provides more support since there is less "padding" on the dorsal aspect of the finger and so the splint is in closer contact with the bone which it is to support. In using this splint, one should not hyperextend the distal interphalangeal joint as has been previously recommended in older textbooks. Full extension is the position of choice when applying the splint, and this position must be maintained for 6 weeks with the splint in place. The splint should never be removed or the finger flexed during this time. The splint should be positioned so that it does not interfere with motion at the proximal interphalangeal joint. Most of these splints are made of flexible metal strips which are available in all emergency centers.

Hairpin Splint

This splint is fashioned out of a thin metal strip or a large hairpin (Fig. 7.39A) and provides excellent protection in fractures involving the distal phalanx of the fingers which generally need no support but do need protection from external injuries, such as comminuted fractures. The hairpin splint provides this protection without allowing any contact between the splint and the skin surface, which might produce pain.

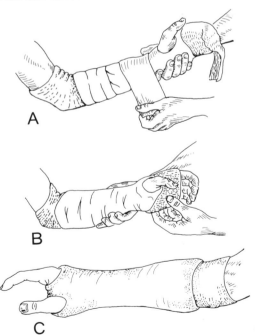

Figure 7.38.   A short arm cast. See text for discussion.

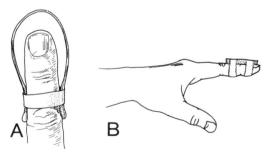

Figure 7.39.   *A.* The hairpin splint is commonly used for comminuted fractures of the distal phalanx. *B.* A dorsal splint applied across the distal interphalangeal joint is used for treating ruptures of the central slip of the extensor tendon or mallet fractures.

Dorsal And Volar Finger Splints

Dorsal and volar finger splints are used in the management of a variety of injuries, the most common being collateral ligament injuries involving the proximal or distal interphalangeal joint or the metacarpophalangeal joint. The splints are fashioned from commercially available metallic splints which have a sponge rubber padding on one side. The splint is cut to the proper size and shaped as desired (Fig. 7.40). When the splint is to be applied for a prolonged period, the metacarpophalangeal joint should be positioned at 50 degrees of flexion and the interphalangeal joint should be flexed to approximately 15 to 20 degrees. This position provides for optimal stretch of the collateral ligaments of the metacarpophalangeal and interphalangeal joints and avoids the problem of contracture of these ligaments as healing progresses. One can test this on himself by extending the long finger at the metacarpophalangeal joint and moving it from side to side. A wide range of motion is noted in doing this; with the finger flexed at 50 degrees at the MP joint, side-to-side motion is markedly reduced because the collateral ligaments are taut in this position. When stress testing shows complete rupture of a collateral ligament, a gutter splint should be used.

Dynamic Finger Splinting

This form of splinting is used commonly in sprains involving the collateral liga-ments of the interphalangeal joints of the hand. This type of splinting is used when there is minimal injury to the collateral ligament or after the collateral ligament has been treated with a splint and requires only moderate support. The most common joint injuries in which this type of splinting is used are stable first and second degree sprains of the proximal and distal interphalangeal joints. The injured finger is splinted to the adjacent normal finger which provides support for the injured digit while permitting motion, primarily of the metacarpophalangeal joint and limited motion of the interphalangeal joint. A piece of felt cut to the proper size is inserted between the fingers and the two digits are taped together as shown in Figure 7.41. This method of splinting is quite good for phalangeal fractures of the toe where alternative methods of splinting would be inconvenient.

Universal Hand Dressing

The universal hand dressing is used in a number of hand problems which present to the emergency center, including infec-

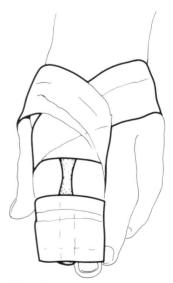

Figure 7.41. Dynamic finger splinting. This type of splinting is used when a collateral ligament is injured only minimally or after the collateral ligament has been initially treated with a splint and requires only moderate support.

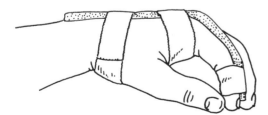

Figure 7.40. A dorsal finger splint. These splints provide support for sprains of the collateral ligaments of the digits; however, they should not be used for fracture management. The metacarpophalangeal joint should be flexed to 50 degrees or greater and the interphalangeal joint should be flexed 15 to 20 degrees.

tions of the hand, serious lacerations, and some forms of tendonitis. The position in which the universal hand dressing immobilizes the hand provides for optimal lymphatic drainage and a functionally resting position for all the joints to facilitate adequate healing. The optimal position in which to immobilize the hand when treating a patient with a hand infection or soft-tissue injury is demonstrated in Figure 7.42A. This position provides 15 degrees of extension at the wrist, 50 degrees of flexion at the MP joint, and 20 to 30 degrees of flexion at the interphalangeal joints with the thumb position as shown. This position permits optimal drainage for swelling, which occurs with virtually all serious hand problems and is a serious limiting factor to adequate healing. To maintain this position in a soft dressing, fluffs are placed between the fingers and thumb as shown in Figure 7.42A. These fluff dressings should extend down to the mid-forearm. This is followed with the application of a gauze roll around the fluffs and between the fingers to secure them in place (Fig. 7.42B). This is followed with an Ace® wrap with holes cut out for the fingers when it is applied. Finally, half-inch tape is applied to hold the Ace® wrap in position. The patient must be advised to elevate the hand above the level of the heart to facilitate the drainage, especially with infections, for which the universal hand dressing has been applied.

Long Arm Posterior Splints

A long arm posterior splint is commonly used in the emergency center to immobilize a number of injuries involving the elbow and forearm. The splint is produced by wrapping a cotton bandage (Webril)® around the forearm from the midpalmar region to the midarm. This is followed by applying a plaster slab to the posterior aspect of the forearm, extending above the elbow with the elbow held in a position of 90 degrees of flexion, and the forearm maintained in a neutral position that is neither supinated nor pronated (Fig. 7.43). A posterior plaster slab applied to the arm should consist of 8 layers of plaster which are wide enough to provide a semicircular dressing around the circumference of the arm as shown in Figure 7.43. This splint can be cut from rolls of plaster or can be made from prefabricated slabs. This plaster is followed by an Ace® wrap to hold the plaster slab in place. A sling should be used after the splint has been applied. There are commercially available splints incorporating the plaster slabs, cotton bandage, and a foam sponging which can be cut to the proper length and applied in a similar fashion.

Anterior-Posterior Splints To The Forearm

Anterior and posterior molds are applied most commonly for the initial management of fractures involving the forearm and wrist in which immobilization must be maintained in a more secure position than with a simple posterior splint and in which, due to anticipated swelling, a cir-

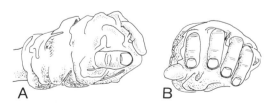

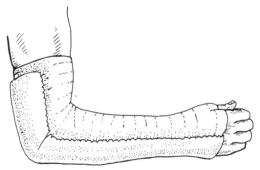

Figure 7.42.   A universal hand dressing consists of fluffs applied between the fingers. This makes for a bulky dressing. The fluffs are then covered by a Kling® bandage, which is followed by an Ace® wrap. See text for discussion.

Figure 7.43.   A posterior plaster splint is applied to the forearm. The splint is applied to the forearm. The splint is extended above the elbow with the elbow flexed to 90 degrees. See text for discussion.

cular cast is not desirable. With these splints, the forearm can be maintained in any degree of flexion, supination or pronation. Stockinette is first applied over the forearm and the hand, and splints are cut to proper length from plaster slabs and applied anterior and posterior to the forearm, as shown in Figure 7.44A. With unstable fractures of the forearm the splint should extend above the elbow flexed at 90 degrees. The arm may be placed in a pronated or a supinated position to stabilize a fracture, depending on the site and position of the fracture which one is supporting. A cotton bandage dressing (Webril)® may be used under the splint; however, if this is done, the bandage should be incised lengthwise to permit swelling of the limb. An elastic wrap is used to hold the splints in position (Fig. 7.44B). A sling should be dispensed to support the forearm after splinting.

Sugar Tong Splint Of The Forearm

The sugar tong splint is commonly used to immobilize forearm fractures, particularly distal radius fractures at the wrist, in patients in whom it is desirable to maintain the forearm in some degree of supination or pronation. The forearm may be placed in a supinated or a pronated position during the application of the splint. A cotton bandage (Webril)® is first applied to the injured limb, followed by a single long plaster slab which extends from the distal palmar crease to the elbow following which it courses around the elbow to the dorsum of the hand just proximal to the metacarpophalangeal joint, thus encircling the elbow joint (Fig. 7.45). The advantages of this splint are that it permits immobilization in a position of pronation or supination without applying a circumferential cast, with its attendant hazards, and is a very simple splint to apply. A sling should be used after application of this splint.

Sugar Tong Splint To The Arm

A sugar tong splint also can be used in the initial management of fractures of the humeral shaft. Humeral shaft fractures are often displaced and, following reduction,

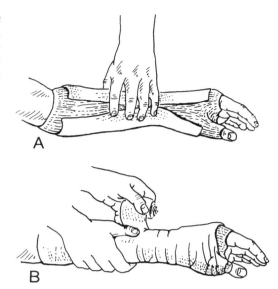

Figure 7.44. An anterior-posterior splint to the forearm. The splint can be extended to make a long arm anterior-posterior splint by extending the slabs to above the elbow. *A.* Stockinette is applied over the forearm. Following this, an anterior and a posterior plaster slab are applied. *B.* The anterior and posterior slabs are held in position with an Ace® wrap.

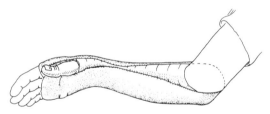

Figure 7.45. A sugar tong splint. See text for discussion.

an assistant may have to maintain position of the fracture while the splint is being applied, as shown in Figure 7.46A. The splint should extend from over the acromion region down the humerus to the axilla, then down the humerus and encircling the elbow joint (extension over the acromion is not properly demonstrated in the diagram). This should be applied over cotton bandage as previously discussed under "Sugar Tong Splints of the Forearm." Following this application the splint is held in place by an Ace® bandage as shown in

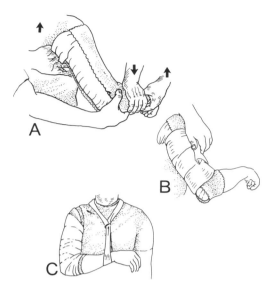

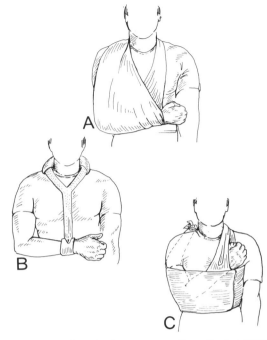

Figure 7.46. A sugar tong splint to the arm or a U-shaped coaptation splint. Webril® is applied to the arm in a one-layer dressing. Following this, a plaster slab is applied, extending from the axilla to the deltoid region. *A.* During this application, an assistant distracts the displaced and overriding segments of a humeral fracture as shown. *B.* An Ace® wrap or an Esmarch's bandage holds the U-shaped splint in position. *C.* A collar and cuff are then used to maintain the elbow in the flexed position.

Figure 7.47. *A.* A common sling. *B.* A collar and cuff. *C.* Stockinette valpeau dressing.

Figure 7.46B, followed by the use of a collar and cuff (Fig. 7.46C).

Types Of Slings

There are three types of slings which are commonly used within the emergency center: a common sling, a collar and cuff, and a stockinette valpeau. These are pictured in Figure 7.47 A through C, respectively. The common sling is the one most often used and is primarily used to support the arm in association with a number of injuries and disorders involving the upper extremity. The collar and cuff is an alternate method used to support the forearm and wrist in patients with humeral fractures treated with a coaptation splint (sugar tong splint to arm) and in those patients in whom a stable humeral fracture requires only the application of a collar and cuff for support. A stockinette valpeau

and swathe (the component which encircles the patient's waist) is used in situations where there is an unstable fracture involving the proximal humerus, which has a tendency to displace due to contraction of the pectoralis major muscle. The position demonstrated in Figure. 7.47C relaxes the pectoralis major and prevents it from displacing fractures involving the proximal humeral shaft.

Application Of A Posterior Splint To The Ankle

This type of splint is commonly used in the emergency center for the initial management of complex ankle sprains and to immobilize fractures of the ankle, foot, and distal tibia until definitive care can be instituted or until swelling subsides. Posterior splints applied to the ankle allow the effective use of ice packs in the treatment of postinjury swelling while providing adequate immobilization of the injured extremity. Stockinette dressing is applied over the leg to cover the area to which the plaster slabs are to be applied and should extend well above the knee and below the toes as shown in Figure 7.48A. A cotton bandage (Webril)® is then applied over the stockinette (Fig. 7.48A), followed by the application of posterior slabs of plaster composed of 8 to 10 sheets. The posterior splint should extend from the toes to below the knee, permitting comfortable flexion of the knee joint (Fig. 7.48B). With the splint properly applied, the patient should be able to flex his knee freely. When posterior splints are used, the foot should be held in 90 degrees of flexion. The stockinette is then folded over the plaster and an elastic wrap applied which secures the plaster to the leg (Fig. 7.48C). When swelling is a significant concern (as with a fracture), the cotton bandage may be incised before the elastic wrap is applied as it may act as a compressive dressing. Posterior splints incorporating the cotton bandage, plaster slabs, and foam sponging are available commercially.

Jones Compression Dressing

A Jones compression dressing is commonly used for soft-tissue injuries involving the knee joint. This dressing provides for immobilization of the limb and a compressive dressing for swelling while permitting some flexion and extension at the joint. The dressing is made by applying a layer of cotton bandage (Webril)® which extends from the groin to just above the

malleoli of the ankle. Following this, an elastic wrap is applied circumferentially from proximal to distal (Fig. 7.49). A second layer of Webril® is then applied, followed by another elastic wrap. This additional layer provides for added support, to maintain uniform compression when the first layer loses its elasticity.

REDUCTION OF SELECTED COMMON FRACTURES

Many of the fractures seen within the emergency center are splinted for immobilization and are referred for definitive care to an orthopedic surgeon. A detailed discussion of fracture management is beyond the scope of this text; however, a chapter on orthopedic procedures would not be complete without discussion of some of the common fractures managed by the emergency physician.

Clavicle Fractures (8, 31)

Clavicle fractures are the most common of all childhood fractures. Overall, clavicular fractures account for 5% of all fractures seen in all age-groups. Eighty percent of all clavicular fractures seen within the emergency center occur in the middle one third of this bone. Childhood clavicular fractures generally require little treatment as rapid healing and full return of function is the usual outcome. Adult clavicular fractures may be associated with complications and, therefore, require a more accurate reduction and closer follow-up to in-

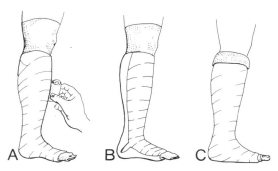

Figure 7.48. The application of a posterior splint to the ankle. See text for discussion. Commercial posterior splints are currently available for use in many emergency centers. The Webril® may be incised longitudinally to permit swelling to occur.

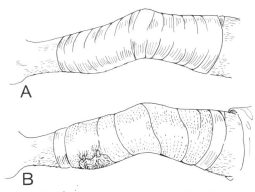

Figure 7.49. A Jones compression dressing.

sure a full return to normal functioning. Adult fractures may be complicated by excessive callous formation and with neurovascular compromise secondary to compression against the first rib. With a clavicular fracture in the midportion, one should examine the patient for and document any neurovascular compromise distal to the injury in the upper extremity.

A figure-of-eight clavicular strap is often utilized in managing these fractures. Commercial devices are available and, when applied properly, they are quite useful in children over the age of 10 years. The family must be instructed in the proper application and adjustment of this device (Fig. 7.50):

1. Pull both shoulders backward tightly as if standing in a military position.
2. Apply the commercial splint around both shoulders as if applying a backpack and tighten the posterior straps as shown in Figure 7.50A.
3. Examine the patient for neurovascular compromise and educate the family as to the symptoms of this complication.
4. Instruct the family in the method of tightening the splint daily. The splint will require frequent tightening and should be worn until the patient can abduct the extremity without pain and there is evidence of clinical union. Children generally require 3 to 5 weeks of immobilization, while adults require 6 weeks or more.

In children a properly applied figure-of-eight clavicular strap which is adjusted frequently is the treatment of choice. Patients must be seen in follow-up to insure proper reduction and maintenance of position. If the child or family is uncooperative and will not utilize the figure-of-eight splint properly, a referral for consideration of a shoulder spica is indicated. While a commercially available figure-of-eight splint can be utilized in the initial management within the emergency center for the reduction and maintenance of position of displaced clavicular fractures in the adult, if after 1 week the fracture is not adequately reduced, the patient should be re-ferred to an orthopedic surgeon for a shoulder spica cast. If the patient is uncooperative initially and will not properly wear and maintain the figure-of-eight strap, referral for a shoulder spica is indicated.

Colles' Fracture (5, 6, 15, 16)

Only simple Colles' fractures can be managed by the emergency physician

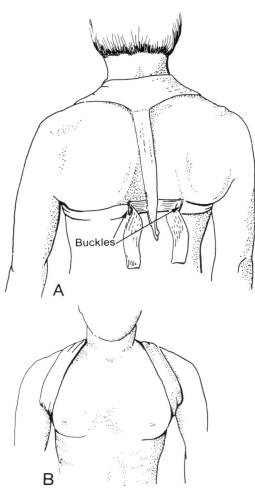

Figure 7.50. *A.* A figure-of-eight clavicular strap. The straps are applied around the shoulders and are adjusted by pulling on the two metal buckles. *B.* The patient should be instructed to hold his shoulders back and his chest out, as if standing at attention, when the straps are tightened.

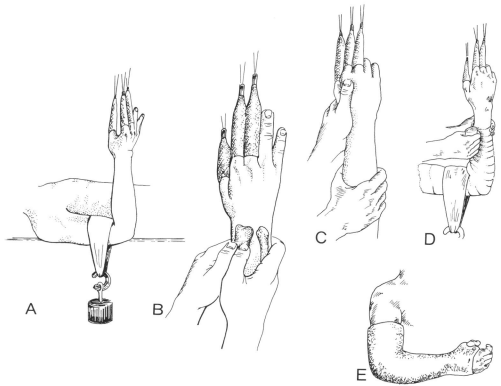

Figure 7.51. The reduction of a Colle's fracture is shown. *A.* Fingers in a Chinese finger trap to disimpact the fracture fragments. *B.* The fracture is reduced by applying a reducing force with the thumbs directing the distal segment volarly, after reversing the mechanism of the fracture by dorsal angulation, until the ends of the fractured fragments come in contact. *C.* Ulnar and volar displacement is corrected. *D.* If the reduction is unstable, the initial portion of a plaster cast is applied while the hand is in traction.

within the emergency center. Fractures of the distal radius and ulna with radiocarpal joint involvement and distal radial fractures with radioulnar joint involvement, in the authors' opinion, should be referred due to the high incidence of associated complications, including secondary joint stiffness, postreduction swelling with secondary compartment syndromes, and cosmetic defects which may follow seriously displaced distal forearm fractures as well as malunion. Only those fractures which are extra-articular involving the distal radius or those involving the distal radius and ulna should be managed within the emergency center by the emergency physician. Colles' fractures, even when managed appropriately, frequently result in

long-term complications. For this reason, only selected Colles' fractures should be treated by the emergency physician. All other distal forearm fractures should be splinted and referred for emergent treatment and follow-up.

The method of reduction of a Colles' fracture is demonstrated in Figure 7.51:

1. The optimal method of anesthesia is a regional block such as the Bier block (discussed in Chapter 3: "Anesthesia and Regional Blocks"). A less effective but acceptable method is to insert a needle into the fracture hematoma after adequate preparation, aspirate the hematoma surrounding the fracture, and inject 5 to 10 ml of Xylo-

caine® into the area. This form of anesthesia will work in most patients; however, it is often incomplete.

2. The recommended method of reduction is with *traction* followed by *manipulation*. Place the fingers in a Chinese finger trap (Fig. 7.51A) and elevate the wrist with the elbow in 90 degrees of flexion. Eight to 10 pounds of weight are then suspended from the elbow for a period of 5 to 10 minutes or until the fragments disimpact.

3. After disimpaction and continuing with traction, apply dorsal pressure over the distal fragment(s) with the thumbs and apply volar pressure over the proximal segments with the fingers (Fig. 7.51B). With the thenar eminence of the physician's hand applied over the fracture site, position the fragment in an ulnar and volar direction to achieve the proper positioning (Fig. 7.51C). When proper positioning has been achieved, the traction weight is removed.

4. The forearm should be immobilized in a position of slight supination or midposition with the wrist at 15 degrees of flexion and with 20 degrees of ulnar deviation. It should be noted that some orthopedic surgeons prefer to immobilize the patient in pronation. The position of the forearm is controversial and, before treatment is undertaken, consultation with the orthopedic surgeon who is to follow the patient is recommended.

5. The forearm should be wrapped in one layer of Webril®, followed by the application of an anterior-posterior long arm splint, sugar tong splint to the forearm or a short arm cast. Short arm splints may be utilized under the following circumstances:
   a. Impacted fracture for which reduction is not necessary.
   b. Stable fracture in elderly patient who needs to maintain mobility of the ipsilateral elbow, whether or not reduction of the Colles' fracture is needed.

NOTE

If reduction must be performed as indicated above, it is best to place the patient, especially children, in a long arm cast.

Displaced Surgical Neck Fractures Of The Humerus (1)

The emergency management of these fractures includes immobilization, ice, analgesics, and emergent referral. If emergent referral is not available in a situation of limb-threatening vascular compromise, reduction can be carried out by the following method:

1. Adequate analgesia for this reduction is best provided under general anesthesia; however, intravenous narcotic analgesics or a high axillary nerve block may be used within the emergency center. With the patient lying supine, the physician should apply steady downward traction to the arm along the long axis of the humerus with the elbow flexed completely (Fig. 7.52A).

2. While maintaining traction, the arm is adducted across the anterior chest and slightly flexed.

3. While traction is maintained at the elbow, the physician places his other

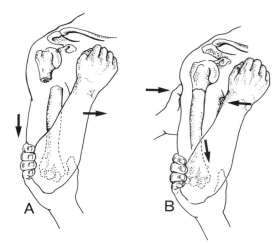

Figure 7.52. The reduction of a displaced surgical neck fracture of the humerus. See text for discussion.

hand around the arm just distal to the fracture site along the medial border of the humerus as shown in Figure 7.52B. The fragments are manually manipulated back into position with lateral forces directed by the physician's fingers and the traction is gradually released.

4. A complete neurovascular examination must be documented before and after any attempt at a manipulative reduction. Following this a sling and swathe dressing may be applied, or a stockinette valpeau and swathe can be used in situations in which there is an unstable fracture of the proximal humerus which has a tendency to displace due to contraction of the pectoralis major muscle. This position allows for relaxation of the pectoralis major. A sugar tong splint of the arm often is applied to aid in stabilization of the fracture in its proper position, and the patient is referred to an orthopedic surgeon.

Supracondylar Fractures Of The Distal Humerus (2, 3, 10, 11, 52, 57)

Supracondylar fractures of the distal humerus are seen often in the pediatric age-group and less commonly in the adult. The acute problem in the initial management of these fractures is to ascertain if there is any impingement on the brachial artery from the displaced fracture fragments (Fig. 7.53). One must assess the neurovascular status of the patient before any attempt at reduction. Reduction of these fractures should be attempted by an experienced physician, especially when vascular compromise is in question. When vascular compromise is not a problem, the patient should be splinted and emergently reduced by an orthopedic surgeon to avoid the delayed complications of ischemic contracture of the distal extremity. When reduction must be performed by the emergency physician, the technique is as follows: The procedure must be performed in a two-step maneuver, and these are described separately.

1. Either an axillary nerve block or a regional Beir block anesthesia may be used to provide analgesia in reducing these fractures (described in Chapter 3: Anesthesia and Regional Blocks).
2. The initial maneuver in reducing these fractures involves extension of the elbow and distal traction on the wrist to disimpact the fracture fragments while an assistant applies proximal countertraction on the upper arm (Fig. 7.54A). After the fracture fragments are disimpacted, the opposite hand of the physician is used to mold the distal segment into its proper alignment with the proximal segment as shown in Figure 7.54A.
3. The second stage in reducing these fractures involves flexion of the elbow with the forearm held in supination at the wrist and posteriorly applied pressure to the distal segment applied with the fingers of the opposite hand of the physician as shown in Figure 7.54B. This displaces the previously disimpacted distal fragment anteriorly into its proper position. Finally, with the thumb of the physician's opposite hand applying a medially directed force to the distal fragment of the humerus and the fingers wrapped around the proximal humerus (Fig. 7.54C), the distal frag-

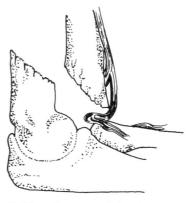

Figure 7.53. Supracondylar fracture of the distal humerus with brachial artery entrapment by the displaced fracture fragments.

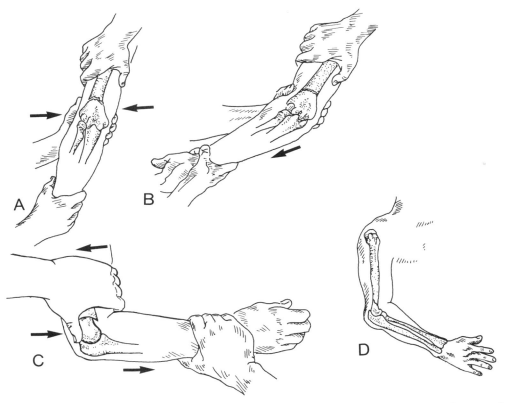

Figure 7.54.   The reduction of a displaced supracondylar fracture of the humerus. See text for discussion.

ment is maneuvered into its final position.

The patient should be placed in anterior and posterior long arm splints. All these patients should be admitted to the hospital for observation for any evidence of delayed vascular complications.

REDUCTION OF SELECTED COMMON DISLOCATIONS

Anterior Dislocations Of The Glenohumeral Joint (37, 47, 48)

An anterior shoulder dislocation is one of the most common problems presenting to the emergency center and represents approximately 50% of all major joint dislocations seen by the emergency physician. The mechanism by which this injury occurs is usually abduction accompanied by external rotation of the arm, which disrupts the anterior capsule and the glenohumeral ligaments. A detailed description of this problem is beyond the scope of this chapter; however, it should be pointed out that emergency physicians always should examine the function of the axillary nerve before any attempt at reduction as this nerve is commonly injured in anterior dislocations (4). This nerve is assessed by testing sensation to pinprick or two point discrimination over the lateral aspect of the deltoid and comparing it with sensation on the uninjured side. In addition, the radial, ulnar, and brachial pulses as well as the integrity of the median, ulnar and radial nerves should be evaluated.

There are many methods of reducing anterior dislocations of the shoulder, several of which will be discussed. Intravenous narcotics and muscle relaxants should be administered before any attempt at reduction. Bag mask, oral airway, and naloxone (0.4 mg), a narcotic antagonist, should be at the bedside of these patients so that any marked respiratory depression can be managed easily. Muscle relaxation is crucial in any attempt at reducing an anterior shoulder dislocation which cannot be reduced by the first technique described below. An alternate method of providing analgesia is by suprascapular nerve block; however, this is not commonly used. The techniques listed below are in order of the authors' preference. The least manipulative maneuvers are first attempted; if these are unsuccessful, one should go on to other methods.

Modified Milch Technique (34, 38)

This technique requires little manipulation and is safe. It has recently been studied and found to require no anesthetic with a high success rate (41, 42). The technique requires gentle, steady external rotation of the shoulder. This is done over several minutes. The patient is told to relax as you progressively externally rotate the shoulder with the elbow flexed. This brings the humeral head out from under the glenoid rim. After external rotation to 90 degrees and reduction are achieved, adduct the arm (41, 42).

STIMSON TECHNIQUE (55)

The Stimson technique is a safe procedure and the treatment of choice in attempting to reduce an anterior dislocation of the shoulder. The patient is placed in the prone position with the arm dependent and a pillow or folded sheet placed under the shoulder (Fig. 7.55). A strap is applied to the wrist or distal forearm and weights are suspended (from 10 to 15 pounds) over a period of 20 to 30 minutes. This time period usually is sufficient for reduction to occur. Muscle relaxation is imperative and the patient must be under constant observation for monitoring of the respiratory status and pulse. Twenty to 30 minutes is usually a sufficient amount of time for displacement of the humeral head, after which either a spontaneous reduction will occur or the examiner may rotate the humerus gently, externally and then inter-

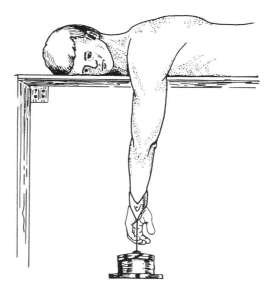

Figure 7.55. The Stimson technique for reducing an anterior shoulder dislocation.

nally, with mild traction; this usually reduces the dislocation.

TRACTION AND COUNTERTRACTION (46)

This method has been advocated for those anterior dislocations which are difficult to reduce by the Stimson technique. In this method, an assistant applies countertraction with a folded sheet wrapped around the upper chest, as shown, and the examiner applies traction to the arm (Fig. 7.56). This maneuver usually dislodges the humeral head, and slight lateral traction on the proximal humerus usually reduces the dislocation.

TRACTION WITH LATERAL TRACTION (46)

This maneuver is similar to the one above; however, in addition to traction along the longitudinal access of the humerus, lateral traction is also applied to the proximal humerus after disimpaction of the humeral head is achieved by the former procedure. The lateral traction is provided by an assistant with a pillowcase folded and wrapped around the proximal humerus as shown in Figure 7.57. (The countertraction shown in Figure 7.56 has

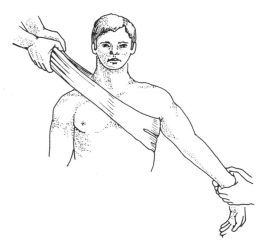

Figure 7.56. The traction and countertraction for reducing an anterior shoulder dislocation. This technique is preferred by many. It has the advantages of being quicker than the Stimson technique and is a safe procedure.

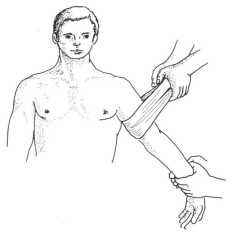

Figure 7.57. Traction and lateral traction. In addition to the folded pillowcase shown above for providing lateral traction, countertraction should be applied with a folded sheet as shown in Figure 7.56. In reducing a difficult anterior shoulder dislocation, traction and countertraction are applied first to distract the humeral head and are followed by lateral traction as shown above.

been omitted from this diagram; however, it should also be applied.) It is important that lateral traction not be applied until the humerus is disimpacted from under

the glenoid. To prevent avulsion injuries during the reduction, the patient must have good muscle relaxation when this maneuver is used.

KOCHER MANEUVER (27, 32)

This maneuver is quite dangerous and is fraught with many complications and should not be used by the emergency physician in reducing anterior dislocations of the shoulder. In our opinion, the Hippocratic technique also should not be used under any circumstances in reducing these dislocations. If the methods described above prove ineffectual in reducing the dislocation, then general anesthesia should be considered and reduction attempted in the operating room. Irreducible dislocations are usually due to soft tissue interposition.

In patients under 40 years of age we advocate the use of a sling and swathe or a shoulder immobilizer for a period of 3 weeks following reduction. In patients over 40 years of age we advocate the use of a sling and swathe for a period of 1 week with range of motion exercises (avoiding abduction and external rotation) to begin within 4 or 5 days following the injury. Once healing occurs, an exercise program to strengthen the subscapularis muscle is advocated to prevent recurrences.

Luxatia Erecta (36)

This is an unusual dislocation in which the humeral head is dislocated inferior to the glenoid. It occurs when the arm is abducted to 180 degrees. The patient presents with the arm raised directly over the head. Reduction is accomplished by applying traction to the arm in line with the deformity, followed by rotation through a 180 degree arc and bringing the arm back to the patient's side.

Sternoclavicular Dislocations (13, 49)

The sternoclavicular joint is stabilized by the sternoclavicular and the costoclavicular ligaments. Complete rupture of these two ligaments permits the clavicle to dislocate from its manubrial attachment.

Dislocations at this joint are either anterior or posterior; by far the most common is the anterior dislocation. Posterior dislocations, although uncommon, may present as a life-threatening emergency due to airway or vascular compromise from the posteriorly displaced clavicle impinging upon the trachea. Patients with a posterior dislocation may present with breathing difficulties secondary to tracheal compression or tracheal rupture. Posterior dislocations occur with serious vascular and pulmonary complications including pneumothorax, laceration of the superior vena cava, and occlusion of the subclavian artery or vein. Approximately 25% of all posterior dislocations of the sternoclavicular joint are associated with tracheal, esophageal, or great vessel injury, which demonstrates the need for early reduction.

Dislocations are reduced as shown in Figure 7.58. A folded sheet is placed between the shoulders, while the patient is in the supine position which serves to separate the clavicle from the manubrium. The arm is abducted and traction is applied by an assistant, as shown in Figure 7.58A. When dealing with an anterior dislocation, while traction is maintained on the ipsilateral arm the examiner pushes the clavicle posteriorly into its normal position. In patients with a posterior dislocation the same maneuver is used; however, the clavicle is pulled forward while traction is maintained by grasping it as shown in Figure 7.58B. In more difficult situations in which the clavicle may not be grasped with the examiner's fingers, a towel clip is used to encircle the clavicle and traction is applied in an anterior direction in a similar manner to that indicated above.

Dislocations Of The Elbow (29, 30)

Elbow dislocations are among the most commonly seen dislocations of the body, second in frequency only to dislocations of the shoulder and the fingers. Posterior dislocations, in which the ulnar olecranon is displaced posteriorly in relation to the distal humerus, account for the majority of dislocations of the elbow. Anterior dislocations are far less common. With pro-

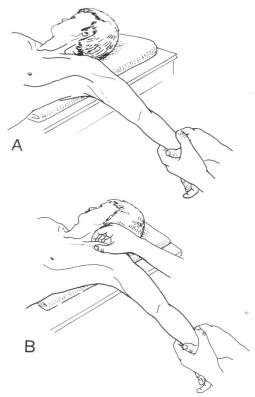

Figure 7.58. Reduction of a sternoclavicular joint dislocation. *A.* A folded sheet is placed between the scapulae as shown. The patient's arm is then abducted and traction is applied. *B.* For posterior dislocation of the sternoclavicular joint, the clavicle is then uplifted back into its normal position. A towel clip may have to be used to grab the clavicle and lift it anteriorly. For anterior dislocations, the clavicle is reduced back into its normal position by posteriorly directed pressure applied over it.

longed delays in reducing these injuries, the articular cartilage is damaged and swelling increases, which may cause circulatory compromise.

Reduction is accomplished after administering an analgesic and a muscle relaxant. The reduction requires gentle traction on the forearm with the elbow in the position of comfort and with the wrist supinated, while an assistant applies countertraction. The olecranon is pulled forward by applying pressure with the right hand and the coronoid process suddenly disengages from under the humerus as shown in Figure 7.59. The elbow is extended only to the degree necessary to disengage the coronoid from under the humerus. The olecranon thus is lifted anteriorly. One should avoid hyperextension in reducing this dislocation. After reduction a long arm posterior splint is applied with the elbow flexed at 90 degrees or more if the arm permits. Swelling sometimes restricts flexion and, during splinting, one should be careful to avoid flexing to the extent that vascular compromise occurs.

Always assess the ulnar and radial collateral ligaments of the elbow for their integrity after reduction. These ligaments are commonly injured in dislocations and sprains of the elbow. A valgus and varus stress test of these ligaments will assess their integrity.

Subluxation Of The Radial Head In Children

This is a common injury, occurring in children between the ages of 2 and 5 years. In children there is little structural support between the radius and the humerus; with

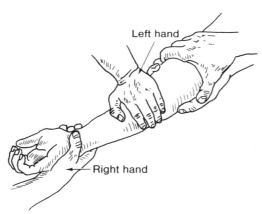

Left hand

Right hand

Figure 7.59. The reduction of an elbow dislocation is shown. An assistant steadies the arm while the physician applies traction with the right hand and downward-directed pressure with the left hand, which reduces the displaced olecranon from its locked position behind the distal humerus. The traction will then bring the olecranon anteriorly. The elbow may have to be extended slightly with this procedure; however, it should never be hyperextended.

sudden traction on the hand or forearm, such as occurs when a parent pulls a child up by the arm to prevent a fall, the annular ligament which attaches the radius to the humerus is pulled over the radial head and lies between it and the capitullum.

To reduce the subluxation, apply direct pressure with the thumb over the forearm in the region of the radial head and slowly supinate and extend the elbow as shown in Figure 7.60. A sudden release of resistance accompanied by a definite click signifies reduction. Roentgenograms should be taken before any attempt at reduction. Older patients should then be placed in a forearm sling for 1 week.

Dislocations Of The Interphalangeal Joints Of The Hand

Dislocations of the proximal and distal interphalangeal joints of the hand are commonly seen in the emergency center and generally are easily reduced. Most dislocations of this joint are posterior dislocations, and the proximal interphalangeal joint is more commonly involved than the distal.

Analgesia is provided by block of the metacarpal or digital nerve to the involved digit. Following this, traction is applied longitudinally in the line of the deformity to distract the articular surfaces of the involved joint. Hyperextension is then applied to permit alignment of the articular surfaces, which is followed by flexion of the joint; this accomplishes reduction. Following reduction the collateral ligaments must be examined by stress tests to ascertain if there is complete rupture. The involved digit should be splinted in a volar or dorsal finger splint, and the patient followed. Dislocations involving the thumb are often difficult to reduce due to entrapment of the volar plate or sesamoids, making this a complex dislocation which requires operative reduction. In attempting to reduce any interphalangeal or metacarpophalangeal joint dislocation involving the hand or foot, when, after two attempts at reduction under good anesthesia one fails, suspect a complex dislocation entrapping soft tissue in the joint.

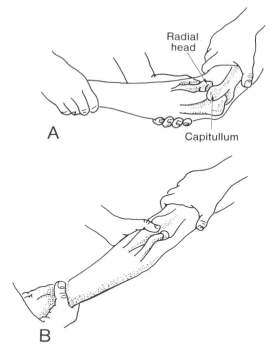

Radial head

Capitullum

A

B

Figure 7.60. Reduction of a subluxation of the radial head in children. *A.* Direct pressure is applied with the thumb over the displaced radial head. *B.* At the same time, the right hand distracts and supinates the forearm while extending the elbow. Usually a "pop" or a "snap" is palpable when the radial head reduces into its normal position.

Hip Dislocations (12, 56)

Hip dislocations require large forces and are frequently associated with acetabular fractures or ipsilateral extremity injuries. All hip dislocations must be regarded as true emergencies and must be reduced early to minimize the incidence of avascular necrosis of the femoral head. Posterior dislocations are far more common than are anterior dislocations. Anterior dislocations of the hip are best managed with early reduction under spinal or general anesthesia. Open reduction is indicated if attempts at closed reduction fail. Emergent referral for reduction is strongly recommended. Posterior dislocations are best managed with immobilization and emergent referral for reduction. If the emergent referral is not available, closed

reduction using the following method should be attempted:

1. The patient should be placed on a backboard and given intravenous muscle relaxants (Valium)® and narcotic analgesics for skeletal muscle relaxation and pain relief.
2. The patient should be lowered to the floor on the backboard, where an assistant immobilizes the pelvis as demonstrated in Figure 7.61A.
3. By pulling up on the distal calf the physician then applies traction in line with the deformity along with gently flexing the knee to a position of 90 degrees (Fig. 7.61B).
4. At this point, gentle but firm pulling of the hip anteriorly by upward traction on the flexed calf will result in reduction in most cases. If this is unsuccessful, reduction should be performed under general anesthesia. If reduction is successful the patient should be admitted for traction, strict non-weight-bearing, and observation.

Stimson's method for reducing posterior hip dislocations is shown in Figure 7.62. This method also may be used; however, the authors' experience indicates a lower success rate with this method than with the technique described above.

Dislocations Of The Knee (25, 28, 51)

Dislocations of the knee represent a true orthopedic emergency, as there is a high incidence of popliteal artery compromise associated with these injuries. Both anterior and posterior dislocations of the knee must be immediately reduced, and a follow-up arteriogram to examine the integrity of the popliteal artery must be performed. A neurovascular assessment should be done before any attempt is made to manipulate this injury. Posterior dislocations appear to be less common than are anterior dislocations.

In reducing these dislocations the examiner applies traction longitudinally in the line of the deformity to the involved extended knee while countertraction is applied above the knee by an assistant, as

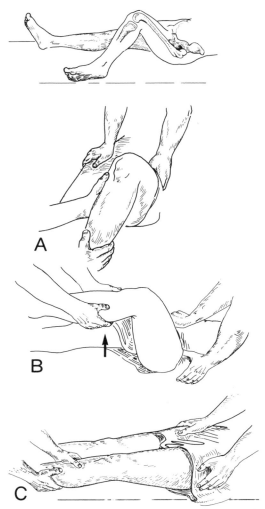

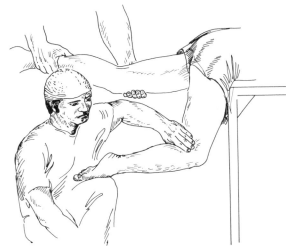

Figure 7.62. The Stimson method for reducing posterior hip dislocations. The patient is placed in a prone position and pressure is applied to the flexed knee directed downward with the foot held against the examiner's knee as shown. The opposite leg is held in extension by an assistant.

Figure 7.61. The reduction of a posterior hip dislocation. *A.* The patient should be lowered to the floor on a backboard while an assistant immobilizes the pelvis as shown. *B.* The physician then stabilizes the patient's foot against his thigh and gently but steadily lifts the flexed knee superiorly as shown with slight external rotation. *C.* After reduction the hip is extended into its normal position.

shown in Figure 7.63A. In posterior dislocations, following disengagement of the articular surfaces and with traction maintained, the examiner rotates his hand to the undersurface of the tibia and displaces it anteriorly into its normal position (Fig. 7.63B). Reduction of this fracture is generally performed without much difficulty;

however, the incidence of associated complications due to the injury itself is extremely high.

Dislocations Of The Tibiotalar Joint (9)

Tibiotalar dislocations are commonly accompanied by fractures involving the lateral or medial malleolus or both. These dislocations are easily reduced by using a muscle relaxant and narcotic analgesic or a regional Beir block for analgesia. The examiner applies longitudinal traction to the ankle, as shown in Figure 7.64, while countertraction is being applied to the leg. After the articular surfaces of the talus and tibia are distracted, the foot is then manipulated back to its normal position. There is a definite "give" when the joint is back in its normal position, which can be both felt and seen as the gross deformity is reduced (Fig. 7.64).

Patellar Dislocations (18, 26, 44)

Patellar dislocations are commonly seen in the emergency center. Patients present with the knee at 20 to 30 degrees flexion

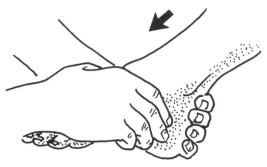

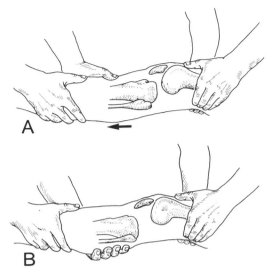

Figure 7.64. Tibiotalar dislocation. Longitudinal traction is applied to disengage the dislocated foot. After disengaging the talus, the foot is then reduced into its normal anatomical position in relation to the tibia.

Figure 7.63. The reduction of a dislocation of the knee. *A.* The femur is stabilized proximally and the leg is pulled inferiorly. *B.* After traction the knee, which is posteriorly dislocated, is then lifted back in its anatomical position.

and the patella usually is laterally displaced. The laterally dislocated patella is reduced by extending the knee while applying medially directed pressure over the patella to reposition it. This is done as a single maneuver. Patellar dislocations frequently relocate spontaneously before the patient arrives at the emergency center.

INJECTION AND ASPIRATION OF SELECTED SOFT TISSUE DISORDERS

De Quervain's Stenosing Tenosynovitis

This condition involves the abductor pollicis longus and extensor pollicis brevis tendons of the first dorsal wrist compartment. The pathognomic test, called "Finkelstein's test," which reproduces the pain is performed by holding the patient's thumb in the palm with the remaining four digits covering it and having the patient make a fist with ulnar deviation of the wrist. This form of tendonitis may be treated with the injection of steroids (triamcinolone, 10 mg) along the tendon sheath, as shown in Figure 7.65. The needle

must be placed along the tendon and not perpendicularly into the tendon. One may instill Marcaine® and a steroid (triamcinolone, 10 mg) along the tendon sheath, which generally provides good relief. Surgical intervention may be required if the condition progresses.

Tennis Elbow

Tennis elbow is an undifferentiated term denoting radiohumeral bursitis and lateral epicondylitis of the humerus. The major features of this syndrome is the localization of tenderness over the prominence of the lateral epicondyle of the humerus (7). Certain severe cases of tennis elbow may require steroid injections. The landmark selected for this injection is the lateral epicondyle. The patient's elbow should be flexed when the steroid is injected (39). The injection is performed in the posterolateral direction and toward the lateral epicondyle. The needle should be inserted laterally along the condylar ridge of the humerus and directed toward the lateral epicondyle. The steroid should be injected at multiple sites at this point. A total of 20 mg of triamcinolone is used along with Marcaine®. Often multiple injections are necessary.

Olecranon Bursitis

The subcutaneous tissue superficial to the olecranon does not communicate with the elbow joint and presents no problems for arthrocentesis, because when it is distended the entire extent of the bursa can be noted subcutaneously from the posterior aspect. The needle should be inserted from the posterior aspect perpendicular through the skin and the subcutaneous tissue and into the olecranon bursa. The indications for aspiration of the olecranon bursa are when one suspects septic bursitis and in some cases of chronic recurrent effusions within that bursa (39).

Subdeltoid Bursitis Or Supraspinous Tendonitis

The optimal injection site for patients with subdeltoid bursitis or supraspinous tendonitis is at the point of maximum tenderness elicited on palpation beneath the acromium process (40). The anterior tip of the acromium is immediately adjacent to the subacromial bursa and is an ideal bony landmark which serves as a guide for injection or aspiration of this bursa. With the arm distracted downward to increase the separation between the bursa and the acromion of the shoulder joint, a needle is inserted just inferior to the acromium and usually enters the bursa. The lateral approach is preferred over the anterior approach to avoid the cephalic vein, as seen in Figure 7.66 (39). Multiple needle punctures aid in relieving pressure from within the bursa. An injection of steroid and anesthetic is then performed.

Stenosing Tenosynovitis

The flexor tendon sheath of the fingers or thumb are usually involved in this con-

dition. The site of predilection in the sheaths is over the palmar aspect of the metacarpal heads. Localization is made easier if the patient slowly flexes the involved digit until a "snapping" of a trigger finger occurs. The site of injection for pain relief is slightly proximal to the point of tenderness. The patient is asked to gently flex and extend the finger and the operator

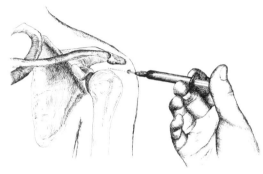

Figure 7.66.   Injection of subdeltoid bursitis or supraspinitis tendonitis. The point of maximum tenderness is beneath the acromium and above the greater tuberosity and the injection should be performed with multiple needle sticks into the bursa to release pressure.

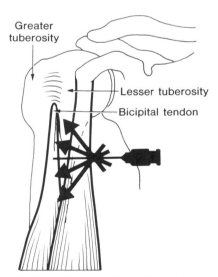

Figure 7.67.   The injection of a bicipital tendonitis involves multiple needle sticks along the tendon sheath. The needle is inserted at one point over the biceps tendon and is directed along the tendon sheath.

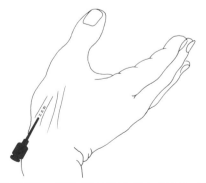

Figure 7.65.   The injection of a tenosynovitis of the abductor pollicis tendon.

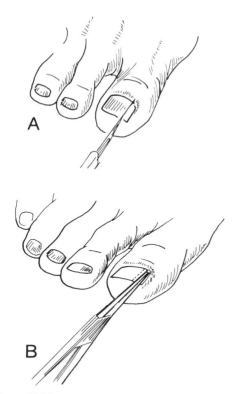

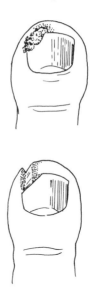

Figure 7.69.   *A.* When granulation tissue covers the distal end of the nail over the ingrown segment, it must be removed. Beneath the granulation tissue is usually a spicule of nail which has grown into the distal nail fold. *B.* A wedge from the distal segment containing the corner of the nail and granulation tissue is excised.

Figure 7.68.   *A.* A #11 scalpel and blade is used to make an incision along the nail. *B.* Following this, one jaw of a hemostat is inserted along the ingrown nail segment, and the segment is grasped firmly. This segment is then detached from the base and the nailbed.

attempts to engage the injection site with the needle tip, and a small amount of steroid is injected (54). The solution should be deposited in the sheath and not in the tendon.

Bicipital Tendonitis

Bicipital tendonitis is a common condition presenting to the emergency center and must be distinguished from pain in the shoulder secondary to subdeltoid bursitis or supraspinous tendonitis. In patients with bicipital tendonitis the point of maximum tenderness is in the groove between the greater and lesser tuberosities of the humerus, which contains the tendon of the long head of the biceps. One can inject Marcaine® into the biceps tendon sheath to differentiate this condition from other causes of pain in the shoulder. If the procedure relieves much of the pain, this can be followed by an injection of steroids.

The patient is asked to externally rotate the arm and abduct approximately 15 to 20 degrees. Locate the point between the greater and lesser tuberosities of the humerus (just medial to the greater tuberosity). Insert the needle from an anteromedial approach and direct the tip toward the tendon lying within the groove between the two tuberosities. Do not inject within the tendon but rather inject in a bandlike fashion along the tendon sheath (Fig. 7.67). The injection is usually followed by significant relief of pain within 10 to 15 minutes.

Ingrown Nails

An ingrown nail is a common problem presenting to the emergency center. The nail most commonly affected is that of the great toe. A number of techniques exist in dealing with this problem. While many surgeons remove one third to one half of the involved nail, it has been our experience that this only delays healing and prolongs discomfort. Only the portion of the nail which is involved should be excised. A digital block should be performed to provide anesthesia for the procedure (see the chapter on anesthesia). A #11 scalpel and blade is used to make an initial incision along the nail as shown in Figure 7.68A. Next, slide one jaw of a hemostat under the ingrown nail segment and grasp it firmly. Move this segment up and down to detach it from the nail bed and remove it (Fig. 7.68B). Cauterize the underlying nail bed with phenol and apply a dressing. Warm soaks are advocated if infection is present. The nail may not grow back for 9 to 12 months. Using this technique, no suturing is necessary and only a small dressing need be applied.

When granulation tissue is the major problem, this can be excised as a wedge along with the distal corner of the nail (Fig. 7.69). A small spicule of nail is usually embedded in the granulation bed and is removed with this wedge resection of the distal corner. This prevents recurrences.

References

1. Adams, J.C., Outline of Fractures. E. & S. Livingston, Edinburgh, 1968.
2. Anderson, L., Fractures. In Campbell's Operative Orthopedics, ed. 5. C.V. Mosby, St. Louis, 1971.
3. Anderson, R., Fractures of the humerus. Surg. Gynecol. Obstet. 64:919, 1937.
4. Antal, C.S., Conforty, B., Engelberg, M., et al., Injuries to the axillary nerve due to anterior dislocation of the shoulder. J. Trauma 13:564, 1973.
5. Carothers, R.G., Berning, D.D., Colles' fracture. Amer. J. Surg. 80:626, 1950.
6. Carothers, R.G., Boyd, F.J., Thumb traction technic for reduction of Colles' fracture. Arch. Surg. 58:848, 1949.
7. Cave, E.F., Fractures and Other Injuries. Yearbook Publishers, Chicago, 1958.
8. Cronwell, H.E., Fractures of the clavicle. J.A.M.A. 90:838, 1928.
9. Detenbeck, L.C., Kelly, P.J., Total dislocation of the talus. J. Bone Joint Surg. 51A:283, 1969.
10. Eastwood, W.J., The T-shaped fracture of the lower end of the humerus. J. Bone Joint Surg. 19:364, 1937.
11. Edman, P., Lohr, G., Supracondylar fractures of the humerus. Acta Chir. Scand. 126:505, 1963.
12. Epstein, H.C., Traumatic dislocations of the hip. Clin. Orthop. 92:116, 1973.
13. Ferry, A., Rook, F.W., Masterson, J.H., Retrosternal dislocation of the clavicle. J. Bone Joint Surg. 39A:905, 1957.
14. Finder, J.C., Post, M., Local injection therapy for rhuematic diseases: A practical guide. J.A.M.A. 172:2021, 1960.
15. Fitzsimmons, R.A., Colles' fracture and chauffeur's fracture. Br. Med. J. 2:357, 1938.
16. Furlong, R., Injuries of the Hand. Little Brown. Boston, 1957.
17. Geiderman, J.D., Dawson, W.J., Arthrocentesis—indications and method. Postgrad. Med. 66:141, 1979.
18. Gore, D.R., Horizontal dislocation of the patella. J.A.M.A. 214:119, 1970.
19. Henny, F.A., Intra-articular injection of hydrocortisone into tempomandibular joint. J. Oral Surg. 12:314, 1954.
20. Hollander, J.L., Intra-articular hydrocortisone in the treatment of arhtirtis. Ann. Intern. Med. 39:735, 1953.
21. Hollander, J.L., Technique of Intra-articular Injection with Hydrocortisone Acetate. Merck & Co., Rahway, N.J., 1953, 22 pp.
22. Hollander, J.L., (ed) Arthritis and Allied Conditions: A Textbook of Rheumatology. Lea & Febiger, Philadelphia, 1969, pp. 380–401.
23. Hollander, J.L., Brown, E.M., Jr., Jessar, R.A., Intra-articular hydrocortisone in the management of rheumatic disease. Med. Clin. North Am. 38:349, 1954.
24. Holzman, R.S., Bishko, F., Osteomyelitis in heroin addicts. Ann. Intern. Med. 75:693, 1971.
25. Hoover, N.W., Injuries of the popliteal artery associated with fractures and dislocations. Surg. Clin. North Am. 41:1099, 1961.
26. Hughston, J.C., Subluxation of the patella. J. Bone Joint Surg. 50A:1003, 1968.
27. Hussein, K.M., Kochers method is 3,000 years old. J. Bone Joint Surg. 50B:669, 1968.
28. Kennedy, J.C., Complete dislocation of knee joint. J. Bone Joint Surg. 45A:889, 1963.
29. King, O.C., Fractures and dislocations about the elbow. Surg. Clin. North Am. 20:1645, 1940.
30. Kini, M.G., Dislocation of the elbow and its complications. J. Bone Joint Surg. 22:107, 1940.
31. Kini, M.G., A simple method of ambulatory treatment of fractures of the clavicle. J. Bone Joint Surg. 23:795, 1941.
32. Kocher, T., Eine neue reductions method fur Schulterverrenkung. Berlin Klin. 7:101, 1870.
33. Krause, W., Quoted in Kling, D.H., The Synovial Membrane and the Synovial Fluid with Special Reference to Arthritis and Injuries of the Joints. Medical Press, Los Angeles, 1938, Chapter 24, 299 pp.
34. Lacey, T., Reduction of anterior dislocation of shoulder by Milch abduction technique. J. Bone Joint Surg. 34A:108, 1952.
35. Landsmeer, J.M.F., Koumans, A.K.J., Anatomical considerations in injection of the hip joint. Ann. Rheumat. Dis. 13:246, 1954.
36. Lynn, F.S., Erect dislocation of the shoulder. Surg. Gynecol. Obstet. 39:51, 1925.
37. McLaughlin, H.L., MacLellan, D.I., Recurrent anterior dislocations of the shoulder. J. Trauma 7:191, 1967.
38. Milch, H., Treatment of dislocations of the shoulder. Surgery 3:732, 1938.

39. Miller, J.A., Jr., Joint paracentesis from an anatomic point of view. I. Shoulder, elbow, wrist, and hand. Surgery 40:993, 1956.
40. Miller, J.A., Jr., Joint paracentesis from an anatomic point of view: II. Hip, knee, ankle and foot. Surgery 41:999, 1957.
41. Mirick, M.J., Clinton, J.E., Ruiz, E., External rotation method of shoulder dislocation reduction. J.A.C.E.P. 8:528, 1979.
42. Parisien, V.M., Shoulder dislocations an easier method for reduction. J. Maine Med. Assoc. 70:102, 1979.
43. Pels-Leusden, Quoted in Kling, D.H., The Synovial Membrane and the Synovial Fluid with Special Reference to Arthritis and Injuries of the Joints. Medical Press. Los Angeles, 1938, Chapter 24, 299 pp.
44. Percy, E.C., Acute dislocation of the patella. Can. Med. Assoc. J. 105:1176, 1971.
45. Roca, R., Yoshikawa, T.T., Primary skeletal infections in heroin users. Clin. Orthop. 144:238, 1979.
46. Rockwood, C.A., Green, D.T., Fractures, J.B. Lippincott, Philadelphia, 1975.
47. Rowe, C.R., Anterior dislocations of the shoulder. Surg. Clin. North Am. 43:1609, 1963.
48. Royle, G., Treatment of acute anterior dislocations of the shoulder, Br. J. Clin. Pract. 27:403, 1973.
49. Salvatore, J., Sternoclavicular joint dislocation. Clin. Orthop. 58:51, 1968.
50. Schmeiden, Quoted in Kling, D.H., The Synovial Membrane and the Synovial Fluid with Special Reference to Arthritis and Injuries of the Joints. Medical Press, Los Angeles, 1938, Chapter 24, 299 pp.
51. Shields, L., Mital, M., Cave, E.F., Complete dislocation of the knee: Experience at the MGH. J. Trauma 9:192, 1969.
52. Spear, H.C., Jones, J.M., Rupture of the brachial artery accompanying dislocation of the elbow or supracondylar fracture. J. Bone Joint Surg. 33A:889, 1951.
53. Sperling, I.L., Hydrocortisone intra-articular use in rheumatic diseases, Mod. Med. 119–123, 1955.
54. Sternbach, G.L., Baker, F.J., The emergency joint: Arthrocentesis and synovial fluid analysis. J.A.C.E.P. 5:787, 1976.
55. Stimson, C.A., An easy method of reducing dislocations of the shoulder & hip. Medical Records 57:356, 1900.
56. Thompson, V.P., Epstein, H.C., Traumatic dislocation of the hip. J. Bone Joint Surg. 33A:746, 1951.
57. Wade, F.V., Batdorf, J. Supracondylar fractures of humerus (a twelve year review with follow-up). J. Trauma 1:269, 1961.
58. Wolf, A.W., et al., Current concepts in synovial fluid analysis. Clin. Orthop. 134:262, 1978.
59. Yehia, S.A., Duncan, H., Synovial fluid analysis. Clin. Orthop. 107:11, 1975.

Otolaryngology, Ophthalmology, Dental Procedures

8

ESOPHAGUS AND AIRWAY FOREIGN BODIES

Only one foreign body impaction in the esophagus is a true emergency, that is, foreign bodies of such bulk that they impact the postcricoid area producing serious respiratory embarrassment or complete occlusion of the airway. In this case, an emergency cricothyroidotomy is needed.

All other esophageal foreign bodies can be removed emergently but do not require immediate intervention within the emergency center. Some foreign bodies, such as safety pins, can cause perforation of the esophagus and in this situation parenteral antibiotics and sedation are advised before attempts at removal. The physician should never try to dislodge the foreign body with a bougie (a device used for esophageal dilatation). The blind passage of a catheter or probing may result in a major rupture of the esophagus. In patients with laryngeal foreign bodies which cannot be dislodged by the Heimlich maneuver (see Chapter 2: "Airway Procedures"), a cricothyroidotomy is needed. Foreign bodies lodged in either one or the other mainstem bronchi is a common problem in the pediatric age-group. These patients usually do not need immediate intervention. Sedation may be necessary, and the patient should be referred for removal of the foreign body under fiberoptic bronchoscopy. A child with a foreign body in the mainstem bronchus should not be turned upside down and slapped on his back; this may dislodge the foreign body into the larynx and cause complete airway obstruction. Some otolaryngologists prefer to use the rigid bronchoscope for removal of foreign bodies in the airway. This procedure is discussed in detail in Chapter 2: "Airway Procedures."

REMOVAL OF FOREIGN BODIES FROM THE EAR

Foreign bodies in the ear are quite commonly seen, particularly in the pediatric age-group. Removal may present an arduous task for the emergency clinician.

The following steps are recommended in removing foreign bodies from the external canal. Removal should first be attempted with irrigation, using water so as not to push the foreign body past the isthmus of the canal, where it may lodge and be very difficult to remove subsequently. A pulsatile flow of irrigation fluid directed against the superior wall of the canal is recommended, similar to the technique used for removal of cerumen impaction. If this does not work, a hook or ear curette may be passed behind the foreign body and extraction attempted (Fig. 8.1). In small children, a general anesthetic may be needed for adequate removal of a foreign body.

Adequate anesthesia of the canal can be achieved by using the four-quadrant block indicated in the chapter on anesthesia. This block will permit instrumentation of the canal, which is almost impossible otherwise. Iontophoresis is a technique by which a local anesthetic solution is dispersed in the canal and tympanic membrane and anesthetizes the canal for re-

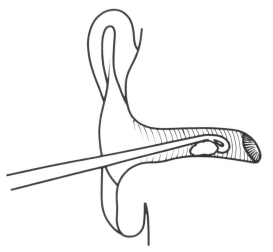

Figure 8.1. Ear curette used for the removal of a foreign body lodged in the ear canal. The first procedure which should be performed is irrigation, using an 18 gauge plastic catheter as indicated in the text. If the foreign body is a pearl and is lodged close to the tympanic membrane, then the patient may need referral for more adequate anesthesia to remove the object.

moval of foreign bodies which are lodged against the tympanic membrane. When a foreign body such as a pearl is lodged against the tympanic membrane and irrigation proves unsuccessful, the patient should be referred to an otolaryngologist who is capable of performing this procedure.

CERUMEN IMPACTION

Cerumen impaction is a common problem obstructing adequate visualization of the tympanic membrane in patients presenting to the emergency center. The cerumen should be softened with either half-strength hydrogen peroxide or Debrox® before removal by irrigation. Irrigation is best performed under direct vision with the plastic cannula of the 18 to 20 gauge Angiocath®, directing the stream gently along the superior wall of the canal. The catheter should be connected to a 30 ml syringe and pulsatile jets of warm water should be used for irrigation. Using this method the returning stream may push the cerumen from behind and out of the canal. If this does not work or if one is dealing with hard wax, a cerumen spoon or curette may be used cautiously. Occasionally a middle ear forceps will prove useful in removing hard balls of wax impacted against the tympanic membrane.

MYRINGOTOMY

Myringotomy is not a commonly performed procedure in the emergency center. The indications for a myringotomy are a markedly swollen, erythematous, tympanic membrane in a patient presenting with a high fever and severe unremitting pain. A local anesthetic is recommended, as indicated in Chapter 3: "Anesthesia and Regional Blocks." An incision should be made in the anterior inferior quadrant of the tympanic membrane (Fig. 8.2). A special scalpel and handle which can be inserted through a metallic earpiece for the procedure is available in routine myringotomy trays. If the special spear-tipped scalpel is unavailable, a 15 gauge spinal needle attached to a tuberculin syringe may be adequate to aspirate the purulent

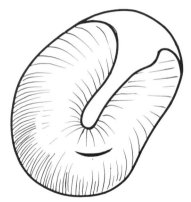

Figure 8.2. An anterior inferior incision is made in the tympanic membrane for drainage of a suppurative otitis media. This avoids injuring the ossicles. See text for discussion.

material. When the purulent material is obtained, it should be sent for a culture and sensitivity; the fluid will spontaneously drain from the middle ear.

INTRAOCULAR FOREIGN BODIES

Most intraocular foreign bodies are metallic shavings. The most common single cause of these is a hammer and chisel. If the removal of metallic particles is delayed, the incidence of endophthalmitis rises sharply after 24 hours (38). Either a burr spud or a 23 gauge needle is used to remove the superficial foreign body of the cornea with a split lamp after adequate topical anesthetic is applied.

Intraocular foreign bodies may be difficult to localize on routine radiographs. When the particle is metallic, localization does not present a major problem; however, with nonmetallic intracorneal foreign bodies much difficulty may be encountered by routine means. Ultrasound and computed tomography (CT) scan of the orbit have been used to localize particles which could not be found by other means (8).

CORNEAL RUST STAINS

Following the removal of metallic foreign bodies from the cornea of the eye, the patient rapidly develops corneal rust stains. These must be removed to prevent permanent staining of the cornea. A 22 gauge needle or a burr spud can be used (1). With either of these instruments a corneal rust stain is *gently* lifted off the cornea with the use of a slit lamp, and normal saline irrigation is used to cleanse the surface. Manipulation increases the chances of secondary infection and also the chance of corneal opacification. Desferal (deferoxamine mesylate) has been used topically and was found to be an excellent siderophilic agent and could completely remove corneal rust stains. This has not been adequately tested, however, and is not currently in common use.

USE OF THE SCHIOTZ TONOMETER

Schiotz tonometry is a commonly performed procedure within the emergency center. The Schiotz tonometer is an instrument used to measure intraocular pressures and is used to diagnose glaucoma. Accompanying the instrument is a series of weights (5.5, 7.5, 10.0, 15.0 g) and a chart converting the units on the Schiotz tonometer to mm Hg. The technique of tonometry is very simple and involves anesthetizing the eye with an appropriate topical anesthetic solution. Place the lowest weight, 5.5 g, on the tonometer. Following this the tonometer is held with the left hand and is rested gently on the center of the cornea as the right hand retracts the lids, as shown in Figure 8.3. Do not apply pressure on the orbit itself; rest the other fingers on the supraorbital and infraorbital ridges. Make sure the tonometer rests on the center of the limbus. Do not press the tonometer firmly against the limbus and leave the side arm freely mobile or erroneous readings will occur. The measurement of the pressure on the tonometer then is translated to mm Hg by use of a chart. If the reading is too low to use the chart, then a higher weight should be applied to the tonometer and the value determined again. The lower the reading on the tonometer, the higher is the intraocular pressure. If the pressure is elevated, then

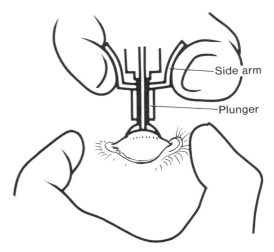

Figure 8.3. Use of a tonometer. Before placement of the tonometer over the cornea, adequate anesthesia of the cornea must be obtained by topical solutions. The plunger of the tonometer will be elevated, indicating the intraocular pressure.

a more accurate value should be obtained using applenation tonometry.

EPISTAXIS

Epistaxis is a common problem presenting to the emergency center. For the emergency physician to thoroughly understand this disorder, a basic understanding of the arteries and veins supplying the nose is mandatory.

The sphenopalatine artery, a terminal branch of the external carotid artery, courses through the sphenopalatine foramen to supply the nasal cavity. It divides into the medial and lateral branches. This artery supplies the majority of the posterior portion of the nose. The anterior and posterior ethmoidal arteries arise from the ophthalmic artery as it enters anteriorly along the crista galli (Fig. 8.4). These arteries course downward and supply blood to the anterior superior portion of the nasal cavity. The arteries supplying the septum form a plexus of vessels anteriorly called Kiesselbach's plexus (Little's area). This plexus, formed along the anterior portion of the nasal septum, is the most common site of epistaxis. Another common site for

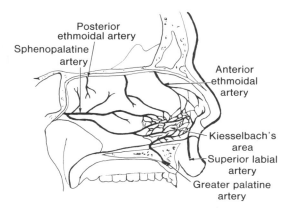

Figure 8.4.   Nasal vessels supplying the septum. (Reprinted with permission of Surgical Clinics of North America. LaForce, R.F., Treatment of nasal hemorrhage. 49:1306, 1969.)

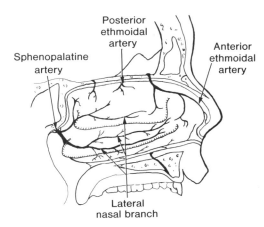

Figure 8.5.   Note the vessels which supply the lateral nasal wall (Reprinted with permission of Surgical Clinics of North America. LaForce, R.F., Treatment of nasal hemorrhage. 49:1306, 1969.)

arterial bleeding to occur is from the anterior superior portion of the nasal cavity supplied by the ethmoidal artery. A third site for arterial bleeding is from the sphenopalatine artery, and these patients usually present with posterior nasal bleeding into the pharynx (17, 27, 37) (Fig. 8.5). The external carotid artery supplies the middle and inferior turbinates via the sphenopalatine artery, while the internal carotid supplies the superior and anterior portion of the nose via the ophthalmic arteries which branch off into the anterior and posterior ethmoidal arteries. The septum thus is supplied by both the external and internal carotid arteries; Kiesselbach's plexus can be thought of as the terminal branches of both the internal and external carotid system meeting on the cartilaginous nasal septum (10, 16, 17).

The venous system also may be the source of epistaxis. A common source of epistaxis is an area of dilated veins in the posterior end of the inferior turbinate called Woodruff's nasopharyngeal plexus. Bleeding from this source occurs particularly in older hypertensive patients and in patients with arteriosclerosis.

One always must consider the etiologies in patients presenting with epistaxis. Cardiovascular factors play a major role, not in the initiation of epistaxis but in the continuation of bleeding (24). Our knowledge of the underlying cause of sponta-

neous nosebleeds remains obscure. In one study involving 1724 cases of epistaxis, 71% of the patients were found to be over 50 years of age. Cardiovascular causes were implicated in 47% of the cases and the cause was undetermined in approximately 30% (24). In the elderly there seems to be a higher incidence of posterior sites of bleeding (9). Specific identifiable causes account for only 10 to 15% of all cases presenting to the emergency center with epistaxis (42). In children with recurrent epistaxis, acute rhinitis or allergic problems may predispose to this difficulty. In the older age-group, hypertension, arteriosclerosis, vascular anomalies, and coagulopathies are the leading causes of recurrent epistaxis (16).

When one sees a patient with epistaxis, the physician must ascertain whether or not the bleeding was associated with a traumatic etiology or whether it was spontaneous. Trauma (including nose picking, auto accidents, falls, sneezing, etc.) accounted for only 13.5% of cases in one large study (16). Most of the bleeding associated with a traumatic etiology is in the anterior portion of the nasal cavity.

The causes of spontaneous bleeding are numerous; the most common of which are listed below.

1. Acute and chronic infections (10, 16, 17). Several severe cases of epistaxis occur in patients with influenza (18). Acute and chronic nasal infections as well as systemic diseases including measles, chickenpox, or nasal congestion associated with an upper respiratory infection all have been documented as causes of spontaneous epistaxis, particularly in children (10, 16–18).
2. Vascular abnormalities. Diseases of the vascular system account for a number of cases of epistaxis such as hereditary hemorrhagic telangiectasias (16, 17).
3. Hypertension, while being an over-diagnosed etiology of spontaneous epistaxis, is, nevertheless, a known cause (17). One must remember that all patients presenting with epistaxis will be anxious and many of them will present with some degree of hypertension. While this requires follow-up, it is uncommon for the hypertension per se to be the etiology of the epistaxis, particularly in the younger age-group.
4. High venous tensions, as occur in emphysema, whooping cough, bronchitis and tumors of the neck, account for some venous sources of epistaxis (17).
5. Coagulation defects account for a small percentage of patients with epistaxis.
6. Neoplasms of the nose or sinus, while being uncommon causes, should be searched for.
7. Other causes include atherosclerosis, Cushing's syndrome, uremia, and scurvy.

In patients suspected of having coagulation defects, appropriate coagulation profiles should be obtained. One should suspect coagulopathies in a patient who gives a history of easy bruising, recurrent nosebleeds without an obvious cause, or a history of bleeding from other sites and, finally, in patients with physical evidence of a coagulopathy or low platelet count such as petechiae.

Treatment Of Epistaxis

The treatment of epistaxis basically includes the arrest of hemorrhage and the search for and treatment of underlying causes.

Equipment (27)

Head mirror
Indirect light with a 150 watt bulb (9, 27)
Nasal speculum
Bayonet forceps
Epinephrine 1:1000 topical
Cotton balls or pledgets
Cotton-tipped applicators
Tongue blades
French Frazier angulated suction catheter
4 × 4 and 3 × 3 gauze
10 inch long umbilical tape, 2 pieces
Small rubber catheter, ½ inch wide
Vaseline impregnated gauze strips
Antibiotic ointment
Nasostat balloon®
10 or 12 French Foley catheter

Technique

1. The patient should be sitting upright with the head bent forward and should be asked to hold the nose pinched for approximately 10 minutes (18). Both the patient and the physician should wear gowns.

NOTE

When bleeding occurs from both nostrils, this almost always is due to blood coming around the posterior portion of the nasal septum and across to the uninvolved side. One should ascertain from which side of the nose the bleeding started first, and this is the side which should be examined for the site of bleeding (10, 27).

2. If bleeding continues, the patient should be asked to blow his nose to remove all clots.
3. With use of a nasal speculum and head mirror, suction all the remaining clots and bleeding.

NOTE

Many of these patients, particularly children, will be apprehensive. The use of morphine sulfate in a dosage of 10 to 15 mg intramuscularly or Demerol® in a dosage of 100 mg for *adults* has been recommended by many authors (17, 29). In the child, a mild sedative hypnotic should be administered. When the bleeding is minimal, the source of bleeding can be discovered before the administration of vasoconstrictors or topical anesthetics into the nose. When trauma is the etiology, one should look at Kiesselbach's plexus, particularly in patients with anterior bleeding. Not uncommonly, a small septal vessel which is bleeding is noted in the anterior portion. When the anterior ethmoid artery is the source of bleeding, one will notice bleeding coming from the anterior aspect of the middle turbinate. This bleeding often is intermittent, and the blood may "trickle" backwards, making it seem like posterior bleeding. When the patient states that the bleeding occurred in the pharynx, first suspect the sphenopalatine artery as the source of posterior bleeding (18). When bleeding is brisk and the source cannot be identified, multiple cotton strips soaked in 4% cocaine and 1:1000 solution of epinephrine should be placed along the floor of the nose. These should remain in place for 5 minutes (10, 13, 17, 18, 27). When the bleeding can be seen to be coming from one site, a cotton pledget soaked in cocaine and epinephrine can be applied to that site to decrease the amount of bleeding, thus permitting cauterization.

NOTE (16, 17)

Silver nitrate sticks are commonly used to chemically cauterize the bleeding point. Persistent or high risk of recurrent bleeding may require electrocauterization. When silver nitrate is used, the applicator should be applied for at least 20 seconds (9). Vigorously bleeding vessels are commonly seen in hypertensives and in patients with arteriosclerotic disease; in these electrocoagulation is necessary. Bi-

polar coagulation such as the Bantan Bovie unit is probably the best type to use (2, 9).

4. Placement of an anterior pack. When a specific bleeding point cannot be identified, but the bleeding is ascertained to be coming from an anterior source, an anterior pack should be placed.
   a. Antibacterial ointment should be squeezed into the plastic package containing the ½ inch wide Vaseline impregnated gauze which is used for anterior packing.

NOTE

A number of authors advise the use of an antibacterial ointment on the pack, since, if it is left in for more than 24 hours, infection is commonly seen (2, 9). Bilateral anterior packs almost never should be used, due to the increased risk of infection and septal damage and ulceration. This is used only when one cannot tell which side, by history or examination, the bleeding is coming from, which is most unusual. In addition to the antibacterial ointment, oral broad-spectrum antibiotics are advised for most patients with posterior packs; some authors advise them for patients with anterior packs as well.

   b. The gauze strips are placed in rows, beginning in the floor of the nose along the posterior aspect and layering the gauze stripping as shown in Figure 8.6. The gauze should be laid down carefully and only after adequate shrinking of the congested nasal membranes and adequate anesthesia has been provided as indicated above.
5. When anterior bleeding continues the following steps may be taken:
   a. A number of authors have recommended the use of Surgigel® or Oxygel® as a packing agent (18). We do not recommend these because they often form a sticky, amorphous mess when left in place (9, 25).
   b. Remove the packing and place cot-

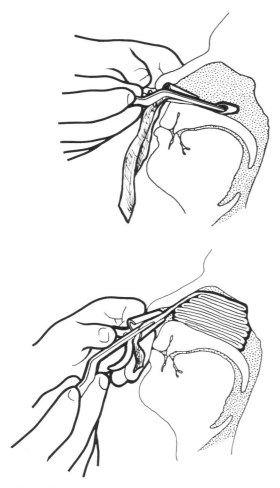

Figure 8.6. Layering of an anterior pack in the nose by placing layer upon layer of ¼ inch Vaseline® gauze packing from the floor of the nose to the superior aspect of the nose. During placement the pack should be periodically "packed" down and compressed against the floor of the nose so that one may build up a tight tamponading pack.

whether the bleeding is coming from under the middle turbinates, suggesting an arterial cause, or from a superior site which an improperly placed pack may not adequately control (24).

c. Heywood (21) has shown that epistaxis due to thrombocytopenia may be difficult to control. He used fresh frozen porcine strips (bacon) thawed and thinned to about 1½ cm in width, mostly composed of fatty tissue and inserted these into the anterior nares of these patients. The duration of the packing varied with the platelet count. All patients in Heywood's study had thrombocytopenia ranging from 5,000 to 16,000, and packing either one or both nostrils with the strips of porcine fat controlled the bleeding in 9 of 11 cases. Others have used the same procedure, although it has not become a routine method by any means. It is postulated by the authors that the bacon in the nostrils promotes hemostasis and diminishes epistaxis by two means: one by the pressure effect and the second because the fatty portions of the porcine tissue may act as a local accelerator of coagulation in the absence of normal platelet numbers. Topical thrombin also may be quite useful in patients with coagulopathies (17).

NOTE

Treatment with drugs. Jacobson (10) successfully treated 300 cases of recurrent or continuous nosebleeds with intravenous estrogens. Patients with familial hemorrhagic telangiectasia may respond to the oral administration of 0.25 to 1 mg ethinyl estradiol daily over a prolonged period of time (18). In males, methyl testosterone in the dosage of 5 to 10 mg daily was added to this regime. The topical application of thrombin and thromboplastin often has been used in cases of diffuse bleeding from the mucous membranes, especially in pa-

ton strips soaked in cocaine and epinephrine solution; these strips are kept in place until the bleeding decreases. A new anterior pack should be placed carefully following this procedure. If bleeding continues, these patients should be checked for a hemorrhagic diathesis. One must try to ascertain tients with acute leukemia and multiple myeloma (17). Neivert (34) found a high incidence of ascorbic acid and vitamin K deficiency in patients with recurrent epistaxis. Nontraumatic, nonirritant nosebleeds occur in approximately one third of children observed over a 15 year period with rheumatic epistaxis (epistaxis occurring during rheumatic fever) (26). This was thought to be due to an increased vascular fragility of the nasal mucous membranes. Vitamin C derived from lemon rind and administered as a tablet increased the capillary resistance, although not to normal levels, and diminished the frequency and severity of rheumatic epistaxis (26). Double-blind studies on the effects of aminocaproic acid (Amicar®), an antifibrinolysin, on recurrent bleeding found that significantly less frequent and severe bleeding occurred among treated patients (42).

Overall, however, drugs have not been proven to work in the acute episode (9). There is no good evidence for carbazochrome salicylate (Adrenosem®), a commonly advocated drug for the control of acute episodes of epistaxis, or Premarin® or epsilon aminocaproic acid being of value in treating patients with acute epistaxis. In later studies using Premarin® and estrogens in a controlled study, there was no effect on the duration of acute epistaxis (15).

d. Surgical interruption of the anterior ethmoidal artery in severe epistaxis due to bleeding at this site may have to be performed in some cases (18, 24, 36). In a large study on arterial epistaxis in which dye was injected into the external and internal carotids, Shaheen found that when the site of bleeding could not be identified, it was reasonable to ligate the external carotid or maxillary artery since that vessel supplied the major portion of the nose (41). In 14% of the cases he examined, the anterior ethmoid was absent unilaterally. Although exceedingly uncommon, there has been a case reported of epistaxis secondary to rupture of an aneurysm of the internal carotid artery which eroded into the paranasal sinuses (39).

e. The Nasostat balloon described below may be of benefit in unremitting anterior bleeds.

6. The packing should remain in place for 5 days and then be removed.

Posterior Bleeding

Posterior bleeding, as indicated above, may be secondary to bleeding from Woodruff's plexus, in which case a cotton pledget moistened with cocaine and epinephrine held snugly below the inferior turbinate may decrease the bleeding (17). The sphenopalatine artery is another common site of posterior bleeding. There are basically two methods which have been described for the treatment of posterior bleeding: the placement of a posterior pack and balloon tamponade. Both of these will be described.

POSTERIOR PACK (Fig. 8.7)

A 3 × 3 gauze bandage is folded lengthwise, rolled tightly until the thick end is less than ¾ inch in diameter and bound tightly around the middle by two pieces of umbilical tape, each measuring approximately 10 inch in length. Umbilical tape is superior to string because it does not cut into the palate (27). Following this a rubber catheter is inserted through the nose and pulled out through the mouth. The umbilical tape is tied to the catheter, and the pack is pulled back into the mouth and into the posterior choani of the nose by pulling on the rubber catheter. The pack lodges securely in the posterior choani of the nose and tamponades bleeding at this point. The umbilical tape then is secured anteriorly by tying it around a piece of gauze to prevent posterior displacement of the pack. An anterior pack is applied on the same side on which the posterior pack was placed, because bleeding may resume at a later time just anterior to the posterior pack due to difficulties in maintaining constant pressure on the sphenopalatine ar-

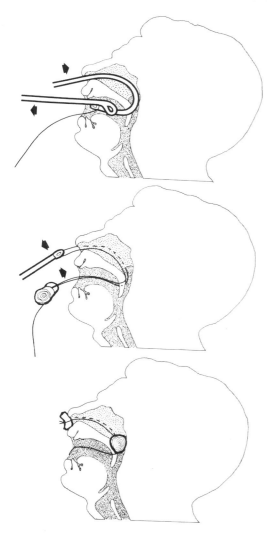

Figure 8.7. Technique of placing a posterior pack. See text for discussion.

tery. Most bleeding can be stopped with a properly placed posterior and anterior pack.

Complications

A number of complications have been described in association with posterior packs. If a string is used rather than umbilical tape, it may cut into the soft palate. Infections of the middle ear have been noted following posterior pack insertion (17). Osteomyelitis of the parasphenoid

following pharyngeal infections from posterior packs also has been described (17). Abscesses in the pharynx following posterior packs may occur.

All patients with a posterior pack in place should be placed on antibiotics. Ventilation-perfusion abnormalities develop with a posterior pack and arterial oxygen may fall 20 to 30 mm Hg; thus, all these patients should be admitted to the hospital (17, 27).

BALLOON TAMPONADE

A number of authors have recommended balloon tamponade rather than a posterior pack due to poor patient tolerance and the complications associated with posterior packs (5, 24, 42, 44). Many nasal balloons have been developed and are currently commercially available. The Brighton and Eschman® balloons function much like a Foley catheter and are held in place by an external balloon which, if accidentally deflated, could result in the entire device and pack slipping posteriorly and blocking the airway. The Nozstop® is a two-balloon device which is bulky and hard to place in the airway and also may block the airway if the outer balloon is deflated. Of all the balloons commercially available, the Nasostat® has been found by the authors and others to be the best designed balloon on the market today (Fig. 8.8) (14). This balloon is designed to act as a self-retaining choanal plug when inflated and will not slip posteriorly due to its being held in position by a permanent noncollapsible bulge in the body of the catheter that impinges on the nares outside the nose. Usually there is no need for an anterior pack with this balloon in place, as it occludes the area where the sphenopalatine artery exits, as well as all sites anterior to the artery.

Technique of Insertion

1. Inflate the balloon to ascertain that there are no leaks.
2. Lubricate the balloon with Xylocaine® jelly and introduce it along the floor of the nose.
3. Inflate the balloon first with approx-

imately 8 ml of air injected very slowly to minimize the discomfort which may occur with the rapid inflation (Fig. 8.9).

4. Inspect the oropharynx for evidence of continuing posterior bleeding. If posterior bleeding persists, more air is slowly injected until either the posterior bleeding stops or the palate is seen to bulge inferiorly into the mouth. If the patient complains of a blocked feeling in the airway, the balloon may be overinflated and air should be withdrawn until the opposite airway is patent.

5. If no bleeding is noted posteriorly and the opposite airway is patent, the air must be withdrawn and measured, and replaced with the same volume of water, since air will leak out over a short period of time.

6. A 2 × 2 strip of gauze is placed be-

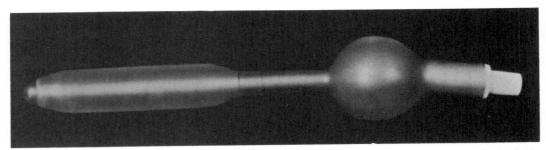

Figure 8.8. Nasostat balloon. (Reprinted with permission of Aspen Systems. Gottschalk, G.H., Epistaxis and the Nasostat. J.A.C.E.P. 5:794, 1976.)

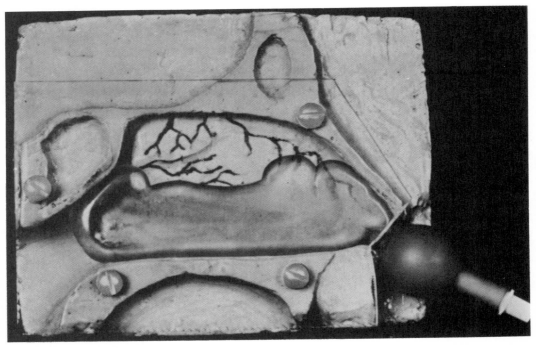

Figure 8.9. Inflated Nasostat balloon. Note that the balloon conforms to the turbinates, thus sealing off posterior as well as anterior bleeding. (Reprinted with permission of Aspen Systems. Gottschalk, G.H., Epistaxis and the Nasostat. J.A.C.E.P. 5:794, 1976.)

tween the nose and the bulb so as to prevent pressure necrosis which may occur. If anterior bleeding continues after the balloon is inflated, it is probably from the ethmoidal artery and an anterior packing placed superiorly in the nasal cavity is indicated. In some patients with a large nasal passage, a larger size Nasostat® may be needed. In patients with continuing ethmoidal bleeding the balloon may be inserted along the floor of the nose, and an anterior pack applied over it and then the balloon slowly inflated to stop the epistaxis (Fig. 8.10).

7. The balloon should remain inflated for 48 hours. Following this period, the balloon may be deflated but should remain in place for an additional 12 to 24 hours. If no bleeding results at this time, the balloon may be removed.

NOTE

When a Nasostat® or other balloon device is not available, one may use a 12 or 14 French Foley catheter (5, 42, 44). The Foley catheter should be inserted along the floor of the nose until it reaches the nasopharynx. The balloon is then inflated with approximately 7 ml of water and is drawn forward until it lodges in the posterior portion of the nose (Fig. 8.11). If bleeding does not stop, an additional 15 ml of water may be added. An anterior pack then is placed anteriorly against the balloon for the same reasons as indicated for posterior pack noted above. This combination has been used to successfully control posterior bleeding (5, 42, 44).

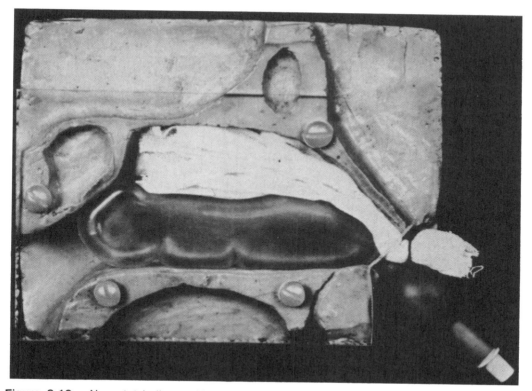

Figure 8.10. Nasostat balloon with an anterior pack placed above it before inflation of the balloon. This is used for bleeding from the anterior ethmoid which cannot be stopped by routine methods. (Reprinted with permission of Aspen Systems. Gottschalk, G.H., Epistaxis and the Nasostat. J.A.C.E.P. 5:794, 1976).

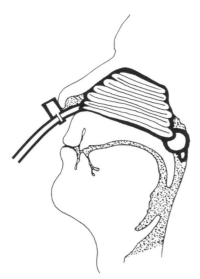

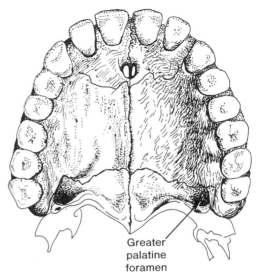

Greater
palatine
foramen

Figure 8.11. When one is dealing with a posterior nasal bleeding, a Foley catheter may be placed into the nasopharyngeal region and an anterior pack then is placed distal to the catheter balloon. The balloon then is inflated and pulled distally, thus forming a tight seal at the site where the sphenopalatine artery exits; this usually stops most posterior nasal bleeding resistant to other forms of therapy.

Figure 8.12. Greater palatine foramen. The technique of blocking the sphenopalatine artery is discussed in the text.

INJECTION BLOCK OF THE SPHENO-PALATINE ARTERY

In the patient who has unremitting posterior nasal hemorrhage, a method has been described for controlling the hemorrhage by blocking the sphenopalatine artery as well as the descending palatine arteries. The patient is placed in a supine position with the mouth opened and the greater palatine foramen is palpated (Fig. 8.12). One must be accurate in locating the foramen since the needle must pass through it to obtain a good block. It is located in the hard palate just anterior to the junction with the soft palate. A slight depression under the palatal mucosa just distal to the third molar can be palpated or can be located with a needle probe. Using a 22 or 23 gauge spinal needle on a 5 ml syringe, inject 3 ml of 2% lidocaine with 1:100,000 epinephrine through the

greater palatine foramen into the pterygopalatine fossa via the pterygopalatine canal. When properly placed, injection here blocks the sphenopalatine artery and also the descending palatine artery. The ideal depth of injection is 28 mm (37), and the needle should be inserted to this depth once within the foramen. The active agent reducing bleeding is epinephrine; lidocaine merely reduces the pain of injection, since the sphenopalatine nerve courses with the artery in the pterygopalatine canal. In one study using this procedure, posterior bleeding was controlled or stopped in 10 of 11 patients within 3 minutes after the block was instilled (37). Authors using this technique advocate that it should be attempted before insertion of any posterior pack, for when bleeding is controlled by this means, the difficulty of inserting a pack and the discomfort of a balloon in place for a prolonged period of time are avoided (27, 37).

Arterial ligation is indicated only when packing or a balloon tamponade have failed.

Figure 8.13 is a useful guide for manage-

Figure 8.13. A schematic guide for the management of and approach to a patient with epistaxis.

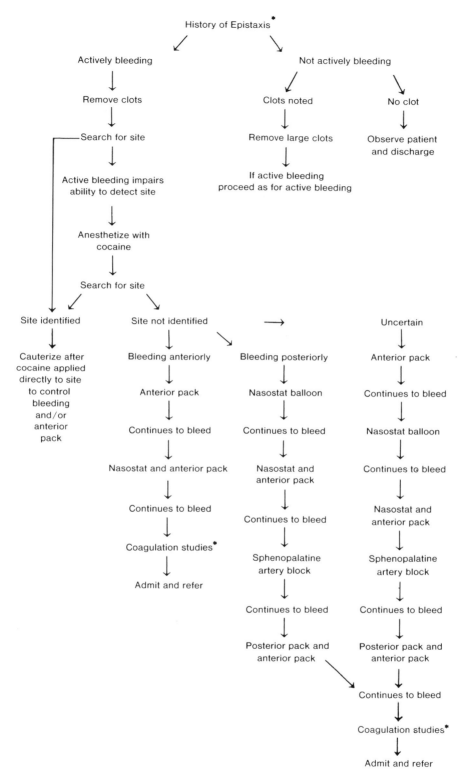

History of Epistaxis [*]

Actively bleeding
↓
Remove clots
↓
Search for site
↓
Active bleeding impairs
ability to detect site
↓
Anesthetize with
cocaine
↓
Search for site

Not actively bleeding
↓
Clots noted
↓
Remove large clots
↓
If active bleeding
proceed as for active bleeding

No clot
↓
Observe patient
and discharge

Site identified
↓
Cauterize after
cocaine applied
directly to site
to control
bleeding
and/or
anterior
pack

Site not identified
↓
Bleeding anteriorly
↓
Anterior pack
↓
Continues to bleed
↓
Nasostat and anterior pack
↓
Continues to bleed
↓
Coagulation studies[*]
↓
Admit and refer

Bleeding posteriorly
↓
Nasostat balloon
↓
Continues to bleed
↓
Nasostat and
anterior pack
↓
Continues to bleed
↓
Sphenopalatine
artery block
↓
Continues to bleed
↓
Posterior pack and
anterior pack

Uncertain
↓
Anterior pack
↓
Continues to bleed
↓
Nasostat balloon
↓
Continues to bleed
↓
Nasostat and
anterior pack
↓
Sphenopalatine
artery block
↓
Continues to bleed
↓
Posterior pack and
anterior pack
↓
Continues to bleed
↓
Coagulation studies[*]
↓
Admit and refer

[*] If the patient has a known coagulopathy or if a coagulopathy is strongly suspected, e.g., uremia, petechiae, easy bleeding, the topical thrombin or pork should be tried early in the course of therapy for all but posterior bleeding.

Figure 8.13

ment of patients presenting with epistaxis to the emergency center.

NASAL FOREIGN BODIES

Nasal foreign bodies can be difficult to remove in a child. Spherical objects such as peas or beads present a special problem as they are hard and smooth and edema with secondary infection develops rapidly. If not removed, the particle may dislodge into the pharynx and result in aspiration.

The initial method for removing a particle from the nose is by the patient forcefully blowing his nose (35). If this method does not work, a hooked probe may be passed behind the object to pull it forward (6, 33). Alligator forceps also have been advocated for removal of particles from the nose (12). When the particle is especially difficult to remove, the following technique is advocated. Place the patient in the Trendelenburg position. A local vasoconstrictor is useful when mucosal edema has developed. A topical anesthetic also should be instilled in the involved nostril. Following adequate anesthesia and constriction of the mucous membranes, the fine wire-loop of an ear curette is bent to form a shallow scoop. The object usually can be spooned out by placing the instrument alongside the object (30) (Fig. 8.14). A technique which has been useful

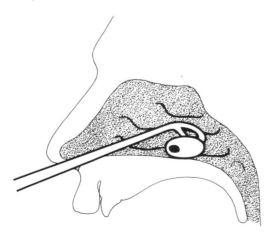

Figure 8.14.   A hooked probe can be used for removal of a nasal foreign body. When the foreign body is too far posterior, techniques described in the text can be used for its removal.

to the authors, particularly in small children with foreign bodies lodged posteriorly, is to place a Fogarty balloon-tipped catheter into the nostril and inflate the balloon. The foreign body may be removed by pulling the inflated balloon forward or the balloon may be used to stabilize the foreign body and a fine wire-loop ear curette or other device as indicated above may be used to remove it. This latter technique is the authors' preferred method for the removal of difficult foreign bodies in small children and infants.

NASAL FRACTURES

Nasal fractures are very commonly seen within the emergency center. The physician first seeing the patient must make an early diagnosis before the development of edema, as this may impair the ability to diagnose a displaced fracture. In children, edema develops very early, while in adults it develops much later. While nasal bones heal by bony union without scar contracture, nasal cartilage does not. Cartilage heals by deposition of scar tissue with contracture that may cause curling and buckling around an organized inflammatory exudate and a chondritis formed during healing. One has a grace period, during which time a reduction of nasal fractures can be done by the emergency physician in the emergency center. This grace period is before swelling occurs. If the patient comes in after swelling is significant, then reduction should be delayed and the patient referred to an otolaryngologist. Reduction of a nasal fracture can be done 7 to 10 days after the swelling has subsided, using a closed technique after the injury. In children, bony fusion may occur earlier and therefore reduction should be done at an earlier time.

We recommend that the following protocol be used in diagnosing fractures of the nose.

1. Look for any deformity or depression of the nasal bone.
2. Palpate the bridge of the nose for any crepitus. One should be cautious not to palpate too vigorously. Fractures

may be present in this area without any obvious crepitation.

3. Examine the inside of the nose after applying 4% cocaine to shrink the nasal membranes. One should look for submucosal hemorrhage or hematoma formation, particularly along the septum and mucosal tears or deviation of the septum or lateral nasal wall. A hematoma of the septum has normal mucosal coloring and is not ecchymotic, making it difficult to identify. A septal hematoma must be identified; missing this diagnosis may lead to the formation of a septal abscess or devitalization of the cartilage and a saddle deformity of the nose. One can palpate the septum and feel a fluctuation over a hematoma.

When a septal hematoma is identified, it should be incised and drained as discussed in Chapter 9: "Plastic Surgery, Principles and Techniques." The technique for drainage through an L-shaped incision is shown in Figure 9.26 in the chapter on plastic surgery. Lateral swelling due to buckling of the lateral cartilage or submucosal hemorrhage also must be found. All of these conditions will present with inability to shrink the mucous membrane with cocaine. If the membranes do shrink with the application of cocaine, one must search for mucosal membrane tears. When a mucosal membrane tear is large and accessible, it should be repaired with plain catgut suture. When one is unable to repair a large defect of the membrane, the area should be packed to prevent hematoma formation.

4. As a final step, radiographs should be obtained. It is reported that only 50% of fractures of the nose are seen on routine radiographs (3, 20).

Nasal fractures can be classified into three categories: 1) Greenstick fractures. In this situation, there is bending of the nasal bones or septum but no complete fracture line is visualized; 2) Linear fracture. Linear fracture may be displaced or undisplaced. When the patient has an undisplaced fracture in good position, the treatment is ice to decrease swelling and analgesia. If there is a linear fracture with either lateral displacement or depression present, the treatment consists of blunt elevation with splinting and/or intranasal vaseline gauze packing; 3) Comminuted fractures. Comminuted fractures of the nasal bones are often open, with mucosal tears exposing the bone. The treatment of these injuries is similar to that of displaced and depressed lateral fractures. The most common fracture seen in the adult is one with lateral displacement or depression of the nasal bone.

An analysis of nasal fractures indicates that patients with greenstick fractures and linear fractures without displacement or depression have a 100% good outcome. Linear fractures with displacement have a 40% good outcome and a 25% poor outcome, while depressed fractures have a 20% good outcome and a 45% poor outcome. In patients with comminuted fractures, only 10% have good results and 70% have poor results (22). These figures are in spite of the usual therapy for the fracture.

Equipment

Asch forceps
Vaseline gauze, ½ inch wide for nasal packing
Bayonet forceps
Anesthetic prep
1% Xylocaine® with epinephrine
5 cc syringe
25 gauge, 1½ inch needle
18 gauge needle
4% cocaine
Cotton balls
Cotton-tipped applicators
Head Light
Prefabricated metal splint, or casting material cut to appropriate shape and size
¼ inch adhesive tape
Tincture of benzoin
Periosteal elevator
Salinger elevator

Technique of Reduction

The physician must have a clear understanding of the anatomy of the nose before reduction of a nasal fracture (Fig. 8.15).

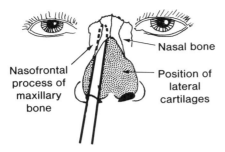

Figure 8.15. Note the anatomy of the nose and the placement of the cartilages.

The nasal part of the frontal bone is posterior and inferior to the nasal bones and adds strength and support to the bony arch of the nose. Therefore, fractures involving the nasal portion of the frontal bone require more uplift and support to prevent postreduction depression of the bridge of the nose. Following reduction the fractures must be splinted and packed properly. Secondly, lateral cartilaginous plates extend upward on the inner surface of the nasal bones and intimately fuse with them, so trauma to the nasal bones often injures these cartilages as well.

The following principles should be employed in reduction of nasal fractures:

1. Anesthesia should be provided by the technique discussed in the chapter on anesthesia.
2. Evacuate any hematomas or effusions and examine carefully for any cartilaginous damage.
3. Reduce the displaced fracture fragments. The bridge of the nose may have to be separated from the nasal part of the frontal bone as shown in Figure 8.15. This is done by inserting the Asch forceps into the appropriate nostril and elevating the nasal bone fragments into proper position by applying outward pressure with the forceps (Fig. 8.16E). The finger placed on the outside of the nose aids in properly aligning the nasal bone (Fig. 8.16B and E). A Salinger forceps is the authors' preferred method of reducing depressed nasal fractures. See Figure 8.16D for description. Adequate anesthesia is essential for this procedure. With an Asch forceps, the nasofrontal process of the maxillary bone may need to be rotated outward if it is depressed, in order for the nasal bones to be properly aligned with it. This is also done with the Asch forceps by applying outward pressure against these processes (Fig. 8.16C). By applying inward pressure with a digit over the laterally displaced segment and with the Asch forceps inserted inside the nose to provide adequate counter pressure, laterally displaced segments can be reduced.

4. A deviated septum is reduced by replacing it in the groove of the vomer with the Asch forceps as shown in Figure 8.16A. See legend to Figure 8.16 for a more detailed description.

5. Following reduction of the nose and septum, the nose should be packed internally on both sides with ½ inch Vaseline gauze to provide internal stabilization of the reduced segments. External stabilization is provided by splints which are made of either dental compound or casting material or by a specially made metal splint which is commercially available, shown in Figure 8.17. The splint should remain in place over the dorsum of the bony arch and cartilage to maintain position for 10 days. Internal splinting should be continued for 5 to 7 days. When a splint is formed from casting material, the splint should be cut out from several sheets of casting material in a shape similar to that of the metal splint shown in Figure 8.17. To secure the plaster splint on the nose, tincture of benzoin is painted on the nose and a strip of adhesive tape ("sticky side up") then is applied to the area where the cast will lie. The cast then is formed and placed in the proper position over the adhesive tape, which aids in keeping it in its proper location. One-quarter inch adhesive strips then can be placed over the casting material in a fashion similar to that shown in Figure 8.17 for the metal splint. Remem-

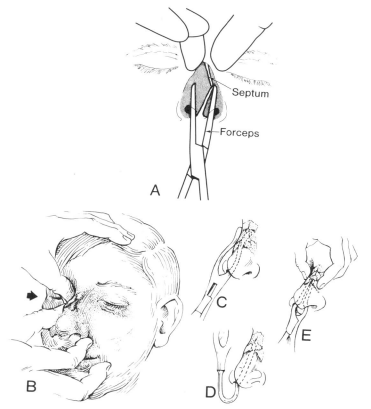

Figure 8.16. An Asch forceps can be used to correct a deviated septum, and a Salinger elevator or the handle of a scalpel can be used to elevate a depressed nasal fracture. One should use the opposite side of the nose for comparison and palpate to adequately reduce these fractures. Manual reduction of laterally angulated nasal fractures often can be done immediately following injury and with only momentary discomfort. (A) An Asch forceps correcting a deviated nasal septum. (B) A finger placed on the outside of the nose can manipulate a displaced fragment back into position. (C) A Salinger or Walsham forceps may be used to correct a laterally depressed fracture. (D) A Salinger elevator (preferred method) can be used to reposition a depressed fragment. (E) A forceps inserted inside the nose can be used to anatomically reposition these fragments. (Reprinted with permission of Williams & Wilkins, Baltimore. R.C. Schultz: Nasal fractures J. Trauma 15:321, 1975.)

ber that with complex nasal fractures, open reduction may be required if one cannot place the fragments together properly.

NOTE

In children, due to the fact that there is less ossification, there is a higher incidence of greenstick fractures, and crepitation may not be palpable even with significant displacement. Less force is required to fracture the cartilaginous structures of the nose, and there is a tendency to form more scar tissue with deformity increasing as the child grows. If the child presents with edema, and the history suggests a fractured nose, the physician should arrange for adequate follow-up even if the radiographs are normal. For children with depressed fractures, the treatment is basically similar to that for the adult with the exception that one must shrink the nasal

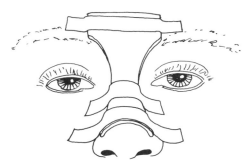

Figure 8.17. Prefabricated nasal splint used for external support of a reduced fracture. This does not provide a great deal of support, and we believe that its major utility is in cautioning the patient against further trauma to the side of the nasal fracture.

membranes with cotton strips saturated with cocaine before any procedure. The cotton should be wrapped around a periosteal elevator, dipped in cocaine and Vaseline®, and used to elevate the depressed nasal arch. The position should be maintained with lateral splints.

HEAD AND NECK ABSCESSES

While abscesses of the head and neck are a relatively common problem seen in the emergency center, only a few can be drained on an outpatient basis. While small superficial abscesses presenting in the anterior triangle (the area anterior to the sternocleidomastoid muscle) may be drained, any deep abscesses in a patient who has torticollis or trismus should be drained in the operating room with the exception of peritonsillar abscesses. There are various potential spaces within the neck which are beyond the scope of discussion in this text. Abscesses may drain or may extend into the carotid sheath or paratracheal region, requiring extensive incisions to promote adequate drainage.

Preparatory Steps In Treating Intraoral Abscesses

It is helpful to rinse the mouth with bicarbonate solution to dissolve excess mucus when dealing with intraoral abscesses, particularly those in the peritonsillar region. After the mucosa is sprayed

with 10% cocaine solution, the site of the proposed incision may be rubbed with a 10% cocaine stick until blanching occurs. Incision then is carried out with the patient in the sitting position and leaning forward whenever possible to avoid pulmonary aspiration of purulent material.

Peritonsillar Abscess

Muller states that while incision and drainage is often done for these abscesses, when compared with immediate tonsillectomy in 186 cases, no problems were encountered with this procedure and a faster return to normal activity was noted (32). Immediate tonsillectomy is recommended by many authors as the treatment of choice for peritonsillar abscesses (4, 31, 43). Other authors also note that it is often hard to obtain adequate drainage of an abscess in the peritonsillar area with a simple stab incision (41). Evidence of loculated nondraining purulent material may be slow resolution of the abscess, trismus, and persistence of pain in patients treated by incision alone. Immediate tonsillectomy assures total evacuation of the purulent matter, and the patient is spared a later admission for an interval tonsillectomy. In view of these data, the emergency physician should review the criteria for immediate tonsillectomy with the referring otolaryngologist. When interval tonsillectomy is elected, the peritonsillar abscesses may be drained within the emergency center. If no trismus or torticollis is present, one can safely assume that there is no extension into the neck. If these are present and are severe, one should consider drainage of the abscess in the operating room.

Technique

1. We advise, before incision and drainage, aspiration with a 20 gauge spinal needle and syringe at the point of maximum bulge in the soft palate.

NOTE

Internal carotid artery aneurysms presenting as acute peritonsillar abscesses have been reported and, therefore, confirmatory needle aspiration is advised in every patient with a peritonsillar abscess (19). Bloody return or pulsatile nature of the lesion should make one suspicious of this diagnosis.

2. An incision should be made superolaterally to the tonsil at the point of maximum bulge in the soft palate and extended slightly laterally (Fig. 8.18). The length of the incision should be approximately 1 to 1.5 cm and should be horizontal. A #11 blade is recommended for the incision, and a Frazier suction tip should be held at the tip of the blade and guided in front of the blade to prevent any aspiration of purulent material. The suction should be continuous, high flow wall suction.
3. Packing generally is not indicated and bleeding is usually minimal. The patient is advised to rest prone or in the lateral decubitus position with the same side down as the side of the abscess. Whenever possible the authors advocate that a peritonsillar abscess not be drained late in the evening before bedtime, particularly in the debilitated patient. Aspiration of purulent material as the patient rolls over into the supine position during sleep may result in a severe infection of the lungs.

NOTE

Approximately 78% of the pathogens found in peritonsillar abscesses are strep-

tococcus (32). In one large series, only 1 patient had *Bacteroides* and 2 patients had *Hemophilus parainfluenzae* and *Enterobacter cloacae,* both of which were sensitive to penicillin. Therefore, the treatment of choice for these abscesses, once drained, is penicillin.

Retropharyngeal Abscesses

Retropharyngeal abscesses can be due to foreign bodies in the pharynx, extension of infections from the ear, or infections in the posterior pharyngeal wall. While drainage has been performed on an outpatient basis under local anesthesia for small high-lying abscesses, admission and drainage in the operating room are recommended by the authors (28). These infections may extend to produce a severe mediastinitis with a high mortality.

Sublingual Abscesses

The sublingual space is localized along the floor of the mouth above the mylohyoid muscle. Intraoral drainage of abscesses occurring in this area is sometimes possible. One must be careful to avoid incision in the posterior lateral region of the floor of the mouth as this contains the lingual artery, vein, and nerve (28).

Technique

1. Anesthetize the roof of the abscess with 1% Xylocaine® with epinephrine. The abscess cavity is opened with a horizontal incision, using a #11 blade under local anesthesia. A Kelly clamp then is inserted into the abscess cavity and opened in order to separate any loculations and promote drainage. These patients usually require some type of sedation or intramuscular analgesia before the procedure. Drains are generally not inserted into the abscess cavity. The patient should be placed on broad-spectrum antibiotics and advised to use mouthwashes with hydrogen peroxide three times daily.

Abscesses Of The Parotid Duct

Parotid duct abscesses are seen in patients who have calculi obstructing the

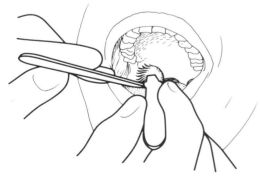

Figure 8.18. Drainage of a peritonsillar abscess. See text for discussion.

orifice of the duct or who have strictures causing stenosis and proximal dilatation. These abscesses should not be drained by probing the external orifice of the duct; drainage should be achieved by direct incision intraorally over the point of maximal bulge of the abscess. Following drainage, the abscess cavity is packed with fine strips of gauze, and the patient is referred to an otolaryngologist for follow-up care.

Aftercare Of Intraoral Abscesses

Following drainage of the abscesses in the oral cavity, the patient should be encouraged to use mouthwashes with half-strength hydrogen peroxide, five times daily until the cavity is healed. The hydrogen peroxide solution aids in breaking up the purulent matter, and the foaming action permits cleansing and debridement of the abscess cavity.

COMMON DENTAL EMERGENCIES

Treatment Of Fractured Teeth

A tooth may fracture at several points. While the emergency physician will generally refer patients with fractured teeth to a dentist, he should be aware of the basic treatment rendered in such injuries. There are seven types of tooth fractures or displacements which may occur (7). These are shown in Figure 8.19 and are discussed here.

TYPE 1 FRACTURE

A type 1 fracture is a fracture involving only the enamel of the tooth. One should apply topical fluoride to the fracture site. There is a possibility that, in the future, pulpal death may occur even with this minor injury. The patient should be rechecked in 3 months.

TYPE 2 FRACTURE

A type 2 fracture involves a fracture of the crown and dentine of the tooth. When calcium hydroxide is available in the emergency center, it should be applied over the fracture site to cover the exposed dentine. When this is not available, clear nailpolish can be used to protect the exposed dentine.

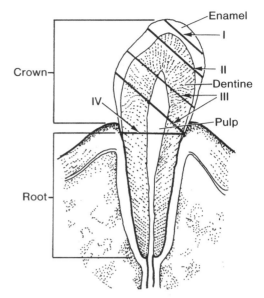

Figure 8.19. Various levels of fracture of the teeth. See text for complete discussion.

While this is frowned upon by some, a coating of clear nailpolish over the exposed dentine will protect it from further injury or contamination from exposure to saliva and air which may lead to pulpitis. A temporary restoration is placed over the cracked tooth by the dentist and a more aesthetic permanent restoration is applied later.

TYPE 3 FRACTURE

A type 3 fracture involves a fracture of the crown, dentine, and pulp. These injuries are divided into three subtypes:

1. *Patients seen within 6 hours.* Calcium hydroxide should be used to cover the pulp. The patient should be referred to the dentist, who will apply a cap to cover the pulp or a dressing of zinc oxide and eugenol paste followed by a temporary restoration.
2. *Patients seen between 6 and 24 hours.* Infection of the pulp probably has occurred by this time. Calcium hydroxide application over the exposed area plus pulpectomy is the treatment of choice, and the patient should be referred to a dentist for this therapy.
3. *Patients seen after 24 hours.* Total

pulpectomy and root canal obliteration are necessary in these cases. Endodontics is usually necessary.

TYPE 4 FRACTURE

In type 4 fractures, there is exposure of the entire pulp. When this type of fracture involves a permanent tooth, endodontic therapy is necessary and a conventional filling is used. When the fracture involves a primary tooth, a total pulpectomy followed by zinc oxide and a eugenol paste filling is preferred.

TYPE 5 FRACTURE

This involves avulsion of the tooth and is a very common injury seen in the emergency center. Time is of the essence in dealing with an avulsed tooth. If the parent calls from home and states that her child has avulsed a tooth, and she has the tooth, she should be instructed to rinse it under warm water and not to scrub the tooth clean and to reinsert the tooth into its normal anatomical position and bring the child into an emergency center. If patient or family is too apprehensive to reimplant the tooth, then place the tooth under the patient's tongue or in an 8 oz glass of water with a teaspoon of salt dissolved. In the emergency center the tooth should be rinsed under warm water and should not be scrubbed as this will remove the periodontal ligament and membrane. This membrane is necessary for adequate repair of the injured tooth. The critical time in which a tooth will usually be successfully reimplanted if adequately treated appears to be 30 minutes. Beyond 30 minutes there is an increased likelihood that the tooth may not be salvageable. When the tooth has been avulsed for several hours, endodontics is usually performed first and then the tooth is reimplanted. If the alveolar socket is fractured at the site of the avulsion, then reimplantation is contraindicated. After the tooth is placed in its normal anatomical position, the patient should be referred.

TYPE 6 FRACTURE

A type 6 fracture involves a fracture of the root of the tooth with or without loss of the crown structure. If the fracture involves the apical one third, the prognosis is good. If the pulp is necrotic, a pulpectomy is necessary. If the fracture involves the middle one third of the root, only a fair prognosis can be given and the tooth may be somewhat loose and need stabilization. A fracture involving the coronal one third of the root has a very poor prognosis and is very mobile. Extraction is usually done in these cases; however, if the root portion can hold a restoration, then extraction may not be necessary. These patients should all be referred.

TYPE 7 FRACTURE

This involves a displaced tooth with no fracture of the crown or root. In these patients the tooth should be wired to the adjacent stable tooth, which provides an excellent splint to keep the loose tooth in proper position. This technique is shown in Figure 8.20.

Any patient with a displaced tooth or an avulsed tooth should be placed on antibiotics due to contamination of the tooth.

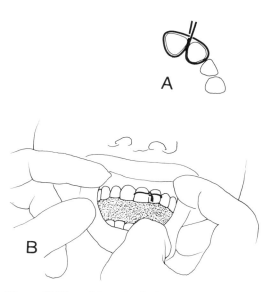

Figure 8.20. A loop technique for temporarily splinting a partially avulsed or loose tooth to the adjacent tooth until dental consultation can be obtained. (A) This view looks up at the tooth from an inferior location. (B) Anterior view.

Postextraction Bleeding

Postextraction bleeding is a very common problem which presents to the emergency center. The patient usually is unable to reach his dentist. When this occurs, the fossa of the extracted tooth should be irrigated with warm saline and all clots suctioned out. A 2 × 2 gauze compress is folded and placed tightly within the socket, and the patient is instructed to bite down firmly over this gauze. The patient should continue biting on the compress for 15 minutes. This usually stops the bleeding if the compress has been placed in the socket rather than over the general region, which will not permit adequate tamponade of the bleeding site. If the bleeding continues, Oxygel® can be inserted into the socket and another 2 × 2 compress applied for 15 minutes. If this is unsuccessful, one should examine to see if bleeding is coming from the alveolar bone. If so, after adequate suctioning of clots, a piece of bone wax should be inserted into the socket and pressed into the alveolar bone. This will usually stop bleeding from a bony site. If none of these methods are successful, as a last resort suturing of the gingiva may be helpful in order to control bleeding.

Postextraction Osteitis (Dry socket)

Patients present with pain over a postextraction site 1 to 3 days postoperatively. This is usually following the extraction of a molar, usually the "wisdom" tooth. The loss of the blood clot in the socket exposes the alveolar bone to air. The patient usually experiences a dull throbbing pain which is accentuated by drinking cool water and breathing in through the mouth. The treatment of this problem is to irrigate the socket with warm saline and pack eugenol-soaked iodoform gauze into the socket. The patient should be given antibiotics and pain medications. *Staphylococcus aureus* is the primary agent responsible for this problem.

References

1. Appelbaum, A., Simplest instrument for removal of foreign body from cornea. Arch. Ophthalmol. 30:262, 1943.
2. Barelli, P.A., The management of epistaxis in children. Otolaryngol. Clin. North Am. 10:91, 1977.
3. Becker, O.J., Nasal fracture: Analysis of 100 cases. Arch. Otolaryngol. 48:344, 1948.
4. Beeden, A.G., Evans, J.N., Quinsy tonsillectomy: A further report. J. Laryngol. Otolaryngol. 84:443, 1970.
5. Bell, M., Hawke, M., Jahn, A., New device for the management of postnasal epistaxis by balloon tamponade. Arch. Otolaryngol. 99:372, 1974.
6. Birch, C.A., Emergencies in Medical Practice. E.S. Livington, Ltd., Edinburgh and London, 1967, p. 185.
7. Braham, R.L., Roberts, M.W., Morris, M.E., Management of dental trauma in children and adolescents. J. Trauma 17:857, 1977.
8. Bronson, N.R., Nonmagnetic foreign body localization and extraction. Am. J. Ophthalmol. 58:133, 1964.
9. Call, W.H., Control of epistaxis. Surg. Clin. North Am. 49:1235, 1969.
10. El Bitar, H., The etiology and management of epistaxis: A review of 300 cases. Practitioner 207:800, 1971.
11. Galin, M.A., Harris, L.S., Papariello, G.J., Nonsurgical removal of corneal rust stains. Arch. Ophthalmol. 74:674, 1965.
12. Gellis, S.S., Kagan, B.M., Current Pediatric Therapy. W.B. Saunders Co., Philadelphia, 1964, P. 88.
13. Giammanco, P., Binns, P.M., Temporary blindness and ophthalmoplegia from nasal packing. J. Laryngol. 84:631, 1970.
14. Gottschalk, B.H., The treatment of epistaxis with the Nasostat. Trans. Am. Acad. Ophthalmol. Otolaryngol. 78:1274, 1974.
15. Grant, J.H., Clinical evaluation of the use of Premarin and the treatment of epistaxis. J. Laryngol. Otolaryngol. 75:909, 1961.
16. Hara, H.J., Severe epistaxis. Arch. Otolaryngol. 75:84, 1962.
17. Hallberg, O.E., Severe nosebleed and its treatment. J.A.M.A. 148:355, 1952.
18. Harpman, J.A., Management of epistaxis other than from Little's area. Arch. Otolaryngol. 75:254, 1962.
19. Henry, R.C., Aneurysm of the internal carotid artery presenting as a peritonsillar abscess. J. Laryngol. Otolaryngol. 88:379, 1974.
20. Hersh, J.H., Management of fracture of nasal bony vault. Ann. Otolaryngol. 54:534, 1945.
21. Heywood, B.B., Davis, R.B., Yonkers, A.J., Treatment of epistaxis with porcine stripped packing. Trans. Am. Acad. Ophthalmol. Otolaryngol. 82:255, 1976.
22. Hurst, A., The importance of nasal fractures. Laryngoscope 70:68, 1969.
23. Jennings, E.R., Glucksman, M.A., Renal vein ligation (letter). J.A.M.A. 213:1905, 1970.
24. Juselius, H., Epistaxis: A clinical study of 1,724 patients. J. Laryngol. Otolaryngol. 88:317, 1974.
25. Kamer, F.M., Parkes, M.L., An absorbent, nonadherent nasal pack. Laryngoscope 85:384, 1975.
26. Kugelmass, I.N., Vitamin P in rheumatic epistaxis.

27. LaForce, R.F., Treatment of nasal hemorrhage. Surg. Clin. North Am. 49:1305, 1969.
28. Levitt, G.W., The surgical treatment of deep neck infections. Laryngoscope 80:403, 1970.
29. Lynch, M.G., Minor surgery of the ear, nose and throat. Surg. Clin. North Am. 31:1315, 1951.
30. McMaster, W.C., Removal of foreign body from the nose. J.A.M.A. 213:1905, 1970.
31. McCurty, J.A., Peritonsillar abscess. Arch. Otolaryngol. 103:414, 1977.
32. Muller, S.P., Peritonsillar abscess: A prospective study of pathogens, treatment and morbidity. Ear, Nose Throat J. 57:46, 1978.
33. Nealon, T.F., Fundamental Skills in Surgery. W.B. Saunders Co., Philadelphia, 1962, p. 179.
34. Neivert, H., Engelberg, R., Pirk, L.A., Nasal hemorrhage: Studies of ascorbic acid, prothrombin and vitamin K. Arch. Otolaryngol. 47:37, 1948.
35. Nelson, W.E., Textbook of Pediatrics. W.B. Saunders, Co., Philadelphia, 1950, p. 915.
36. Oppenheim, H., Uhde, G., Shapiro, R.L. et al., Surgical interruption of the anterior ethmoid artery in severe epistaxis. Arch. Otolaryngol. 56:448, 1952.
37. Padrnos, R.E., A method for control of posterior nasal hemorrhage. Arch. Otolaryngol. 87:85, 1968.
38. Percival, S.P.B., A decade of intraocular foreign bodies. Br. J. Ophthalmol. 56:454, 1972.
39. Polcyn, J.L., Roth, G.R., Epistaxis from rupture of aneurysm of internal carotid artery (letter). J.A.M.A. 213:876, 1970.
40. Schultz, R.C., Nasal fractures. J. Trauma 15:319, 1975.
41. Shaheen, O.H., Arterial epistaxis, J. Laryngol. Otolaryngol. 89:17, 1975.
42. Stell, P.M., Epistaxis. Clin. Otolaryngol. 2:263, 1977.
43. Templer, J.W., Hollinger LD, Wood RP II, et al., Immediate tonsillectomy for the treatment of peritonsillar abscess. Am. J. Surg. 134:596, 1977.
44. Wadsworth, P., Method of controlling epistaxis (letter). Br. Med. J. 1:506, 1971.

Plastic Surgery Principles and Techniques

9

SKIN ANATOMY AND FUNCTION

Skin Structure

The skin is composed of an epidermal and a dermal layer, the thicknesses of which vary in different parts of the body. The epidermis of the palm and soles is quite thick, measuring 0.4 to 0.6 mm. The skin in the remainder of the body ranges in thickness from 0.075 to 0.15 mm. The dermis consists of fibroelastic connective tissue, containing both collagen for strength and elastic fibers for stretch and flexibility. The thickness of the dermis varies from 1 to 4 mm and is greatest in the back, followed by the thigh, abdomen, forehead, wrist, and scalp, and is least in the eyelid. Dermal thickness varies inversely with the age of the patient.

The color of normal human skin is related to the number, size, type, and distribution of melanocytes. The clinical applicability of this fact is discussed later in this chapter.

Normal Repair (28, 43)

In the normal process of wound repair, the injured vessels at the wound edge thrombose and nearby vessels dilate. Platelets and white cells adhere to the epithelial lining, and leukocytes migrate into the area of injury. Within a few hours, the edge of the injured tissue is infiltrated by granulocytes and macrophages. The tissue thus becomes overladen with highly metabolically active leukocytes which are replaced in a few days by fibroblasts which have migrated from the perivascular connective tissue.

In the first 8 days following a laceration, the wound has little inherent strength and is held together by blood vessels crossing the wound, a fibrous coagulum, and wound epithelialization. Each of these processes will be discussed separately.

After a wound the process of *neovascularization* begins early. Angiograms have shown that within 10 hours after a laceration there is relatively sparse vasculature and the wound edges appear no different from the rest of the surrounding skin (60). At 3 days the number of vessels increase around the wound, and there is some vasodilatation. By the third or fourth day the new blood vessels are seen bridging the wound space of primary wounds, and in open wounds a rose-colored hue can be noted where the first few vessels appear. By the fifth day an occasional new vessel can be seen crossing the width of the wound. At 7 days there is a marked increase in the number of vessels around the wound, and new vessels are seen bridging the gap. In fact, when a patient returns for suture removal, e.g., after 7 days, there is an increased vascular hue around the edges of the wound that is often so intense it is mistaken for an infection! New vessels join with existing ones from the other side and join the cut vessel ends in a skin graft, if one has been used over the wound. Subsequently there is a gradual diminution in the wound vasculature so that by 21 days the wound has returned to normal appearance. Capillary vessels decrease within the scar over a period of approximately 6 months.

When one looks at the different suture materials used in repair of wounds and the effect on vascularity, there is no difference between wounds closed with nylon, chromic catgut, plain catgut, or even tape (60). However, the effects of *tightly tied* sutures were striking. By the third day, tightly tied wounds showed an absence of blood vessels. After 7 days, completely avascular areas, up to 3 mm in size, were noted around the suture (60). Histologic sections showed that microinfarction and necrosis had been produced in the tissue surrounding tight sutures. Mattress sutures were much more likely to devascularize the wound than were simple or continuous sutures, unless extreme care was taken in tying the suture loosely.

Within a few days the *leukocytes* present in the wound are replaced by macrophages, which debride the injured tissue, stimulate fibroblast migration and activation, and initiate the process of neovascularization. When fibroblasts replace the majority of the white cells, collagen synthesis by fibroblasts begins. Newly formed collagen appears in the healing wound as early as the second day, reaching its peak rate of synthesis by the fifth to the seventh day. Collagen continues to be synthesized for 6 months to 1 year; however, at the same time as it is being formed it is also being degraded, as the initial collagen is highly disorganized. If this restructuring of collagen were not to occur, the patient would develop a hypertrophic scar. The most rapid rate of increase in the *tensile strength* of the wound occurs by the *third week,* and at this time the wound has its greatest mass. Paradoxically, while the strength of the wound is increasing during the first 7 to 10 days due to the low tensile strength of the wound, dehiscence is more likely to occur at this time than at 3 weeks.

Epithelial cells multiply at the wound edge and migrate across the wound to form a protective surface. Within 12 hours after a laceration, epithelial repair begins with the migration of basal cells over the incised dermis. The proliferation of epithelial cells bridges the gap of the wound and acts as a barrier preventing bacterial penetration of the skin. The time for completion of epithelial bridging is affected by the technique of closure. *Eversion* of the skin edges permits epithelial bridging of the laceration to occur within 18 to 24 hours. End-to-end approximation of the skin edges results in an additional 12 hour delay in the formation of an epithelial bridge. If the wound edges are inverted, the bridging is completed 72 hours after closure.

AXIOM

Inversion of the wound edges results in a threefold increase in the time it takes for epithelial bridging to occur.

Downward growth of the epithelial cells occurs not only at the incision site but also at any interruption of the skin, such as a suture tract. This invasive epithelium begins to regress by 10 to 15 days after a laceration and leaves behind a small keratinized epithelial "spur," commonly known as a suture puncture mark. If percutaneous *sutures* are *removed* before the *eighth day,* invasive spurs of epithelium regress leaving no discernible mark. After that time a permanent scar results in a crosshatched or "railroad track" appearance of a wound. In thin skin, i.e., eyelids, epithelial tracks can form in less than 8 days. The severity of "spur" formation is affected by the region of the body at which the laceration occurs. Skin of the eyelids, soles, and palms seldom show suture puncture scars, unlike the back, chest, upper arms, and lower extremities where these marks are common. The size of the needle and the suture play an insignificant role in the development of these suture puncture marks.

Wound contraction occurs with wound healing. The force of contraction is applied by the myofibroblast. Contraction will continue until the force generated by the open wound is equalized by the tension of the surrounding skin. This is due to the movement of full-thickness skin toward the center of the skin defect by the drawing in of surrounding normal skin. A wound thus becomes smaller if permitted to contract. In some areas, like the face, contraction may pull and distort normal skin. In wounds in which grafting is appropriate, coverage with a full-thickness graft greatly diminishes the force of contraction.

FACTORS AFFECTING NORMAL REPAIR (28)

Drugs

Many factors have a significant effect on normal wound repair which the emergency physician must be aware of both for therapy and for prognostic purposes. When administered within 3 days after injury, steroids can cause problems in repair and are able to suppress the inflammatory response necessary for proper wound healing (43). Polymorphonuclear leukocytes and macrophages fail to enter the wound and fibroplasia is suppressed. However, steroids alone rarely halt repair unless given in large doses. In open wounds the effect of steroids is much worse than in closed wounds, since open wounds require more tissue healing than do primarily closed wounds. Contraction and epithelialization of open wounds take longer with steroids. Anti-inflammatory steroids begun after injury inhibit repair considerably less than do steroids started just after wounding. Vitamin A can be administered therapeutically in selected individuals to stimulate healing when steroid suppression of wound healing is a factor. Vitamin A facilitates the migration of macrophages into a wound, which is important for the initiation of wound healing and is inhibited by glucocorticoids. In addition, poor vascular regeneration in steroid-treated patients is reversed by vitamin A. The dose of vitamin A is 25,000 U/day and is safe and effective over a period of weeks. Topical vitamin A (1000 U/gm) is used with good results when applied three times per day in patients with nonhealing wounds, particularly steroid ulcers. If *topical or systemic vitamin A* is given, the effects of steroids can be partially overcome.

Wound repair is also inhibited by sex hormones. *Estrogen* depresses collagen synthesis and thereby mildly decreases tensile strength of wounds. *Progesterone* increases neovascularization and oxygen supply to the wound, increases inflammation, but inhibits collagen synthesis. When estrogen is added to progesterone, neovascularization is reduced to normal and thus the total effect is a marked decrease in wound repair. Therefore, progesterone depresses collagen synthesis markedly, and a combination of progesterone and estrogen depresses collagen synthesis even more markedly. Most females, however, have no problem with repair during pregnancy or while ingesting oral contraceptives.

Aspirin, phenylbutazone, and *vitamin E* inhibit inflammation, and this effect is reduced by vitamin A. Vitamin E has been dispensed in over-the-counter preparations advertized as an agent which decreases scar formation when applied topically over a wound. Vitamin E appears to decrease scar contracture; however, this has not been adequately proven.

Vitamin C is essential in the synthesis of collagen, and deficiencies in this vitamin impair wound healing. *Colchicine* interferes with microtubule function and slows collagen transport from the cell to the extracellular space.

Associated Conditions

Diabetics heal poorly. The function of white cells is impaired during episodes of hyperglycemia, and minor infections (including infections which are remote from the wound site) impair healing. The impaired microvasculature and neuropathy which ensues during diabetes decrease sensation, and cutaneous ulcers may develop. Major infections occur more easily in the diabetic than in the nondiabetic patient. For these reasons it is important to avoid anemia, hypoxia, and hypovolemia during the process of repair in the diabetic with wounds. Other factors which decrease collagen synthesis are infection, associated traumatic injuries, hypoxia, uremia, advanced age, and circulatory impairment.

Region

Certain areas of the body heal better than others, depending on skin thickness, pigmentation, and location. Thick skin heals more poorly than thin skin. Wounds over the back, chest, and shoulders tend to heal with more scarring than do wounds of the eyelids (40). Darker skin tends to heal more poorly than light skin because melanin deposition may occur at the wound site. In addition, hypertrophic scars and keloids occur more with thick and dark skin. Oily skin has a greater tendency for scar formation. Certain regions heal with a much thicker scar regardless of meticulous care. This is particularly true for lacerations over the sternum and lower extremity. Also, patients with skin disorders obviously will heal poorer than those with normal skin.

Abnormal Repair (28, 42)

KELOIDS

A keloid is a large, firm mass of scarlike tissue composed of homogeneous, eosinophilic bands of collagen mixed with fibers and fibroblasts. Keloids can originate from a wound or from a skin lesion such as acne. The hypertrophic tissue extends beyond the original wound and the epithelium tends to be darker than the normal skin. Keloids tend to occur over areas of increased skin pigmentation and are more common in wounds over the ears, waist, arms, elbows, shoulders, and especially the sternum.

Certain individuals are predisposed to keloid formation, and the patient usually can give a history of forming keloids. Keloid formation is more common in black patients.

A number of theories exist as to the cause of keloids. Some authors feel they are due to excess melanocyte-stimulating hormone (MSH) (47) corroborated by the observations that darker skinned patients form keloids, that keloids are rare in the palms and soles where melanocytes are rare, and that keloid development is enhanced during puberty and pregnancy when MSH is stimulated. Some authors feel that keloids are due to increased tension on the wound edges (47).

To decrease keloid formation, we advocate a closure which provides the least tension on the wound edges and a pressure dressing over the wound. All patients who have a tendency to form keloids should be followed closely; when the wound is in a conspicuous region, these patients should be referred to a plastic surgeon and he should be consulted during their initial presentation to the emergency center for aftercare considerations. Intradermal corticosteroid injections have been used to suppress MSH secretion and may even cure small keloids by accelerating collagen lysis. These injections are placed in the upper dermis and a pressure dressing is applied. Larger lesions can be excised and the wound grafted and irradiated during the first 24 hours of excision and resuturing. Another alternative is to inject the wound edges with a corticosteroid at the first sign of a keloid formation and, as an adjunct, apply a firm pressure dressing during the healing period.

HYPERTROPHIC SCARS

Hypertrophic scars are bulky scars which remain within the boundaries of the wound. They occur more around joints and areas of motion or tension. Keloids rarely resolve spontaneously, whereas hypertrophic scars tend to develop to a peak size and often regress over a period of months to years.

There are two theories for the pathogenesis of a hypertrophic scar. One is that a continuous inflammatory response occurs due to infection, which causes more connective tissue formation. Another theory states that it is due to tension on the wound edges. Incisions which cross flexion creases often become hypertrophic, and one must be particularly careful in dealing with these wounds.

In patients with a tendency to form hypertrophic scars, the application of a *pressure dressing* and *splinting* may be preventative. A firm pressure dressing at the level of capillary pressure (2 mm Hg) causes diminution of the mass of collagen and probably retards the synthesis of collagen by diminishing circulation. It often takes months of splinting and pressure to aid in the prevention of hypertrophic scars. Small scars may be treated with anti-inflammatory steroids, and radiation has been used.

MECHANISM OF WOUND INJURY
(28)

Wounds may occur as a result of three types of forces: shear forces, tension forces, and compressive forces. A wound from a sharp instrument, such as a knife, results in a classic example of a *shear* injury. These wounds do not have a great deal of associated soft-tissue damage around the laceration. The surface area of the tissue contacted by the wounding instrument is small, and tissue failure is obtained with a small amount of energy. *Tension* is another mechanism for producing a wound, e.g., a flat object striking the tissue which overlies a bony prominence. This results in a contusive injury to surrounding tissue around the laceration. In *compressive* injury, two equal forces are oriented toward each other and result in a stellate-type laceration, such as, with a hard round object (e.g., rock) striking a bony prominence (e.g., skull). The energy required (and dispersed into the tissues) for compressive forces to result in lacerations is greater than that for shear or tension wounds. Damage occurs to the wound edges and is associated with a reduction in blood flow and a hundredfold increased susceptibility to infection!

AXIOM

Wounds which are due to compressive forces, e.g., a stellate laceration, are associated with a hundredfold increased susceptibility to infection as compared with those due to shear forces, e.g., a knife.

SUTURE MATERIAL AND ADJUNCTS FOR WOUND CLOSURE

Skin Tape

Skin tape may be used to close superficial wounds or deeper wounds once the subcutaneous dermal layers have been approximated by absorbable suture material. Skin tape should not be used in widely separated wound edges. The tensile strength of the surgical tape must be sufficient to maintain wound approximation during healing. Weak tapes will not resist pull at the wound edges and will tear, permitting the wound to separate. Adding reinforcing rayon filaments to the backing of the tape may increase tensile strength fourfold (15). Skin tape comes in many sizes: ⅛ inch, ¼ inch, and ½ inch wide strips which are approximately 2 to 3 inches in length. Before skin tape is used, the skin must be cleansed with acetone or alcohol to remove all oils and particles which may cause the tape to form a poor contact with the skin, even though the skin has been scrubbed with an iodophor.

Contaminated wounds whose edges were approximated by suture material had a higher infection rate than did contaminated wounds whose edges were taped (13). Irritation of the skin by tape can be correlated in part with the degree of tape occlusivity which leads to accumulation of fluid underneath the tape, promoting tissue maceration and bacterial growth. The microporous tapes which are now used have interstices which permit moisture to be absorbed, and a dry skin surface is maintained below the tape. Tape closure will not work well in some areas, such as the skin of the axilla, palms, and soles. In addition, tape closures should not be used in areas where there is much moisture, such as over flexor surfaces of joints. Tape closure should not be used on crush-induced injuries in which there is a laceration. The optimal lacerations which can be closed with skin tape are wounds that are secondary to sharp instruments.

Ideally skin tape should be applied for 2 to 3 weeks. In patients with oily skin, the tape may loosen in 7 to 9 days rather than the usual 2 to 3 weeks or cause sebaceous duct inflammation (15, 56).

The *advantages* of skin tape are as follows:

1. No anesthetic is needed.
2. No suture marks are left when the tape is removed.
3. No skin reactivity occurs.

4. They can be left in place for a long time beneath casts.
5. Saves time in both application and removal.

The *disadvantages* of skin tape are as follows:

1. The tape does not adhere well to oily or wet skin.
2. The tape does not provide for eversion of the wound edges and can actually produce inversion when used in wounds which are deeper than the dermis.
3. A child may remove the tape prematurely.
4. The tape cannot be applied to skin over joint surfaces or wounds which are under significant tension when closed.

WHEN TO USE SKIN TAPE FOR CLOSURE

Skin tape can be used in lacerations which extend only partially through the dermis. These wounds are not widely separated and can be easily approximated with the use of skin tape. Skin tape can also be used in the closure of full-thickness lacerations which are small and are oriented such that they are parallel to skin tension lines, resulting in very little separation of the wound edges. One should not use skin tape in closing lacerations which are in regions of the body where there is excessive motion such as over joints, eyelids, and fingers. Skin tape is especially useful in those wounds in which the edges are cleanly incised and "come together" naturally without tension.

Skin Clips And Staples

Skin clips are no longer in use and have been replaced by skin staples. The staples provide for good approximation of the wound edges. They do not come in contact with the skin surface and do not leave suture marks when removed. If there is tension on the wound, then the skin clips or staples may leave marks. The steel used is inert and, thus, causes less tissue reaction than do most sutures and is associated with a low incidence of wound infection in uncontaminated wounds (28). The staples, however, seem to have a damaging effect on local tissue defenses. Stapled wounds seem to be more susceptible to infection than are taped wounds. This increase of susceptibility to infection mitigates against the use of staples in superficial wounds that are contaminated, which is the most common type seen by the emergency physician (25). When using skin staples, one must close the subcutaneous tissue first. Staplers on the market today come as disposable units, with about 35 staples in each unit.

The *advantages* of staples are as follows:

1. A wound can be closed more rapidly with staples than it can with sutures.
2. They are easier to place than are sutures.
3. Placement of staples requires less skill than does placement of sutures.

The *disadvantages* of staples are as follows:

1. They are more expensive to use.
2. Wounds closed with staples are more susceptible to infection.
3. They do not permit eversion of the wound edges, particularly in irregular lacerations.

Staples are best used in clean wounds which are linear and located in areas which are not easily contaminated such as the back, arms, and thighs. They have not gained popularity within most emergency centers.

Wound Adhesives

A word should be said about wound adhesives, although they are not in popular use at the present time. The best known wound adhesive is methyl 2-cyanoacrylate. This is a very powerful adhesive which undergoes a process of polymerization and is thereby converted from a liquid to a solid state. A small amount of water is needed to catalyze this reaction and enough is usually present in the air. One requirement in using wound adhesives is absolute hemostasis. The adhesive is applied as a thin layer between the wound edges and the edges are approximated and held ½ to 3 minutes. Numerous reports advocating the use of cyanoacrylate to repair wounds say their use should not include skin closure because the polymer acts as a barrier between the opposing edges of the wound, which prevents apposition and delays healing (42). One can be certain that new adhesives will be developed and undergo study in the future.

Suture Material

Sutures are divided into two general categories: *absorbable* and *nonabsorbable*. Those sutures which undergo degradation in tissues rapidly and lose tensile strength within 60 days are referred to as absorbable sutures. Those sutures which maintain their strength for longer than 60 days are referred to as nonabsorbable sutures. Chromic catgut, polyglycolic acid (PGA, Dexon®) and Vicryl® are absorbable sutures; silk, cotton, nylon, Dacron and polypropylene (Prolene®) are examples of nonabsorbable sutures. In many situations, it is a matter of choice regarding which suture material one chooses to use in closing a particular wound. There are some universal principles which apply to suture choice, however, and these will be discussed. Absorbable suture is used in situations in which one would prefer to have a substance which is totally absorbed and in situations in which continued strength is not important beyond 3 to 4 weeks. Nonabsorbable suture is generally used in skin and facial closure, whereas absorbable is used in subcutaneous and mucosal closures (Table 9.1). PGA, an absorbable suture, loses its tensile strength more rapidly than does chromic catgut. After 28 days, PGA exhibits no residual tensile strength but chromic catgut of comparable size retains its strength at this time (22).

The tensile strength of a suture depends on the size of the thread and the material of which it is composed. The tensile strength varies with the square of the diameter of the thread. If one doubles the diameter, the strength is quadrupled (61). The tensile strength of a knot is about 70% of the strength of either strand entering the knot (61). Size for size, the weakest suture material is catgut. Catgut is an irritant to the tissues, forming a zone of acute inflammatory reaction. Thus, one should use the smallest suture with the necessary strength to obtain wound closure (23). The exact mechanism of absorption of absorbable sutures remains unclear, but it is postulated to be due to the action of tissue esterases (77).

A strong suture material for delicate closures is 6-0 nylon. A heavier suture material, such as 4-0 nylon, may be used in areas of the body where tissues are thicker and added strength is needed, such as in the back, arms, and legs.

Monofilament nylon and polypropylene are used in skin closure, since they are the most inert substances and cause the least tissue reaction, thereby producing the least amount of scarring. Silk, on the other hand, is highly reactive and is not used in skin closure unless it is to be removed in 2 or 3 days (77).

A suture is basically graded according to its tissue reactivity, knot holding capability, capillary or wick action, tensile strength and cost (Table 9.2). Tissue reactivity indicates the degree of inflammatory response which the suture material induces within the tissue. Catgut, for example, induces more tissue reactivity than does PGA. Knot-holding capability is very important, particularly in areas where

Table 9.1.   Sutures Used in Various Tissues

Suture	Tissue
Nylon (Ethilon) Polypropylene (Prolene) Silk Mersilene	Skin
Chromic gut PGA (Dexon®), Polyglactin 910 (coated Vicryl)	Subcutaneous
Polypropylene (Prolene) Nylon (Ethilon)	Pull-out subcuticular
Polyglactin 910 (coated Vicryl) (not for prolonged hold) Silk Dacron	Fascia
Plain gut	Mucosa

Table 9.2.   Grading of Various Suture Materials

Suture	Tensile Strength	Wick Action	Infection	Reactivity	Comments
Nylon	+++	0	0-+	+	Minimal, transient acute inflammatory reaction, very strong, least infectivity, poor knot-holding ability, requires 6 knots.
Polypropylene	+++	+	0-+	+	Minimal, transient acute tissue reactivity, very strong, nonabsorbable, easier to tie and holds knot better than nylon, requires only 3 knots, no tissue ingrowth, excellent for skin and for a pull-out suture.
Silk	+++	++++	++++	++++	Knots very well, easy to sew, more tissue reaction to this suture material than to others.
Mersilene® Dacron	+++	++	+	++	Slight erythema and induration at suture site has been reported in 2% of cases, a good overall suture, easy to tie and holds knot well.
PGA (Dexon®) Vicryl®	+	++	+	++	PGA has a very low infectivity rate. In rats 2 weeks after implantation of Vicryl® approximately 55% of its tensile strength was lost. This should not be used where tensile strength is needed for prolonged periods.
Chromic gut	++	+	++	+++	Gut causes more tissue reactivity than do other absorbable sutures commonly used. While it is absorbed faster, it tends to retain its tensile strength better. Due to its tissue reactivity, it is not preferred except in mucosa or muscle closure.

there is much motion such as the tongue. Some suture materials such as nylon have a poor knot-holding capability, while others such as Vicryl® and silk maintain their knots superbly. Capillary or wick action relates to the amount of tissue fluids a suture material can absorb. Sutures such as silk have a high capillary action, while others such as nylon have a low capillary action. The greater the capillary action, the greater are the chances for bacterial infection around the suture. Tensile strength is an important property in a suture since those materials with a high tensile strength permit one to use a smaller suture than do those with a lower strength. In both the absorbable and the nonabsorbable suture class, there is a further division into monofilament and braided suture to be discussed later.

SUTURE SIZES

The (largest) suture available is (#5.) Smaller sizes are available, decreasing to #1 to be followed by #0. The most commonly used sizes in the emergency center are 4-0, 5-0, and 6-0, in order of descending size. There are few indications in the emergency center for suture material larger than 0. The size of suture used to close a wound will vary according to the material with which it is made. For example, a smaller size of Dexon as compared with chromic catgut can generally be used to close a wound since Dexon has greater tensile strength than does chromic catgut.

NONABSORBABLE

The nonabsorbable sutures are characterized by their generally greater tensile strength and low tissue reactivity when compared with the absorbable sutures. While there are many nonabsorbable sutures used, they can be classified into four categories: silk and cotton (organic), braided synthetics, monofilament synthetics, and wire (see Table 9.3). A braided suture is one in which there are multiple filaments which make up the strand of suture, whereas in a monofilament suture there is only one filament forming the strand.

Cotton is the oldest nonabsorbable su-

ture and is not used in emergency medicine nor for that matter in general surgical practice.

Silk is a braided suture and has many advantages as well as disadvantages regarding its use in the emergency center. Silk has the best knot-holding ability of any available suture material. It is more pliable and easier to handle than most sutures and ties easily. Silk stays securely tied with three knots, while other suture material requires five or six knots for an equal degree of security and takes more time and effort to tie. The disadvantages of silk are that, being a braided suture, the braids provide a place for the "lodging" of bacteria and, in the infected wound, actually protects the bacteria from attack by the body defenses (74). In infected wounds, bacteria form a small cystic area around the silk and eventually form an abscess. Teflon has been used to fill these

Table 9.3 Nonabsorbable Suture Material

Braided	Monofilament
1. Silk	1. Nylon (Ethicon)
2. Cotton	2. Polypropylene
3. Dacron	a. Prolene
a. (1) Untreated	b. Ethicon
(plain)	
(2) Dacron	3. Steel
(Deknatel®)	
(3) Mersilene	
(Ethicon®)	
b. (1) Impregnated	
with Teflon	
(2) Ethiflex (Eth-	
icon®)	
(3) Tevdeu	
(Deknatel®)	
(heavy)	
(4) Polydeu	
(Deknatel®)	
(light)	
c. (1) Treated with	
silicone	
(2) Ti-Cron®	
(Davis &	
Geck)	
d. (1) Coated with	
Polybutilate	
(2) Ethi-bond	
(Ethicon)	
4. Nylon (Neurolon)	
5. Steel	

interstices but this adversely affects knot tying and handling and also does not prevent bacteria from "lodging" in the wound (74). Silk also has the disadvantage of causing more tissue inflammatory reaction than any other nonabsorbable suture material. Its use in the emergency center is generally restricted to suturing the tongue, because silk will not unravel in the tongue.

All the synthetic sutures have many properties in common. They have good retention of tensile strength over many years and are generally inert in uninfected tissue. The braided synthetics are generally less reactive than silk and are stronger than silk in the same size range. The braided synthetics include Dacron® polyester, Dacron® impregnated with Teflon,® and nylon, all of which are much less reactive than silk. They have the disadvantage of being somewhat more difficult to handle than silk.

The monofilament synthetics most commonly used in the emergency center are nylon and polypropylene. The monofilament sutures are inert, do not shelter bacteria, and heal without stitch abscesses in a contaminated wound. These sutures maintain their strength well. Nylon is more difficult to handle and tie and holds knots poorly, whereas polypropylene holds its knot and is as easily tied as many of the braided synthetics. These are the most commonly used suture materials in the emergency center, where the physician is dealing with a contaminated laceration rather than a surgical incision in most instances. One must remember to place five or six knots when using either nylon or polypropylene, particularly over areas where there is significant motion.

Wire is rarely, if ever, indicated in the emergency center. It is stiff and has no real advantages over the monofilament sutures. It is hard to knot and actually is not tied but twisted.

ABSORBABLE

The absorbable suture materials used in the emergency center are plain gut, chromic gut, Dexon® (PGA) and Vicryl® (Table 9.4). These are all absorbed in 3 to 6 weeks by an inflammatory reaction pro-

duced around the suture; thus, all absorbable sutures produce some tissue reaction (77). While the above is true for sutures which are smaller than 4-0 size, suture material which is larger than 4-0 may last as long as 3 to 4 months before absorption occurs. In addition, the rate of absorption and loss of tensile strength is dramatically worsened by infection. Different tissues absorb these sutures at varying rates, and thus mucous membranes would absorb sutures faster than would fascia and muscle. The rate of absorption, depending on the tissue, can vary from 2 weeks to 6 months (Table 9.5) (74).

Catgut is one of the most commonly used suture materials; however, in the emergency center Vicryl is becoming more popular. Catgut is made of collagen from the submucosal layer of the small intestine of sheep and the serosal layer of cattle small intestine. The smaller the caliber, the faster it is absorbed. The collagen in the catgut is digested by collagenase and thus causes a significant tissue reaction as noted earlier; therefore, these materials should not be used in skin closures.

Chromic catgut is soaked in chromic acid salts which are similar to the substances used in tanning leather and permits the catgut to retain its strength for 2 or 3 weeks (77) with about 90% absorbed in 30 days and complete absorption by 50 days (28). Plain catgut loses its tensile strength in 1 or 2 weeks and the chromic acid causes retention of the suture for a longer period, causes less tissue reaction

Table 9.4.   Absorbable Suture Material

1. Plain gut
2. Chromic gut
3. Dexon (PGA)
   (polyglycolic acid)
4. Vicryl
   (Polyglactin 910, Ethicon)

Table 9.5.   Time of Absorption of Absorbable Sutures

Suture	Absorption Time
Plain gut	7 to 14 days
Chromic gut	20 to 40 days
Coated Vicryl	60 to 90 days

initially, and increases the tensile strength of the suture.

Both the chromic catgut and the plain catgut are packaged wet because drying damages them and causes the suture to become friable. Although gut treated with chromic acid will absorb slower, it must be remembered that the chromium is lost after about 10 to 20 days and the suture produces a marked exudation in the tissue thereafter and is rapidly absorbed.

Dexon® and Vicryl® are synthetics and retain strength for 3 or 4 weeks (28). Their dissolution is more predictable than that of catgut, with less tissue reaction than catgut. Vicryl® is totally absorbed in 80 days and Dexon® in 120 days. Chromic catgut is absorbed much faster.

NEEDLES

There are two types of needles: tapered and cutting. A needle is classified according to its shape, its cross-section, its point, and whether it has an eye. In emergency practice, there is virtually no need for an eye needle which produces large cutaneous holes. A swaged needle* does not produce a larger hole than is necessary and is the type needle that is used in the emergency center. With regard to shape, there are two shapes of needles: straight and curved. The straight needles are placed in tissue with the hand, and the curved needles are used with a needle holder. The curved needles most commonly used are the ⅜ circle needle and the ½ circle needle, which is the most commonly used in general surgical practice. Cutting needles at one time were made with the "cutting edge" placed along the line of stress (the line of pull of the suture material) into the tissue, and the "cutting edge" on the inside diameter of the curved needle. This placement caused the hole to enlarge as the two opposing edges of the tissue were brought together. Presently, cutting needles are of the reverse cutting type (Fig. 9.1). This type of needle does not place a "cut" along the direction of the

suture's line of stress, does not produce an enlarging hole in the wound, and the "cutting edge" is on the outside diameter of the curved needle. Cutting needles are used when going through tough tissue such as skin and fascia. The taper needle is a needle with a round cross-section, it does not cut tissue, and it is used in vascular work and fine mucosal closures (Fig. 9.1). Packages of suture material will state "cutting needle" even though it is in fact a reverse cutting needle, since their use is so common that the word "reverse" has been dropped in labeling.

A number of different needle types and sizes are used in the emergency center. The emergency physician should be familiar with some basic information to intelligently select the proper needle and size. There are basically two varieties of needles—cuticular and plastic. Cuticular

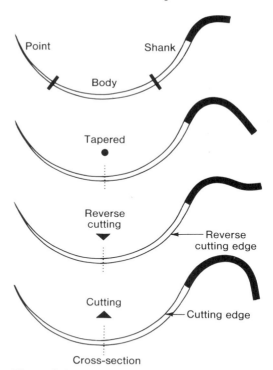

Figure 9.1. Needles used in suturing. See text for discussion. Note that with the reverse cutting needle the "base of the triangle" is in line of suture pull as it passes through tissue, thus avoiding enlargement of the hole as suture tension and wound edema ensue.

---

* In this needle the thread is attached directly to the needle without a hole, and the needle is the same diameter as the thread.

needles are honed (sharpened) 12 times. Plastic needles are designed for cosmetic closures and are honed 24 additional times to cause less trauma when penetrating the tissue. Cuticular needles come in various series: C (cuticular) and FS (for skin). Plastic needles also have a letter designating the series: P (premium or plastic) and PS (plastic surgery). Within the series of a particular brand of sutures, a number coming after the letter indicates the needle size *within that series*. They are not cross-related, thus a PS-6 needle is not necessarily the same size as an FS-6. The larger the number, the smaller is the needle size within a series. Thus a PS-1 is larger than a PS-3.

SUTURE MATERIALS AND RISK OF INFECTION

The chemical composition of the suture material is an important determinant of early infection. The greatest incidence of infection encountered in tissues is with cotton or silk sutures (27). Nylon and polypropylene sutures have a lower infection rate than any other nonabsorbable suture. Of the absorbable sutures, PGA has produced the least inflammatory response in contaminated tissues (27). Plain gut elicits less infection in contaminated tissues than does chromic gut in the same tissue. When one looks at other nonabsorbables, nylon and polypropylene have been found to elicit the least infection rate in contaminated tissue, and the infection rate is actually lower than that with metallic sutures (3). Infection rate in contaminated tissues containing either nylon or polypropylene does not differ.

When one compares monofilament to multifilament sutures, interesting findings have been noted. It requires 10^6 *Staphylococcus pyogenes* per gram to elicit purulence and to form clinically significant infection when monofilament sutures are placed in a contaminated wound (28). When braided silk sutures are used, however, the number required is reduced to 100 staphylococci (28). Silk sutures have been found to potentiate infection 10,000 fold when compared with nonbraided nylon (29). The infection rate of contaminated tissue containing braided nylon is lower than that with any other multifilament, nonabsorbable suture. In general, tissues with knotted multifilament sutures have a higher infection rate than do monofilament sutures. When an inert material is used to cover a filament of Dacron, it is found to play no part in altering the rate of infection. Since silk and cotton are found to have a higher rate of infection than any other nonabsorbable suture, silk should never be used in a contaminated wound. Regarding the lower infection rate with nylon and PGA sutures, it has been found that the degradation products of both of these materials are potent antibacterial agents (28).

THE WOUND AND SUTURE MATERIAL

Wounds which are parallel to the natural lines of the face and parallel to the flexion or extension lines above the joints heal better and with decreased scarring. Whenever possible, surgical incisions should be made parallel to these lines. Studies have shown that there is little difference in suture marks between absorbable and nonabsorbable sutures; it is the method of closure which determines the suture mark (53). *Suture marks* are largely preventable by early removal of the sutures and by following the principles and techniques which are outlined later in this chapter. As a general rule, 5-0 Vicryl® is used for subcutaneous closure and 6-0 nylon for skin (52, 72, 75). Some authors have recommended 6-0 chromic gut for the closure of skin in small children to avoid suture removal (75). When using this material the suture must be kept moist, e.g., with bacitracin ointment or Vaseline® gauze, for early dissolution of sutures to occur. Divided muscle may be approximated with 4-0 chromic gut (52, 72). Special types of wounds are discussed later in this chapter.

Tools For Suturing

A few tools are necessary for optimal closure of wounds. These include the Webster needle holder with jaws designed to hold 6-0 suture material, two skin hooks, and #11 and #15 Bard-Parker scalpel blades. Two types of scissors are necessary: an Iris scissors for use on the skin and a suture scissors (75) (Fig. 9.2).

INSTRUMENT HOLDER

For ideal eversion of wound margins, the needle of a suture should enter the skin at a 90 degree angle or more. This angle is difficult to achieve if the instrument holder is grasped by the thumb and third finger. The needle holder should be held in the palm, providing greater flexibility in the angle of entry into the skin.

FORCEPS

Toothed forceps are used in subcutaneous fascia and thick muscle fascia. An Adson forceps is a fine-toothed, atraumatic forceps used for skin. A smooth forceps has no teeth and is used for grasping gauze sponges or tissue that may be perforated and is not used for skin (Fig. 9.3).

SCALPEL BLADE (Fig. 9.4)

The configuration of the cutting edge of a scalpel blade is designed to accomplish specific tasks. Three types of blades are in current use in the emergency center. These include a #10 blade which is predominantly straight except for its curved distal end. The scalpel handle with this blade should be held like a violin bow in order that the long straight cutting edge of the blade contacts the skin. One sweep of the

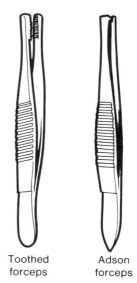

Figure 9.3.   A toothed forceps and Adson forceps.

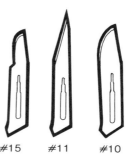

Figure 9.4.   Various blades. A #15 blade is used for fine precision work, a #10 for larger incisions, and #11 for stab incision.

blade results in a deep straight incision. Holding a #15 blade in the same manner prevents the cutting edge from contacting the skin. A #15 scalpel and blade should be held like a pencil (Fig. 9.5). This blade is used for precise, short incisions which often must follow an irregular anatomic landmark. When using these blades the physician must learn to cut to the desired depth with one sweep of the blade, which will result in a wound which is more resistant to the development of infection. A #11 blade is used in emergency medicine for a stab incision, such as incision of an abscess or cricothyrotomy.

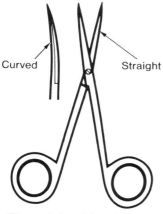

Figure 9.2.   Iris scissors.

SKIN HOOKS

Skin hooks are ideal for picking up wound edges. When one gains experience in their use, they can be used with greater ease and produce less trauma to the tissue than does a forceps. A skin hook is a needle-pointed instrument which enters the wound edge from its undersurface, thus producing a very small puncture rather than compressing the wound edge as one would do with a forceps (Fig. 9.6).

TRAUMATIC WOUNDS (GENERAL PRINCIPLES)

Contaminated Wounds—Preparation

INFECTION-POTENTIATING FRACTIONS IN SOIL

Soil has four major components: inorganic materials, organic matter, water, and air. The major component is inorganic minerals. The organic content of soil, ranges from 1 to 7% and is restricted primarily to topsoils. In swamps, bogs, and marshes, there is an increase in the organic content (98%). The organic component is chemically very reactive.

Fractions of soil with large particle sizes have small surface areas and low levels of chemical reactivity. Silt particles are smaller than sand with a surface area and chemical reactivity three to four times

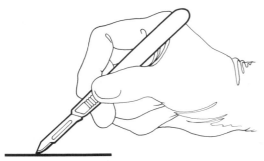

Figure 9.5. A #15 scalpel and blade should be held like a pencil, with the point directed downward as shown. When the #15 blade is held like the #10 blade then the belly of the blade rather than the sharpened point (which is the cutting edge of this blade) is in contact with the skin edge to be incised.

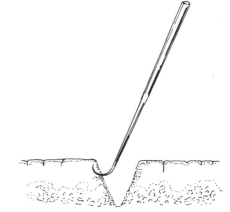

Figure 9.6. A skin hook is preferred over a forceps, as it causes no trauma to the wound edge. It takes practice to become skilled in handling a skin hook.

greater than that of sand. The inorganic component of soil with the smallest particle size is clay. Clay containing minerals has a large surface area. These large exposed surfaces of clay are associated with high levels of chemical reactivity.

Sterilized samples of topsoil and subsoil consist mainly of inorganic matter which impair the ability of a wound to resist infection. Wounds contaminated by 5 mg of sterile soil require only 100 bacteria to elicit purulent discharge (28). When the soil is fractionated, the fractions found to potentiate infections reside predominantly in the clay and organic components. These "infection-potentiating" fractions (IPF) in soil have a number of effects. These fractions inhibit leukocytes from ingesting bacteria. The surface of clay and other organic particles are anionic and surrounded by cations. Soil IPF have considerable impact on nonspecific humoral factors, and exposure of fresh serum to IPF eliminates bacteriocidal activity. All therapeutic measures should be directed at physically removing the IPF of soil from the wound.

BACTERIAL CONTAMINANTS AND INFECTION

The skin has varied numbers of bacteria in different areas of the body. In most regions the bacterial colonization is limited to the outermost layer of the skin, which is composed of a sloughing mass of dead cells. Beneath this layer is the stratum corneum which is composed of tightly packed cells, providing an effective barrier against bacterial invasion.

Over most body surfaces the density of the bacterial population is low, measuring only a few thousand or less organisms per square centimeter. The number of organisms on the palms and dorsum of the hand is sparse, numbering only in the hundreds per square centimeter. Most of these organisms on the hands reside beneath the distal end of the nail plate or adjacent proximal or lateral nail folds (24).

The type of bacteria contaminating a wound is less important than the number of bacteria in the development of infections. The infective dose of aerobic bacteria in wounds in healthy tissue has been determined to be 10^6/gm or greater. When the bacterial counts are below this level the wounds will heal without infection except in the presence of sutures when small numbers of bacteria 10^4/gm can produce infection (27, 28, 43a). The critical number of anaerobes that will elicit soft-tissue infections has not been documented.

Covering the surface of the skin with an *occlusive cover* promotes skin hydration which encourages bacterial growth. A dramatic *increase in bacteria* is encountered with such occlusive dressings. Wounds to be covered with dressings should have an ointment such as Vaseline® gauze or bacitracin over the wound to preclude hydration of the skin but still prevent desiccation of the wound margin.

SHAVING OF HAIR AROUND WOUNDS

The shaving of hair around wounds in areas where there is much hair growth has been advocated as beneficial in decreasing the source of bacterial contamination. Studies by Seropin and Reynolds (70) demonstrated that the infection rate of surgical patients after razor preparation was 5.6% compared with a rate of 0.6% after use of a depilatory agent, due to the trauma inflicted by the razor. It also was shown that skin shaved with a recessed blade was more resistant to bacterial contamination. We recommended that hair removal be performed only when it will interfere with wound closure and then only by either scissors or shaving with a recessed blade (19, 70). Never shave the eyebrows.

ANTISEPTICS AND WOUND PREPARATION (116)

There are many types of antiseptic solutions commercially available for use on the skin around lacerations. The ideal agent must be safe and fast-acting, with a broad antibacterial spectrum and a substantial effect after removal. This ideal antiseptic should be capable of reducing the number of organisms in intact skin following a single application.

Presently, the *iodophors* are the best known agents for providing good antimicrobial activity and cleansing with little tissue toxicity or damage. These agents are complexes of iodine which possess a broad spectrum of activity against fungi, viruses, gram positive and gram negative bacteria. There are three general categories of iodophors in clinical use: solubilized inorganic elemental iodine, as tincture of iodine; iodine complexed with various surfactant compounds; and iodine complex. Iodine compounds are very stable, do not stain, have no odor, and are less irritating to the tissues than is tincture of iodine. After contact with wounds, these complexes release iodine slowly, resulting in prolonged activity. These complexes are basically composed of iodine plus an organic molecule. The most commonly used forms in the emergency center are as a solution or as a soap, e.g., Betadine®.

Mercury compounds have been commercially available for a long period of time; however, these agents are unacceptable for use in the emergency center. Organic mercury (Methiolate®) penetrates the skin very little, is bacteriostatic, and is not effective against spores. In addition, these agents may sensitize the skin.

pHisoHex®, a soap, has been shown to cause central nervous system damage in neonates and its use in the emergency center in wound preparation is discouraged.

Alcohol cleans the surface of dirt and oils; however it is not an effective antiseptic. Alcohol has been widely used as a skin disinfectant due to its ability to remove lipids from the skin surface and its bacteriocidal action. The action of alcohol as a disinfectant, however, is restricted due to its inability to kill spores at normal temperatures and, for this reason, is not reliable as a skin disinfectant. Alcohol is active against gram positive and gram negative organisms. Ethanol is most effective at concentrations of 50 to 70%. Isopropyl alcohol is significantly more active than ethanol, is less volatile, and is more commonly used for skin disinfection.

Hydrogen peroxide in a 3% solution is a very weak disinfectant whose primary use is in the cleansing and debridement of wounds. When hydrogen peroxide is applied to tissues, oxygen is rapidly released by tissue catalases and the germicidal action is brief. It is also toxic to tissue in open wounds.

Quaternary ammonium salts are dilute solutions of cationic surface-active agents with organically substituted ammonium compounds. Gram positive organisms seem more susceptible than gram negative to these salts. Gram negative pseudomonas are resistant to quaternary ammonium compounds and actually may grow in these solutions. These agents are not safe for use in surgical wounds. They contain toxic anionic detergents that damage the tissue defenses and potentiate the development of infection. Contaminated wounds subjected to topical treatment with these agents develop more infection than do contaminated wounds subjected to 0.9% saline (28). Benzalkonium chloride (Zephiran®) is a quaternary ammonium salt which is a fast-acting bacteriocidal agent with good penetration into wounds. It is antagonized by soap and tissue fluids; during its use, benzalkonium chloride forms a film, and bacteria remain intact under this protective film. The bacteriocidal action of these agents is slower-acting than the iodine preparations.

Pluronic F-68 (Shurclens®) is a surfactant which has little or no local or systemic toxicity. This agent meets many of the criteria of an ideal agent wound cleanser. Experimental studies (67) show that this agent prevents the development of infection and, when used around the wound as well as in the wound, did not result in any significant damage to cellular components of the blood, wound healing, or resistance to infection. In a clinical trial involving 1000 patients, it was decided that this was the agent of choice, when compared with iodinated solutions and normal saline. The cellular damage produced by various antiseptic solutions is shown in Table 9.6.

DEBRIDEMENT

Debridement is an essential part of preparing a traumatic wound for closure. It removes bacteria and tissue heavily contaminated by IPF in soil and protects the patient from invasive infections. It removes permanently devitalized tissues which impair the ability of the wound to resist infections. All devitalized tissue left in a wound damages and potentiates infection (39). There are three mechanisms by which devitalized soft tissue enhances infection. The devitalized tissue acts as a culture medium, promoting bacterial growth. This tissue inhibits leukocyte phagocytosis and provides an anaerobic environment within the wound which also acts to limit leukocyte function.

In ascertaining the margin of devitalized tissue, one often must use clinical judgment. Within 24 hours after injury there is

Table 9.6. Cellular Damage Produced by Various Antiseptic Solutions (11a)

Antiseptic Solution	% Cellular Damage Resulting when no Saline Irrigation is Performed Later	% Increased Cellular Damage after Subsequent Saline Irrigation
Alcohol	100	100
Hydrogen peroxide	100	90
Ordinary soap	90	25
pHisoHex	25	5
Distilled water	5	0
Polyvinylpyrrolidone iodine (1%)	5	0
Saline solution	0	0

a sharp demarcation, often apparent, between the devitalized skin and the viable skin. The margin to excise on a wound is based on the region of the body and the appearance of the tissue as well as the degree of maceration and contamination. Facial wounds require little debridement as compared with wounds of the lower extremity, because of the high vascularity of the region. A technique which has been used to demarcate the area for debridement in a devitalized wound is to apply a fluorescein dye to a gauze pack and pack the wound. Complete excision of the stained (devitalized) wound margins will minimize debridement of uninjured tissue. Alternately one can excise a wound until active bleeding is noted, indicating viable skin. The best debridement includes high-pressure irrigation followed by limited ex-

cision of any loose bone or edges of tissue which clearly are not viable (Fig. 9.7). Periosteum and other specialized tissue such as tendons should be saved unless severely contaminated (39). The decision whether to close a wound primarily or secondarily is to a large extent based on the adequacy of initial debridement and the location of the wound. If there is any question about the adequacy of debridement of a badly contaminated wound, it is best to do a delayed primary closure, rather than risk the chance of infection. Facial wounds almost always can be closed primarily after initial wound care. This debridement is aided by irrigation with copious amounts of isotonic sodium chloride.

In *abrasions,* deep "ground-in" particles of dirt may be embedded in the wound following accidents such as falls on dirt

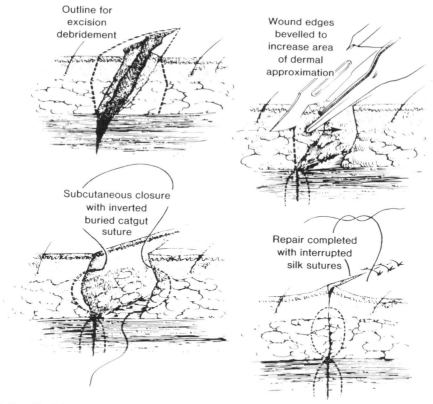

Outline for excision debridement

Wound edges bevelled to increase area of dermal approximation

Subcutaneous closure with inverted buried catgut suture

Repair completed with interrupted silk sutures

Figure 9.7.   Excision of the macerated edges of a traumatic wound. Angulating the blade bevels the wound edges so that a subcutaneous closure will result in eversion of the edges, permitting no tension on the epidermis and dermis. (Reprinted with permission of R. E. Straith, J. M. Lawson, The Subcuticular Suture. Postgraduate Medicine 292:164, 1961.)

roads. If these particles are left in place, they lead to what is called a traumatic tatoo. A *Traumatic tatoo* represents particles of dirt that have remained embedded in an abrasion and have epithelialized. Most of the particles are superficial and immediate removal is the procedure of choice. Removal may be aided by a surgical scrub brush or a sterile toothbrush after adequate field block or regional nerve block anesthesia (1) (Fig. 9.8). Xylocaine® gel 5% applied for 5 to 10 minutes over an abrasion can work extremely well in providing adequate anesthesia for this procedure. Alternately T.A.C. (see section on anesthesia for wounds) can be used. The point of a #11 scalpel blade will aid in removing deeply seated particles from the abrasion. A sterile, hard, natural-bristle toothbrush can be used with either sterile saline or surgical soap. One should rinse and blot the area frequently until all pigment has been removed. Tar embedded in wounds may be removed easily with the use of Vaseline® or Neosporin® ointment, mayonnaise, or lastly with acetone (20a).

Leave the abraded areas open and cleanse the involved area with a mild detergent four times per day. The use of a topical antibiotic ointment is advocated (1) and the lesion usually heals in 2 or 3 weeks. Alternately, an antibacterial impregnated gauze dressing may be used (Xeroform®) over the wound. Traumatic tatoos of the explosive type (as opposed to the abrasive type discussed above) leave the pigment deposited deeply in the central focus of the abrasion (1) and may require dermabrasion.

MECHANICAL CLEANSING (IRRIGATION)

Irrigation of a contaminated wound is an excellent means of removing soil and bacterial contaminants and should be performed routinely on all traumatic lacerations with the exception of those which are caused by a sterile instrument. The force of the irrigating solution must exceed the adhesive forces of the contaminants; therefore, one must provide enough force in the irrigating stream to dislodge the particles.

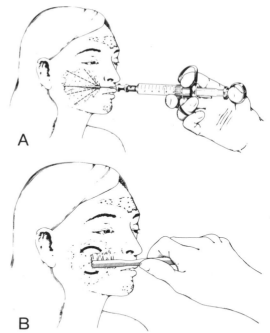

A

B

Figure 9.8. *A.* Technique for anesthetizing a traumatic abrasion with embedded particles. *B.* Removal of the particles with either an ordinary toothbrush or a bristle brush used for scrubbing hands. The tip of a #11 blade can be used to remove deeply embedded or larger particles. (Reprinted with permission of Williams & Wilkins. Agris, J., Traumatic tatooing. J. Trauma 16:799, 1976.)

The amount of hydraulic force needed to dislodge a particle is decreased as the velocity of the irrigating stream is raised. Large volumes for extended times are required when small syringes are used. Irrigation has been studied and the data in the authors' opinion show that the preferred method of irrigation which causes the least tissue injury from too high an irrigating pressure and the maximum particle dislodgement is obtained by using a 35 mm syringe with a large bore needle or plastic cannula such as a 16 or 18 gauge (57, 66). This technique provides approximately 8 pounds of pressure per square inch. Pressure below this level is considered low-pressure irrigation and above is referred to as high-pressure irrigation (Fig. 9.9). The concern that high-pressure irrigation would result in increased tissue injury is

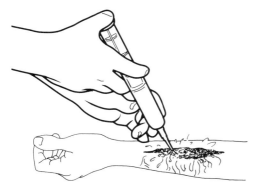

Figure 9.9. Irrigation of a traumatic wound decreases the bacterial content significantly and dislodges particulate matter from the wound. A #16 or #18 gauge needle or plastic cannula attached to a 35 cc syringe is ideal for providing proper irrigation pressures. See text for discussion.

true. One must weigh the effect of contaminated particles remaining in the wound against the risk of tissue injury. Concern that high-pressure irrigation forces particles deeper into wounds is not true. Low-pressure irrigation is most effective in dislodging relatively large particles from wounds. Direct scrubbing of a wound with a gauze sponge soaked with saline does not decrease the incidence of infection and does impair the ability of the wound to resist infection.

CONTAMINATED WOUNDS, DELAYED CLOSURE AND ANTIBIOTICS

The optimal time in which to repair a traumatic laceration without an increased risk for infection generally is regarded as less than 6 hours (5, 39, 55). With oral antibiotic coverage, the time for primary closure can be extended to 14 to 16 hours (5, 55). Proper cleansing of the wound and debridement include removal of all foreign bodies and nonviable tissue. Mechanical debridement and irrigation are the best means of assuring a clean wound with the least tissue destruction (23, 55). Hemostasis, closure of the dead space, and approximation of the wound edges without tension are vital. For an excellent repair, adequate wound immobilization with a properly applied pressure dressing is es-

sential in assuring a good result (5). One should keep strong antiseptics away from the injured tissues. Substandard results are due mostly to a failure to remove foreign material and to a failure to excise irregular devitalized edges (56).

Indications for antibiotic therapy after wound closure remain controversial. The length of time a wound has been open and the level of contamination play an important role in the decision-making process. The effect of topical antibiotics is limited by the fibrinous coagulant which surrounds the bacteria and prevents contact with a topical antibiotic. Indications for antibiotics are affected by the mechanism of injury. Shear forces secondary to glass or a knife are responsible for most lacerations and these wounds are highly resistant to infections, requiring 10^6 organisms per gram of tissue to produce infection (68), whereas compression injuries resulting in stellate lacerations weaken the local tissue defenses and increase the susceptibility to infection (68). When the risk of infection is high, we advocate oral antibiotic therapy for the first 3 to 5 days after suturing (34).

The earliest sign of infection is tenderness at the wound edges (5, 55). Remember that erythema may occur with normal healing. Later lymphangitis and swollen, tender regional lymph nodes develop, followed by systemic signs of infection in severe cases. If suppuration develops, some or all of the sutures should be removed. In less cosmetically important areas such as the trunk or extremities, a more conservative approach for heavily contaminated wounds is to leave the wound open for drainage and simply cover it or pack it with saline gauze dressings, changing them every 6 hours for the first 2 or 3 days and perform a delayed closure to decrease the risk of infection (5). It has been shown that the optimal time to suture a contaminated wound by a delayed closure is the fourth day (65). It is at this time that the tissue reaches peak resistance to infection.

Anesthesia For Wounds

Three anesthetic agents are in current use for providing local anesthesia: procaine (Novocain®), bupivicaine (Marcaine®), and lidocaine (Xylocaine®). Of these, the agent which is by far the most commonly used is Xylocaine with or without epinephrine 1;100,000. Anesthesia by local infiltration is the method most commonly employed in most emergency centers today. Regional nerve block or field block anesthesia is the optimal method to use when one is dealing with anything other than a small laceration. This method provides for less tissue damage at the laceration site and avoids the inadvertent introduction of more contaminants into the injured tissue. Cleansing the wound of bacteria, soil contaminants, and debris as well as surgical debridement of infected wounds cannot be effectively accomplished without anesthesia. Lidocaine is the most commonly employed local anesthetic agent used. Loss of sensation occurs within 5 minutes and lasts an average of 97 to 156 minutes (2). Lidocaine does not exhibit antimicrobial activity and does not damage the local wound defenses. The addition of epinephrine, a potent vasoconstrictor, overcomes the vasodilating effects of lidocaine. The reduction of blood flow induced by epinephrine limits the clearance of the anesthetic agent from the tissue and prolongs the duration of anesthesia by up to 50%, permitting an increased dosage of lidocaine without toxicity. The toxic dose of lidocaine containing epinephrine (1:100,000) is 7 mg/kg and one should not exceed 500 mg total or 50 ml of 1% lidocaine. When using lidocaine without epinephrine, 4.5 mg/kg is the toxic dose and one should not exceed 300 mg or 30 ml of 1% lidocaine. Epinephrine does impair tissue defenses, which mitigates against its use in heavily contaminated wounds (2, 17). This must be tempered by the fact that epinephrine does reduce bleeding and therefore decreases the chance of hematoma formation. Hematoma formation increases the chance of infection. Epinephrine is a strong vasoconstrictor and decreases bleeding; however, it should never be used in lacerations of terminal structures such as the fingers or toes. In the usual circumstance, a 1 or 2% solution of lidocaine should be injected through a 27

gauge needle. Some fibrous tissues, such as scalp or scar tissue, require a 22 gauge needle for infiltration and may require longer periods of time for anesthesia than other tissues (71). While one can inject the wound from within, the optimal method is a field block or a regional block (55). Infiltrating the wound edges swells the edges and makes a cosmetic closure more difficult. As mentioned earlier, regional block anesthesia is the preferred technique as it is removed from the wound site and thus avoids contamination of the wound.

Patients with an overdose from an inadvertent intravenous injection of lidocaine will develop nausea, vomiting, headaches, transitory excitement, apprehensiveness, and/or convulsions. Secondary signs are an irregular pulse (which may be rapid or slow), hypotension, and a decrease in tidal volume. Patients allergic to Xylocaine® will tolerate procaine. (See Chapter 3: "Regional Anesthesia.")

Procaine has an onset of action of 3 to 10 minutes as well as a duration of less than 1 hour, and a maximum dose of 700 mg or 10 mg/kg. Bupivicaine also has an onset of 3 to 10 minutes, with a duration of action of 4 to 12 hours, making it useful where prolonged anesthesia is desirable.

Table 9.7 summarizes the various agents used and indicates the onset of action as well as the duration of anesthesia. A new topical local anesthetic agent has been tested in minor lacerations; this is a combination of tetracaine 0.5%, adrenaline 1:2000 solution, and cocaine 10% (TAC). This composition of TAC yields an average dose of cocaine 590 mg/5 cc and tetracaine 25 mg/5 cc. This agent was not tested in lacerations of the pinna or other end organs such as parts of the ear, the penis, or the digits, due to the possibility of compromising their vascularity. Mucosal lacerations were not anesthetized with this agent because of the increased vascularity of the mucosa which accelerates the absorption of these anesthetics and increases the risk of toxic accumulations of their side effects. This agent was studied in 158 patients and compared with lidocaine with epinephrine (62). Most of the patients who were tested were chil-

Table 9.7. Onset of Action and Duration of Various Anesthetic Agents

Drug	Concentration (%)	Approximate Relative Potency	Onset Time (Min)	Reappearance of Pain Sensation (Min)
Procaine	1	2	7 ± 1	60–90
Mepivacaine	1	4	4 ± 1	120–240
Prilocaine	1	4	3 ± 0.6	120–240
Lidocaine	1	4	5 ± 1	90–200
Tetracaine	0.25	16	7 ± 2.5	180–600
Bupivacaine	0.25	16	8 ± 3.2	180–600

dren with small lacerations. The time required for surgical repair for patients matched for age and length of lacerations were essentially identical for older children. For children under 5 years of age the time required for repair of lacerations using TAC was significantly shorter than for the lidocaine with epinephrine group. The anesthetic agent (TAC) was applied after completion of wound preparation. The TAC was applied topically with a saturated sterile 2 × 2 inch gauze pad with firm pressure for a minimum of 10 minutes. Five cc of TAC was applied to all wounds under 3 cm in length and an additional 5 cc was applied for each increase in length of 3 cm. (62) The authors' experience with this agent has shown it to be useful, particularly in children and in cleansing abrasions.

Hemorrhage And Hemostasis

A wound hematoma almost always is associated with controllable bleeding which has been inadequately controlled. In a patient with a bleeding wound, *direct pressure* with a 4 × 4 pad should be applied over a broad area. If bleeding continues to be uncontrolled, pressure over a proximal artery may be used. A blood pressure cuff can be inflated above systolic pressure when bleeding is a problem. Diffuse oozing from a wound often accompanies coagulation defects. Bleeding also may be a particular problem in patients with excessive ingestion of aspirin or other anticoagulants.

Ligation of the bleeding vessel with a small hemostat is advised (5). When there is not a single vessel causing the bleeding and the patient is generally oozing from the wound and direct pressure does not result in subsidence of the bleeding, then a compress soaked in epinephrine often is helpful. However, a reflex hyperemia after the epinephrine solution is metabolized may be associated with more bleeding subsequently. In small cavities, one may use a *fibrin* or *gelatin* foam pad or topical thrombin. These agents are particularly useful in the oral cavity. If all these measures fail in a patient with diffuse oozing, the wound is packed and an elastic compressive bandage is applied over the site. Proximal control of the bleeding is achieved with the use of either a blood pressure cuff inflated to above systolic pressure or digital pressure over a proximal artery. Pressure should be maintained for 15 to 20 minutes. The pack should be removed gently, followed by deflation of the cuff. This procedure usually yields a dry field which can be closed. A pressure dressing must always be applied following a wound repair, wherever possible.

BASIC PRINCIPLES IN WOUND CLOSURE

LINEAR SCARS AND SKIN TENSION LINES (Figs. 9.10 and 9.11)

A number of skin tension lines have been described, some of which are relevant to the emergency physician in considering the repair of lacerations, in determining the cosmetic outcome of a scar, and in planning the revision of a laceration. Skin lines are divided into static and dynamic skin tension lines. The natural *static skin tension lines* are partly dependent on the natural characteristics of dermal fibers and partly on the pattern in which they are woven. Clinical evidence of these tension lines in the skin is the retraction of skin edges noted around a laceration, when the laceration is perpendicular as

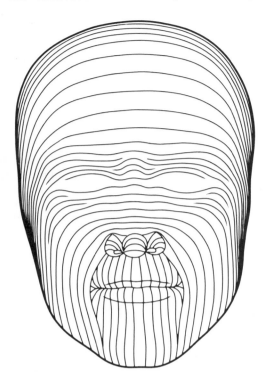

Figure 9.10. Lines of skin tension on the face. Elective incisions or modifications of existing wounds should be performed along these lines. See text for discussion.

opposed to parallel to these lines of tension. Wounds which result in a wide scar occur from strong opposing static skin tensions. When there is minimal separation of the wound edges, repair occurs with a fine scar.

Wrinkle lines or *dynamic skin* tension lines result from the contraction of the muscles underlying the skin (10, 69). These lines cross at right angles to the long axis of the muscles and are caused by contraction of these muscles (10, 11, 69, 71). The skin is attached to the underlying muscles by fascia, causing the skin to be thrown into accordion-like folds or lines at right angles to the direction of the muscle (69). Scars become adherent to the underlying tissue, so they least interfere with skin dynamics if placed transversely across muscles and joints and in the same lines as wrinkles (49). Optimally the scar then becomes an exaggeration of the normal

skin tension lines (49). In the face the wrinkle lines are called lines of facial expression; more recently, the term *relaxed* skin tension lines has been used in discussing elective incisions and the prognosis of wound healing (10). These are similar to wrinkle lines in most instances but not in all cases. Wrinkle lines are primarily influenced by muscle pull, whereas other factors enter into relaxed skin tension lines. On the forehead, vertical contraction of the frontalis demonstrates the relaxed skin tension lines. In the elbow, transverse relaxed skin tension lines are noted on the anterior and posterior aspect (10). Langer's

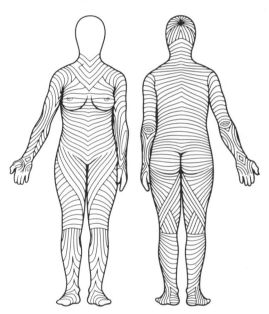

Figure 9.11. Skin tension lines. In the male, the semicircular lines over the deltoid region extend down over the breasts, producing curved radial lines as opposed to the horizontal lines demonstrated above in the female. Authors vary in their descriptions of the posterior skin tension lines. Kraissl (49) states that the skin tension lines meet in the scapulae and that the latissimus dorsi and trapezius produce a vertically oriented semicircular pattern rather than the more horizontal pattern over the posterior shoulder and thoracic region. Karissl also feels that the skin tension lines are transversely oriented along the entire lower extremity from the hip to the foot, similar to those shown above in the calf region.

lines referred to in standard texts are inaccurate, have little practical use, and should not be used, as they do not consider the effect of dynamic skin tension on a healing scar (10, 11, 49, 69).

When possible, skin should be incised parallel and never perpendicular to the normal tension lines and relaxed skin tension lines (71) to produce the most inconspicuous scars. Revisions can often be done in a laceration by the use of "Z-plasty" as early as 2 months after injury (11), but 6 months is preferable.

TENSION AND LAYER-BY-LAYER CLOSURE

Close each layer separately: periosteum, fascia of muscles, and subcutaneous fascia. Layered repair should be carried out with sutures which are snug but do not strangulate the tissue (52). When muscle is divided, one should use a two-layer closure to approximate it (52).

Before considering special situations, several axioms can be derived from the principles discussed above.

AXIOM

Use the smallest suture needed to approximate the edges of a wound.

AXIOM

Use small sutures placed closer together rather than larger sutures placed further apart.

AXIOM

Edema occurs after closure so only approximate the edges, do not strangulate the tissue.

AXIOM

Use forceps as little as possible; skin hooks, when one learns to handle them properly, offer the best means of handling a wound edge.

In general, an irregular wound should be perceived as a "jigsaw puzzle," i.e., if the most complicated section is closed first, then the remainder is closed more simply. If the laceration is jagged, the margins can be excised and removed, resulting in a linear laceration which can then be closed more easily.

RELATIONSHIP OF SUTURE TO THE WOUND EDGE

When placing a skin suture, the needle should pass perpendicular to the wound edges as shown in Figure 9.12. If the needle passes tangential to the surface of the skin, more tissue will be encompassed by the suture loop near the surface than will be encompassed deeper down, resulting in inversion of the wound edges. When the wound edges are difficult to evert, then the needle may be passed at an angle

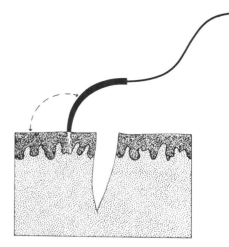

Figure 9.12. The needle should pass perpendicular to the skin.

greater than 90 degrees to the skin. When the suture loop thus formed is closed, the tissue at the bottom of the loop comes together first (since more tissue is enclosed within the bottom of the suture loop by this technique), resulting in the pushing of the more superficial tissue upward and eversion of the wound edges.

Sutures should be placed close to the wound edges. The farther from the skin edges a suture is placed, the greater the force needed to approximate the edges and the greater the tension within the tissue enclosed by the loop of suture. Edema develops in a wound during the first 48 hours after injury and tightens the sutures further (40). Tension in a wound is divided into intrinsic and extrinsic (18). Intrinsic tension within a suture loop is produced by an "inward" constricting tension within the wound (Fig. 9.13). Extrinsic tension on a wound is the pulling tension or the outward force which maintains the wound edges separated. Subcutaneous sutures tend to decrease the extrinsic tension from the skin sutures and permit early removal of the latter, leaving little or no scarring (18). In certain wounds, tension sutures should be placed to remove the extrinsic tension from the wound edge and prevent scar spread (20).

Large "bites" result in large suture marks due to the constricting effect of the suture (intrinsic tension) on tissue vascularity (Fig. 9.14). It is much better to use more sutures placed closer together (75). Sutures

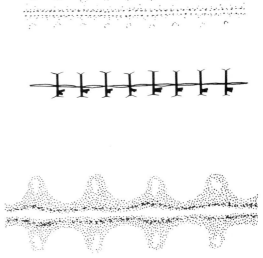

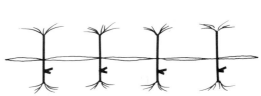

Figure 9.14. Sutures should be placed closer together taking smaller "bites." Large suture bites result in larger, thicker suture marks due to the constricting effect resulting in increased intrinsic pressure within the suture loop.

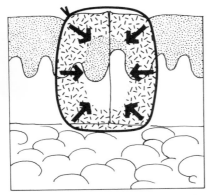

Figure 9.13. Intrinsic tension within the wound produced by a suture loop. See text for discussion.

should enter 2 to 3 mm from the edge of the wound, roughly equal to the skin thickness (5). The sutures should be placed about 3 to 5 mm apart. In the face, even more meticulous care is needed for ideal healing. Never encompass more than 2 to 3 mm of tissue on either side of wounds on the face. The maximum amount of tissue encompassed by a single suture on the face, as a general rule of thumb, should be 4 mm between the entrance and exit sites on the two sides of the wound (52).

Horizontal and vertical forces act on wound edges, causing them to gradually flatten (75). Eversion of the wound edges helps in overcoming these forces. Eversion of the wound edges is most important in areas where the laceration lies perpendicular to the relaxed skin tension lines due to the greater tendency for "spread" of the scar with these lacerations. In addition, slight eversion of the skin edges compensates for contracture of the scar which always follows any wound healing (5). If the edges persist in being inverted the result will be an unaesthetic, depressed scar.

The methods of everting the edges include the following:

1. With thick skin, incise the edges so it overhangs the perpendicular (Fig. 9.7 and 9.15). Thus, when the suture is placed, the top of the skin will come together before the bottom, causing eversion.
2. Reflection of the wound edge when placing the suture will aid in incorporating more tissue in the lower half of the suture loop than in the top, which will cause eversion of the edges when closed (Fig. 9.16).
3. Buried sutures placed in the manner shown in Figure 9.15, which incorporates the lower part of the dermis within the loop, also aids in providing eversion of the edges.
4. Adequate undermining is essential for eversion and is described in the next section.
5. In those wounds where the edges persist to invert following a simple closure, then a vertical mattress suture is indicated (5).

TIMING OF CLOSURE

The timing of a closure is vitally important and has been discussed in more detail in a previous section. *Primary closure* is generally performed in a wound less than 6 to 8 hours old, the exception being in the face where, if the wound is clean, closure can be safely performed up to 24 hours later (28). If the wound is clean, and the patient happens to be ingesting oral antibiotics at the time of injury, then the wound may be repaired primarily within the first 24 hours. The antibiotics should be continued for 3 days following the suturing. For delayed closure the area is debrided and a dressing of fine mesh saline absorbant gauze is applied. Antibiotics should be administered, and the wound closed when clean. In the delayed repair, few subcutaneous sutures should be used as there is an increased risk of infection

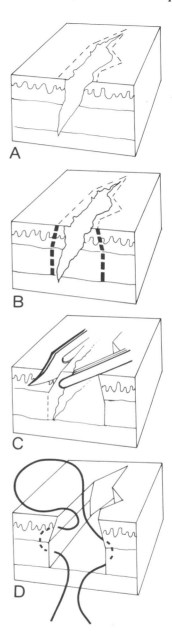

Figure 9.15. *A.* Excision of the macerated edges of a traumatic wound. *B.* Incise the edges so that the surface of the wound overhangs the perpendicular. This permits approximation of the top of the surface of the wound before the base of the wound and allows eversion of the wound edges. *C.* This is best done with a #15 or #11 blade. *D.* A buried suture going through the deep dermal layer.

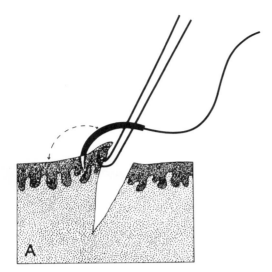

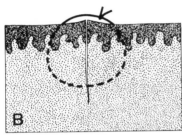

Figure 9.16. *A.* Reflection of the wound edge permits passage of the needle so that it incorporates more tissue at the base of the suture loop than at the top and aids in eversion of the wound edge. This is especially useful in thin skin over wrinkle lines or creases which tend to invert. In this figure the skin hook is shown reflecting the wound edge. *B.* This technique incorporates more tissue in the lower half of the suture loop than in the top and pemits eversion of the wound edges when the suture loop is tied.

with more sutures. Always do a delayed repair rather than risk a high chance of infection in severely contaminated wounds, particularly in wounds caused by compressive forces. (See the section "Contaminated Wounds, Delayed Closures and Antibiotics.")

Four days post-injury is the ideal time for delayed wound closure (65).

UNDERMINING

The *extrinsic tension* on a wound is the "pulling" tension of a wound outward to maintain separated edges (Fig. 9.17). This tension varies with the direction of the laceration in relation to the skin tension lines. Undermining involves the separation of the skin and attached superficial subcutaneous tissue from deeper subcutaneous tissue and fascia (Fig. 9.18). Undermining is important because it relieves extrinsic tension. The amount of undermining necessary to close a laceration is approximately double the width of the gap of the laceration at its widest point (75).

AXIOM

The amount of undermining necessary to close a laceration has been determined to be approximately double the width of the laceration at its widest point.

This gap is largely determined by the orientation of the laceration to the skin tension lines. For example, a 1 cm wide laceration should be undermined 1 cm on both sides of the wound. Undermining is also important in allowing the eversion of the skin edges as well as in relieving the extrinsic tension from the skin sutures, thus aiding in obtaining a small scar (see discussion on eversion in the section on "Relationship of Suture to the Wound Edge").

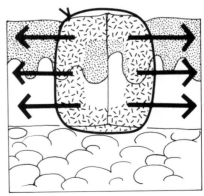

Figure 9.17. Extrinsic tension on a wound. See text for discussion.

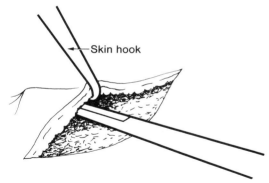

Figure 9.18. Undermining involves the separation of the skin and attached subcutaneous tissue from the deeper subcutaneous tissue and fascia. This is done in a natural tissue plane in order to relieve some of the extrinsic tension on the wound edge.

The techniques of undermining are as follows:

1. Undermining may be performed by multiple connecting stab incisions with a #11 blade. Likewise a pair of iris scissors placed between the skin and the subcutaneous tissue and opened repeatedly will undermine a wound easily (75), as shown in Figure 9.18. This method is preferred by the authors. The tunnels thus formed are then connected at the appropriate level (75).
2. Undermining could be performed with the belly of a #15 blade in a manner similar to that described above (75).

CLOSURE OF DEAD SPACE

Condie and Ferguson (13a) demonstrated that obliteration of the dead space by the use of subcutaneous sutures reduces the rate of infection in *clean* wounds. In heavily contaminated wounds, suture closure of the dead space should be avoided whenever possible. Only a minimum number of sutures should be placed in the subcutaneous layer as the infection rate increases progressively in these wounds with more sutures. Closure of the dead space should be performed with "buried" sutures (Fig. 9.19), and one should use a minimum number of sutures (56).

Absorbable buried sutures are best in wounds that are not clean. Permanent deep sutures placed in contaminated wounds are frequently "spit out" weeks or months later.

AXIOM

Closure of the dead space will relieve surface tension and, thus, decrease scar spreading, particularly when the laceration is perpendicular to the skin tension lines or the orientation of the muscles.

Closure of the dead space is best done with the least number of sutures and with just enough tension to approximate the tissue. The greater the number of sutures used, the greater is the infection rate.

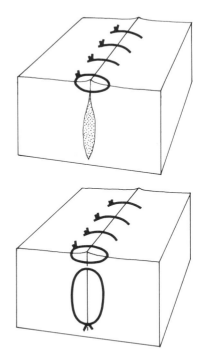

Figure 9.19. Closure of the dead space with buried sutures. The least number of sutures necessary to close a subcutaneous space should be used.

BASIC SUTURING TECHNIQUES

Instrument Tie

Only the instrument tie is discussed here (Fig. 9.20). This is the tie most commonly used in the emergency center for simple closures. For our discussion, the suture will be divided into two parts, the end close to the needle, termed "needle end," and the end far from the needle, termed the "free end." Two loops or a "double-throw"* of suture from the needle end (one loop shown in diagram for simplicity) are wrapped around the distal portion of the needle-holder and the free end of the suture is grasped and pulled through the loop thus formed. The free end should be kept short before pulling through the loops to form the first knot, otherwise too much suture material will be discarded with each instrument tie. The next suture loop is wrapped around the needle-holder in the opposite direction and pulled in a direction opposite to the first tie to form a square knot. After all the knots are placed squarely, the mass of knots should be shifted out of the center of the wound and to one side to decrease tissue reaction of the wound.

Simple Closures

SIMPLE INTERRUPTED

Simple interrupted sutures are the most commonly used suture in the emergency center. The proper technique for this suture in order to provide eversion and good apposition of the wound edges is quite difficult to master. To assure the best results in placing the simple interrupted sutures:

1. One should take equal volumes of subcutaneous tissue from both sides. In wounds in which there is unequal thickness on one side, the subcutaneous tissue should be brought over from the thicker to the thinner side

---

* Two loops are used to fix this half-knot in place and resist the extrinsic tension of the wound in the interim, before the square knot is finished. Occasionally three loops may be needed with nylon.

before approximation of the skin as discussed in the general section.
2. The needle should enter the skin edge at an angle of 90 degrees or greater (see Fig. 9.12) and the angle of exit should ideally be the same as the angle of entrance.

AXIOM

The closer the needle to the wound edge, the greater is the control on the ultimate position of that edge.

When eversion is difficult to achieve in a wound, eversion of the edges may be obtained by passing the needle at a more acute angle than perpendicular to the skin, thereby taking a wider bite of subcutaneous tissue from the base of the wound than from near the skin edge (see Fig. 9.16). When the stitch is tied, the tissue at the base of the suture loop will come together before the tissue at the surface, thereby uplifting and everting the wound edges. In addition, before tying the first knot one should lift up on the stitch ends in order to more accurately oppose the wound edges. When nylon is used, at least four knots should be placed in order to be certain that unravelling does not occur. With Prolene®, Vicryl, or silk, one can use three knots to secure the suture in place.

The needle should be held by the needle-holder about halfway along the length of the needle. If held too near the end where the suture attaches to the needle, the needle may bend when passed. Always follow the curve of the needle. If one needs to pass the needle at a more acute angle, do not do so by bending or pushing on the needle but rather by lifting the edge of the skin with the forceps or skin hooks and/or by entering the skin at a greater angle. If a more acute passage is needed (in the intertriginous space between the fingers or toes) a one-half circle needle should be used.

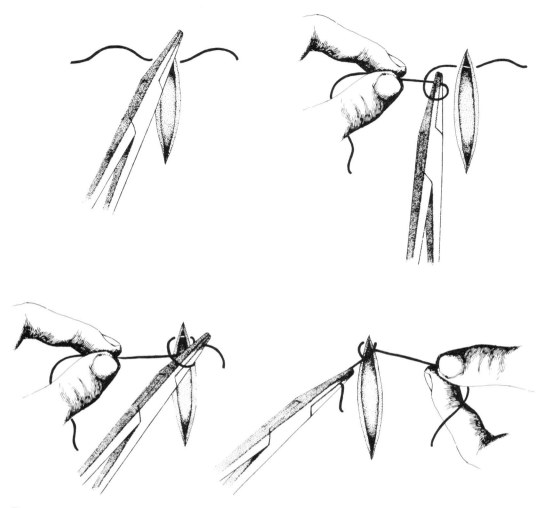

Figure 9.20. The instrument tie. Two loops of suture are wrapped around the distal portion of the needle-holder and the free end of the suture is then grasped and pulled through the loop thus formed. A third suture loop is wrapped around the needle-holder in the opposite direction and pulled in a direction opposite to the first tie to form a square knot.

OPEN LOOP SIMPLE INTERRUPTED

This tie is a modification of the simple interrupted in which the same basic technique is used with the exception of tying the knot. Introduced by Joseph Walike (75) the open loop simple interrupted suture is formed by using a knot as described under "Instrument Tie." On the first limb of the knot, tighten a *double throw* only until the suture lies flat against the skin surface. The second limb of the knot is a single knot *square* to the first which is tightened until the suture starts to deform the ends of the first double throw thus creating an *open loop* (Fig. 9.21). A third single throw made square to the second throw completes the knot and, if properly tied, the loop will not close no matter how tightly the third throw is secured against the second. If the second and third throw are not square, a granny knot will result and the loop will close. Six-0 nylon used for this suture requires only three knots to secure the suture, rather than the usual 4 or 5.

The open loop technique has many advantages. If swelling occurs about the wound, the knot has some spring and will yield rather than cut into the tissue. The open loop technique also facilitates suture removal when sutures need to be placed very close to the wound edge. The scissors are simply placed into the loop and when the loop is cut open the knot unravels. A major difficulty with this method is that, in closing some wounds, "perfect" approximation is achieved after the first double throw only to be followed by deforming the apposition of the edges when the sec-

ond part of the knot is placed and secured. This problem is a common one, particularly in areas where the skin is thin and there is little subcutaneous supporting tissue such as on the back of the hand.

INTERLOCKING SLIP KNOT

In a crying infant it may be difficult to insert the point of a scissors under the knot to remove sutures. The interlocking slip knot introduced by Lucid (53a) facilitates removal. The technique of placing this knot is shown in Figure 9.22. One can remove the suture with one hand without scissors. To remove, simply pull the longer end and then, if necessary, the shorter end.

CONTINUOUS OVER AND OVER

This suture is not commonly used in emergency medicine; however, if one becomes proficient in its use one can achieve as adequate a closure as with the simple interrupted. It does have some disadvantages. There is more epithelialization of the suture track with this stitch, especially if the stitch is not removed early (28). Inclusion cysts may form in 3 to 4 weeks after the removal of these sutures (28). The stitch is most commonly used in the scalp, where lacerations and resulting scars are

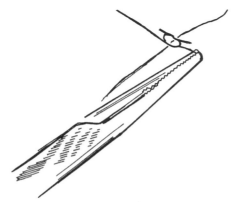

Figure 9.21. Open loop simple interrupted suture. See text for discussion.

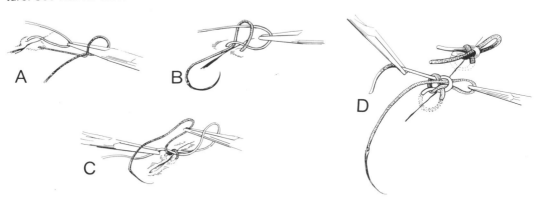

Figure 9.22. Interlocking slip knot. *A.* Make a loop around the needle-holder with the free end of the suture material. *B.* Grasp the needle end of the suture material and pull through the loop and tie against the skin of the wound. *C* and *D.* Grasp the needle end of the suture material with the needle-holder and pass it through the loop while applying countertraction to the free end of the suture material. To remove the suture, pull the long end and then, if necessary, the short end. One of the resulting tails of the suture may be trimmed at the skin edge before pulling it through the wound. (Reprinted with permission of Williams & Wilkins. Lucid, M.L., The interlocking slip knot. Plast. Reconstr. Surg. 34:200, 1964.)

covered by hair and cosmetic repairs are not as necessary as elsewhere on the body. The primary advantage of this suture is the rapidity with which it can be placed, and it is especially useful in patients with multiple lacerations. The technique is shown in Figure 9.23A and B.

In a continuous over and over suture, the first stitch is placed similarly to a sim-

ple interrupted stitch (Figure 9.23A-*a*). Instead of being cut, the suture is passed as a continuous running stitch (Figure 9.23A). Each time it is passed through the skin to form a loop of the continuous stitch, the needle should be passed perpendicular to the skin edges similarly to the technique used in placing a simple interrupted stitch. This will aid in achieving eversion of the wound edges with this technique. The end of the wound is then approximated in similar fashion and the suture is tied as a simple interrupted stitch (Fig. 9.23B). An alternate method of placing a continuous over and over suture is shown in Figure 9.24.

CONTINUOUS SINGLE-LOCK STITCH

This suture may cause less epithelialization of the suture tract while maintaining the advantage of a running suture. In placing this suture a simple interrupted suture is first placed as with the continuous running stitch. This long end of the suture is then held taut and the needle is passed through the skin just as in the continuous over and over stitch, but on coming

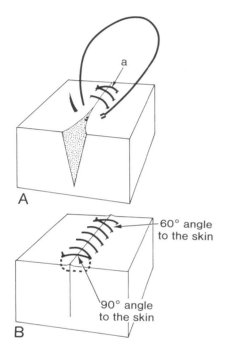

Figure 9.23. The continuous over and over suture. *A.* This continuous suture is begun with a single suture which then is tied to anchor the rest of the suture. The needle should be passed perpendicular to the skin edge and the suture threads should lay perpendicular to the wound margin to maximize the effect of the suture on extrinsic wound tension as with the simple interrupted suture. *B.* To finish and tie off this continuous suture, grab the loop formed at the free end after insertion of the needle through the skin. Grab the loop at its mid-point with the needle holder and pull on this loop. It will come together as if it were a single thread. Tie the needle end of the suture material and this "looped" free end as one would tie a simple interrupted suture. When one is proficient with this suture, eversion of the skin edges is quite adequate.

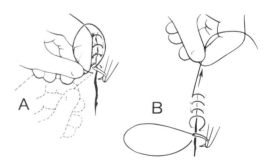

Figure 9.24. *A.* Conventional method of running a suture. *B.* By maintaining the initial cut end of the suture long, it can be used as a holding stitch. The advantages of this are: only one point need be held throughout the entire process of placing a continuous suture, thereby negating the continuous motion of regrasping with every stitch placement; the danger of forming a pursestring at the end of the wound; and the possibility of having placed sutures with altering tension along the wound. (Reprinted with permission of Surgery, Gynecology and Obstetrics. Noe, J.M., A technique for placement of a continuous suture. 150:404, 1980.)

out on the other side the needle passes *in front* of the thread (Figs. 9.25B and 9.26). Once again, in placing the next stitch the suture is held taut to maintain approximation of the sutured edges. As with the continuous over and over, in the final stitch the terminal suture is also tied as a simple interrupted stitch.

This is a superior stitch to use when one desires to close the skin with a running stitch. It provides for a more secure and regular apposition of the wound edges and less epithelialization of the tracts than does a continuous over and over since it combines basically the simple interrupted with the continuous over and over stitch. It has the disadvantage of taking somewhat longer to place the stitch than does the continuous over and over.

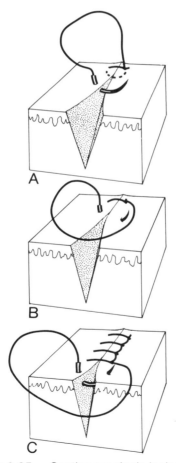

Figure 9.25.   Continuous single lock stitch.

Mattress Closures

The mattress stitches all have in common their ability to secure good apposition and to produce the least amount of tension on the wound edges since the basic principle in all mattress closures is that one provides a "two in one" closure. The "outside stitch" pulls in the wound to relieve tension from the edges and provides a "tensionless repair," and the "inside stitch" secures perfect apposition.

VERTICAL MATTRESS

This suture is unsurpassed in its ability to provide eversion of the wound edges. It provides the best apposition and the best control of the wound edge. One can alternate this suture with a simple interrupted in large wounds and save time. The major disadvantage in this stitch is the time that it takes to place. The technique is shown in Figure 9.26. The vertical mattress suture is basically a double suture, the first stitch of which is made by passing the needle more widely separated from the wound edges and deeper into the wound than usual (Fig. 9.26A). When the wound edges are approximated, this first suture loop will relieve the extrinsic tension from the wound edges and promote better healing. For the good cosmetic effect the second loop is made by passing the needle back through the epidermis and lower dermis close to the wound edge, taking a small bite of skin from both sides and approximating the edges (Fig. 9.26B and C). The suture is then tied and approximates the subcutaneous tissue (with the first suture loop) and the skin edges (second suture loop).

LOCKED VERTICAL MATTRESS STITCH

The locked vertical mattress stitch was introduced by Condon (14). In some patients, e.g., obese or elderly patients in whom there is diminished elasticity of the skin, approximation of the skin edges with a vertical mattress often is done by applying excessive tension to the deep portion of the suture. This excessive tension results in increased inflammation around the suture site and increased pain and scar-

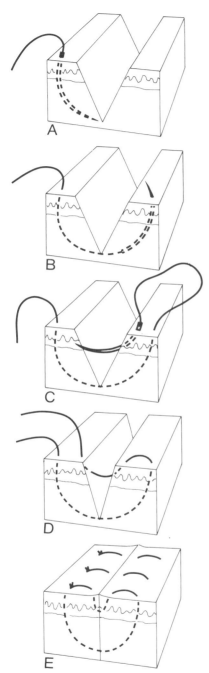

Figure 9.26. Vertical mattress stitch. See text for discussion.

ring, producing the "railroad track" appearance of the healed wound. The locked vertical mattress obviates this tendency to

apply excessive tension. Once locked, the edges of the skin remain approximated without tension. The deep portion of the suture can then be tied loosely.

The technique is as follows (Fig. 9.27). The needle goes in 1 cm or more from the margin of the wound, the distance approximately equal to the depth of the wound. After being brought out with a similar bite on the far side of the wound, the needle is then returned taking a very minute bite of skin at the wound edge (Fig. 9.27A). The needle end of the suture is then passed back through the loop formed on the far side of the wound, thus forming a locked portion of the stitch as shown in Figure 9.27B and C. The locking end of the suture is drawn taut to bring together the margins of the skin without any tension in the deeper portion of the wound. The two free ends of the suture are then tied loosely. To remove the suture, one needs to cut the end farthest from the knot and pull on the knot.

HORIZONTAL MATTRESS

The major advantage of this type of mattress stitch is that it reinforces the subcutaneous tissue by pulling it together across the length of the wound (Fig. 9.28C) and prevents stretching of the scar. Stretching is prevented by the fact that the horizontal mattress stitch removes more extrinsic tension from the wound margins than other stitches due to its placement along the axis of the wound. It is more rapidly placed than the vertical mattress and requires fewer stitches to close a wound of similar length than would be required should a vertical mattress be used. The disadvantage is that while some eversion of the wound edges is provided, it is more difficult to achieve. The technique' is shown in Figure 9.28.

HALF-BURIED HORIZONTAL MATTRESS

This stitch is very commonly used in emergency medicine. It is especially useful in closing a flap when the corner has limited vascularity and perhaps questionable viability. If one uses a routine simple in-

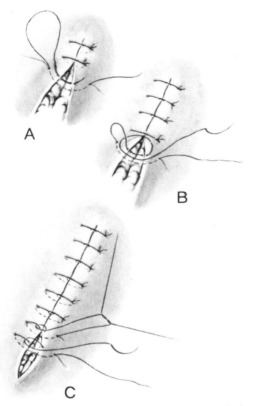

Figure 9.27. Locked vertical mattress stitch. *A.* Take a deep bite of the skin and subcutaneous tissue. The distance from the wound margin at which the needle enters should be approximately the same as the distance and depth at which the needle crosses the wound. The needle is brought out from the opposite side of the wound and is returned with only the most minute bite of skin being taken at the edge of the wound. *B.* The end of the suture is then passed back through the loop on the far side of the wound. This forms the locked portion of the stitch. This step is easily accomplished by passing the needle and suture back through the locking loop. *C.* The suture is drawn taut to bring the margins of the skin together without any tension in the deeper portion of the wound. (Reprinted with permission of Surgery, Gynecology and Obstetrics. Condon, R.E., Locked vertical mattress stitch for skin closure. 127:839, 1968.)

terrupted stitch in approximating the corner to the opposite side, it may damage the skin and cause vascular compromise due

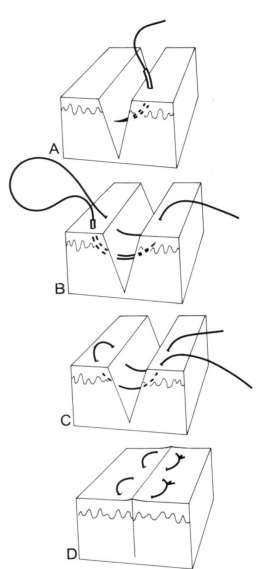

Figure 9.28. Horizontal mattress stitch. *A.* The needle was passed ½ to 1 cm away from the wound edge deeply into the wound. *B.* The needle is then passed through the opposite side and reenters the wound parallel to the initial suture. *C.* One must enter the skin perpendicularly to provide some eversion of the wound edges and must enter and exit both the wound and skin at the same depth, otherwise "buckling" and irregularities occur in the wound margin. *D.* The suture loop is then tied as shown.

to the tension on the suture (Fig. 9.29). In placement of the half-buried horizontal mattress, the suture is buried in the flap so it may hold a thin flap in place without tension or vascular compromise. It is useful in closing a V-shaped wound and prevents necrosis of the tip of the V, which may occur with a simple interrupted suture. The technique of placing this stitch is shown in Figure 9.30. The needle is passed through the lower dermis at the same level through the skin edges of both the V-shaped flap and the parent skin edge from which it came, as shown in Figure 9.30A. There are numerous situations in which this stitch can be used, some of which are shown in Figure 9.31.

CONTINUOUS HORIZONTAL MATTRESS

The continuous mattress is not commonly used in emergency medicine. It has the advantage, like the horizontal mattress, of providing good apposition with less tension on the wound edges by pulling only the subcutaneous tissue of the wound. The stitch has the added advantage that it is rapidly placed. The stitch is placed equidistant on either side of the edges of a laceration and then is tied (Fig. 9.32). Apposition is not as good with this stitch as with other sutures and for this reason it is not recommended for routine use.

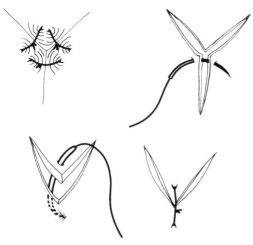

Figure 9.29. Simple suture producing vascular compromise at the V-shaped tip.

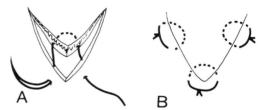

Figure 9.30. Half-buried horizontal mattress stitch. This minimizes the vascular compromise at a corner flap. See text for discussion.

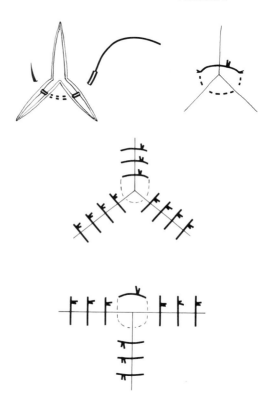

Figure 9.31. Half-buried horizontal mattress stitch used to approximate the center of a T-shaped laceration, a Y-shaped laceration, and a stellate laceration.

Subcutaneous And Buried Sutures

SUBCUTICULAR

The major advantage of this closure is that it provides superb cosmetic results when done properly. It requires more time and skill, however, to master. There is no possibility of suture marks since no sutures pass into the skin surface. The stitch

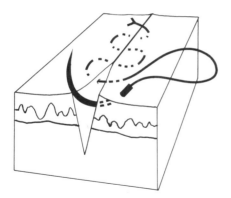

Figure 9.32. Continuous mattress stitch.

is placed by passing the suture horizontally, as shown in Figure 9.33, through the dermis in small bites of about 0 5 cm. One must adequately undermine the wound edges to achieve a good result (71). The stitch is alternated from one side to the other (Fig. 9.33). There are several points that should be mentioned in placing this suture. One must maintain the same depth and level of placement of the suture in the opposing sides of the dermis (71). The exit and entrance sites of the needle on the opposing sides of the dermis should be at the same level. The entrance of the needle into the dermis may be backed up a little from the exit on the opposing side; however, this is not completely agreed upon to yield the best results. If the wound is very long and one elects to use this closure, then the suture should be placed every 2 inches. The continuous subcuticular suture is anchored at the start and finished in the same fashion noted for continuous over and over (see text and legend to Figure 9.23). A good suture material to use in this closure is 5-0 or 6-0 nylon.

After completing the continuous subcuticular suture, one can add a simple interrupted suture or skin tape over the wound to secure more complete apposition or eversion of the wound edges.

An alternate method of using the continuous subcuticular was presented by Noe (63a). The initial suture is left long and is used to hold and stabilize the wound while the subcuticular suture is placed. The terminal ends are then taped securely in place (Fig. 9.33).

Subcuticular stitches should be left in place for a minimum of 7 days.

BURIED SUBCUTANEOUS STITCH

This suture is similar to the simple interrupted, but the suture is placed in such a manner as to bury the knot to avoid any irritation by the knot on the dermis of the skin edge. This suture is used to overcome tension at the wound edge from below and, thus, decrease the chance for vascular compromise and scar spreading. One should use this suture in the superficial layers under the skin surface and not necessarily in the deep fascial closure, where a simple interrupted suture can be used or one of the running sutures described above.

To place a buried stitch, pass the needle up from under the lower margin of the subcutaneous tissue on one side and then carry it over to the other side, passing the

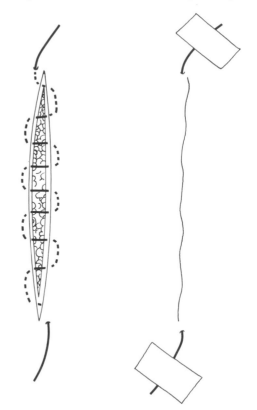

Figure 9.33. Subcuticular stitch. See text for discussion.

needle from above toward the lower portion of the wound as shown in Figure 9.34. This inverts the knot to avoid excessive tension at the wound edge.

An alternate method first introduced by Straith (71) which permits more eversion of the wound edges is one in which the edges of the wound are excised as shown in Figure 9.35A. The subcutaneous stitch

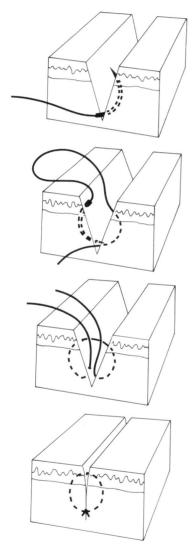

incorporates a piece of the lower dermis and takes a wider bite on the dermal side than on the deeper portion of the wound (Fig. 9.35B and C). This provides for eversion of the skin edges when the suture is tied since the lower dermis comes together before the subcutaneous tissue (Fig. 9.35D). This method, once mastered, is superior for closure of wounds and results in a wound whose skin edges can be apposed with skin tape, producing excellent results.

Reinforcing Sutures

FOR WOUNDS UNDER TENSION

As discussed earlier, the mattress suture is good for closing wounds and for decreasing the tension on the wound edges. When there are very widely separated wound edges and closure cannot be accomplished without producing significant tension on the edges, the wound can be reinforced with either a button stitch or tape as shown below. The buttons are sterile buttons which are present in most operating suites. A straight needle and 0 silk is usually used to place the stitch. One should not try to achieve apposition of the wound edges with this stitch but rather approximation to a point where the wound can be closed without significant tension by another technique. The reinforcing sutures should remain in place long after the skin sutures are removed, until adequate time has passed for the wound to gain strength. We have found this most useful in very elderly patients whose skin is thin and friable with no elasticity who present to the emergency center with wide gaping lacerations of the lower extremity. Closure of these wounds results in tearing through the tissue and is fruitless until the edges are brought closer together (Fig. 9.36). Table 9.8 lists the various basic closures and their advantages and disadvantages.

ADVANCED CLOSURES

The rotation of advancement flaps is quite useful when dealing with injuries sustained where there is significant tissue loss making end-to-end approximation of the wound edges impossible. It is critical

Figure 9.34. Buried subcutaneous stitch. This is particularly useful when approximating the subcutaneous tissue just beneath the skin edge, as it prevents irritation of the skin edge by the knot.

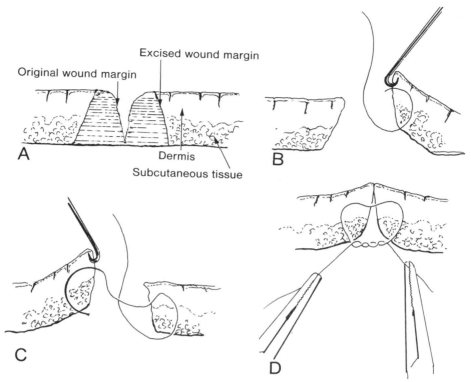

Figure 9.35. *A.* Bruised skin edges are sharply excised. The skin is then undermined above the fascia. *B.* Buried suture passing up through the dermal layer of the skin. Notice that the suture emerges from the near skin edge taking a larger "bite" from the dermal portion of the wound than the subcutaneous portion. *C.* Suture is then passed through the far skin edge. Path of the suture is a mirror image of the opposite side and emerges above the fascia in the undercut area. *D.* The knot is then tied as a double-hitch knot to prevent slipping. Illustration shows eversion of the skin edges over the previously buried sutures. (Reprinted with permission of Postgraduate Medicine. Straith, R., The subcuticular suture. 29:166, 1961.)

in performing these closures that there be adequate undermining. All of the area underneath the skin being rotated or advanced must be undermined as well as the skin edges around the avulsed segment. Adequate undermining cannot be overly stressed. When to use one type of closure as opposed to another is often a matter of preference; however, it is guided by location of the wound, how adherent the skin is to the underlying surface, and the shape and type of wound.

The "Dog Ear" (Fig. 9.37)

To correct the "dog ear" that occurs when one side of a sutured wound ends up longer than the other, one should do the following:

1. Make a superficial marking incision at a 45 degree angle to the line of the laceration.
2. Incise this marking with either a straight iris scissors or a #15 blade (Fig. 9.37A).
3. Undermine the area.
4. Trim off the excess skin (Fig. 9.37B) of the "dog ear" so that the "dog ear" repair will fit in the area of skin that was excised.
5. Suture the wound (Fig. 9.37C).

Z-Plasty

Z-plasty is used to change the orientation of a wound to produce a better scar. This is most commonly used in the initial closure of a clean wound which extends

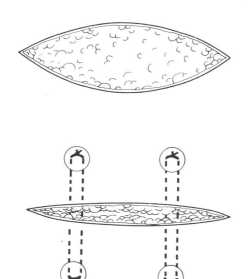

Figure 9.36. Reinforcing sutures for wounds under tension which cannot be closed. These are particularly useful in elderly patients who have pretibial lacerations which are widely gaping and in whom the skin is too atrophic to approximate without the suture cutting through the skin into the wound.

vertically across the flexion crease of a joint or the mucosa of lower lip.

The Z-plasty can be made at various angles to the original laceration, depending on the amount of lengthening one desires. The most common angle used is 60 degrees, which increases the wound length by 75%; the 45 degree angle Z-plasty increases the length of the wound by 50%; and the 30 degree Z-plasty increases the length of a laceration by 25%. Thus with a Z-plasty one must increase the length of a laceration to overcome the effects of wound contracture as well as change the orientation of the wound. The Z-plasty performed at an angle of 60 degrees is the most commonly used, because an increase in the length of a wound by 75% has been found in clinical practice to be optimal for preventing contractures at most sites. A Z-plasty can be performed in changing lacerations which run vertically across flexor creases such as the wrist, antecubital fossa, and popliteal fossa and vertical lacerations coursing across the anterior surface of the ankle. Z-plasties obviously in-

crease the size of the wound by increasing the wound length. Z-plasty should not be done in dirty wounds since they also decrease the blood supply, and therefore the possibility of infection is greater. Normally, Z-plasty should be deferred for secondary scar release and reconstruction. Many scars will not need release even though at the time of primary closure it would appear this would be necessary.

The technique of performing a Z-plasty is shown in Figure 9.38. Undermining is crucial in obtaining a good result. The angle desired should be measured and a line drawn with a skin-marking pencil to accurately plan the incision. A 60 degree angle is measured at the ends of the original laceration and the line is extended at this angle from both ends, forming a "Z." The line should be extended to the point where it meets with a similar line drawn at the same angle from the opposite end, thus forming a diamond-shaped figure (Fig. 9.38A). The stippled area (Fig. 9.38A) is then undermined. With a #15 blade an incision is made carefully along the drawn lines, extending from the ends of the original laceration marked *a* and *b* in Figure 9.38A. The two Z-shaped flaps thus formed are then elevated (Fig. 9.38B) and transposed as shown in Figure 9.38A and B. The Z-plasty is then closed (Fig. 9.38C).

Closing A Defect

SQUARE

To close a square defect, an advancement flap may be needed. Two parallel incisions should be made approximately two times the length of the side of the square (Fig. 9.39). The stippled area should be undermined widely and small "burrows" triangles should be excised at the ends of the incision which are one half the length of one side of the original square. These triangles should be equilateral triangles. The flap should then be advanced as shown in Figure 9.39 to cover the defect. The edges are approximated using simple interrupted sutures with the corners closed with half-buried mattress stitches. This method obviously works only with small defects.

Table 9.8.   Basic Closures and Their Advantages and Disadvantages

Suture	Advantages	Disadvantages
Simple interrupted	Permits good eversion of the wound edges. Is commonly used and can be applied rapidly.	Proper technique to provide eversion of edges requires practice to master. Eversion is not as good in difficult wounds as with other techniques. Does not relieve extrinsic tension from the wound edges.
Continuous over and over	Can be applied rapidly to close multiple lacerations and large wounds.	Apposition of the wound edges and eversion are more difficult to achieve. Inclusion cysts may form.
Continuous single-lock stitch	Can be applied rapidly. Apposition of the wound edges is more complete than with the continuous over and over stitch. Less epithelialization of the tracts.	Apposition of the wound edges is not as perfect as with the simple interrupted unless the procedure is mastered well.
Vertical mattress stitch	Unsurpassed in its ability to provide eversion of the wound edges and perfect apposition. Relieves tension from the skin edges.	Takes time to apply. Produces more cross-marks.
Horizontal mattress stitch	Reinforces the subcutaneous tissue. Relieves extrinsic tension from the wound edges more effectively than does the vertical mattress.	Does not provide as good apposition of the wound edges as does the vertical mattress.
Half-buried horizontal mattress	Relieves intrinsic tension and vascular compromise when approximating the tip of a flap.	Takes skill to master proper technique in order to provide perfect apposition of the wound edges.
Continuous mattress	Can be rapidly placed in order to approximate large lacerations in cosmetically unimportant areas.	Does not provide good apposition of the wound edges or eversion.

ALTERNATE METHOD

An alternate method of closing a defect is to rotate a flap from alongside the wound. The following dimensions must be measured out and drawn with a skin pencil:

Angle A = A′
Line BC = B′C′
Line CB′ = C′B″

Then B′C′ and C′B″ are incised, undermined, and rotated as shown in Figure 9.40.

Approximating the Edges of a Laceration with Grossly Unequal Lengths (Fig. 9.41)

The width of the laceration is measured from its widest point AB, and an equilat-eral triangle is excised from the center of the longer side such that the base of the triangle C′D′ is equal to the length of A′B′, and the laceration is undermined and closed as shown in Figure 9.41. The small vertical incision does not result in significant scarring.

Closure of an Ellipse

Elliptical defects placed over areas where the skin is adherent to the subcutaneous fascia may not permit approximation of the edges by simple means. A defect as shown in Figure 9.42A can be closed by excising the margins of the wound to form an ellipse (Fig. 9.42B). The ends of the ellipse are then extended to form an S pattern (Fig. 9.42B). The area is widely undermined as shown in Figure

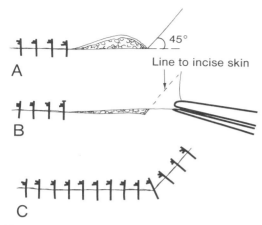

Figure 9.37. The dog-ear. See text for discussion.

9.42C. This permits approximation of the ends of the ellipse. The ellipse is then closed by bringing together the subcutaneous tissue with buried sutures. These buried sutures should be placed at the periphery of the undermined area to approximate the edges of the ellipse in a stepwise fashion as the subcutaneous layers are brought closer and closer together. The final result is a laceration which is S-shaped and can be closed with little tension on the wound edges (Fig. 9.42D). The wound is then closed with a simple interrupted stitch (Fig. 9.42E).

Closure of Defect with a V-Y Advancement Flap

The V-Y advancement flap is used for repair of fingertip lacerations and is called the Kutler procedure. It is used to close an area where there is an elliptical defect (Fig. 9.43A). The wound margins are first excised as shown in the stippled area to form an elliptical wound. A V is then incised at a distance equal to slightly greater than the width of the elliptical defect at its widest point (Fig. 9.43A). The ellipse is then closed with simple interrupted sutures after adequate undermining is performed (Fig. 9.43B). Following this the V-shaped incision is closed as a Y (Fig. 9.43C).

Closure of a Rectangular Defect

A rectangular defect is closed by removing a skin triangle at both ends. The length

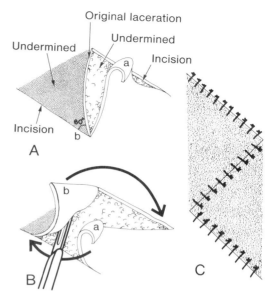

Figure 9.38. Z-plasty. Shown above is a 60 degree Z-plasty. The stippled area is the area which is undermined. *A.* Point *a* should be transposed to the position shown in *B.* Point *b* should likewise be transposed as shown above. The end result is a laceration in which the orientation of the wound is changed from its original configuration to one that is parallel to the relaxed skin tension lines or skin creases. It also lengthens the laceration, thus decreasing the effective contracture.

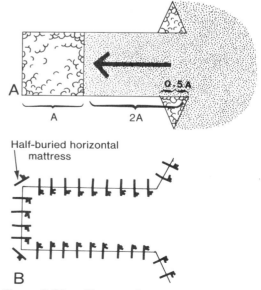

Figure 9.39. Closure of a square defect. See text for discussion.

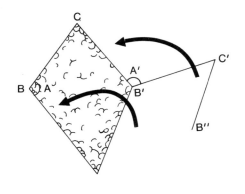

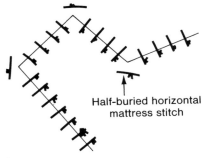

Half-buried horizontal
mattress stitch

Figure 9.40. Closure of a diamond-shaped defect. This technique is especially useful in areas where the skin is tightly opposed to the underlying subcutaneous tissue preventing advancement of a freed flap. See text for discussion.

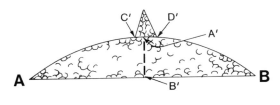

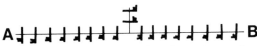

Figure 9.41. Approximating the edges of a laceration with grossly unequal lengths. See text for discussion.

from the base to the apex of the triangle A'B' should be equal to the width of the rectangle AB. The wound is then undermined and closed as shown in Figure 9.44.

Closure of a Triangular Defect with a Rotation Flap

A triangular defect can be closed with a rotation flap. The base of the triangle should be extended in a wide circular fashion as shown in Figure 9.45. The arc is extended as if to form a complete circle from the base of the triangle. The arc should be extended so that points A and D are at exactly the same level. The arc is then extended further so that the triangle with the dimensions described below can be formed. In converting a wound into the form a triangle, try to place the base of the triangle in such a position as to permit the secondary incisions to fall into favorable skin tension lines. Curved incisions can be made to extend from one or more sides of the triangle. In excising the triangle, the

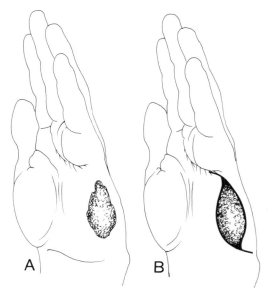

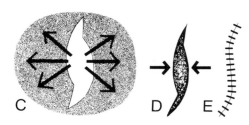

Figure 9.42. Closure of a wide ellipse. See text for discussion.

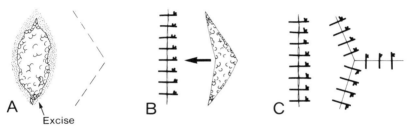

Figure 9.43. Closure of a defect with a V-Y advancement flap. See text for discussion.

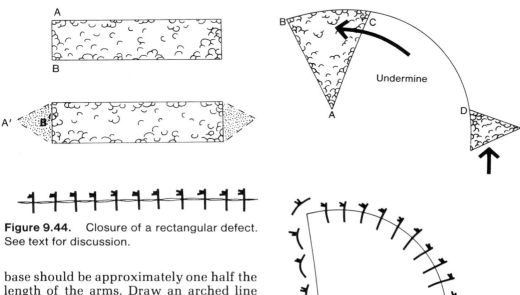

Figure 9.44. Closure of a rectangular defect. See text for discussion.

Figure 9.45. Closure of a triangular defect with a rotation flap. See text for discussion. Note that half-buried horizontal stitches are used in areas where vascular compromise may be present.

base should be approximately one half the length of the arms. Draw an arched line extending from the base of the triangle, which is approximately four times as long as the area it is to close. Rotation of the flap thus created is facilitated if this line is drawn beyond a line extending from the apex of the triangle perpendicularly. After undermining, close the triangle by approximating point c to point b. This will create a "dog-ear" which is then removed by creating a burrows triangle. The defect is undermined and closed as shown in Figure 9.45.

An alternate method is shown in Figure 9.46. This alternate method is used when a triangle cannot be excised from the end of the arc, due either to cosmetic considerations or to a region which does not permit enough room for excision. An arc is extended from the base of a triangle similarly to that previously described and ends at the same level as the point of the triangle (C), so that point a and point c are at the same level. Point b is then marked on the arc so that the length of ab is equal to half the length of the base of the triangle. The area is undermined and point a is sutured to point b and the original triangular defect is closed (Fig. 9.46B and C). This alternative, however, cuts into the base of the flap and may compromise the flap's blood supply.

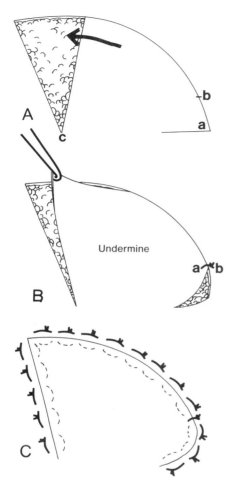

Figure 9.46. Alternate technique for closure of a triangular defect. Here, half-buried horizontal mattress stitches are used throughout the closure.

The Interpolation Flap

The authors feel that this flap should be commonly used in emergency medicine to close a defect. In this case, the defect, an oval, must be redrawn with a marking pencil over the site adjacent to it which is to be used as in Figure 9.47A. The flap and tissue adjacent to it are incised and then undermined as in Figure 9.47A. The base of the flap must have a good vascular supply for the flap to survive. The flap is then rotated (Fig. 9.47A and B), which results in approximation of the upper half of line ab to line cb. The defect is then closed

using half-buried horizontal mattress sutures as shown in Figure 9.47C.

REPAIR OF SPECIFIC TYPES OF WOUNDS

Closure Of Wounds Of Unequal Thickness

To approximate the edges of a wound in which the opposing sides are of unequal thickness, one should undermine both edges in the subcutaneous tissue plane at approximately the same depth. Following this, a "flap" of subcutaneous tissue is brought from the thicker side to the thinner side beneath the area undermined. This "subcutaneous closure" serves to elevate the depressed wound edge and permits good approximation of the wound.

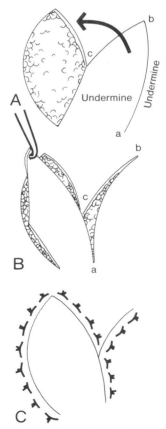

Figure 9.47. Interpolation flap. See text for discussion.

Tangential lacerations can be closed in a number of ways, depending on the site and the length of the laceration. An important factor is the angle at which the tangential wound is made. When the angle is not acute, resulting in a laceration such as the one shown in Figure 9.48A, the optimal method of closure is to change the wound into a perpendicular laceration by excising the margins as shown in Figure 9.48B. This should not be done on the face.

The subcutaneous tissue is then undermined, and the wound edges approximated (Fig. 9.48C). When the angle of the tangential laceration is acute, then the subcutaneous tissue should be approximated, following which the deep dermal layers are brought together on the opposing edges of the wound—using either a buried suture or a half-buried horizontal mattress closure. The superficial dermis and epidermis can then be approximated with skin tape, since sutures placed at this site usually result in overriding of the wound edges. A pressure dressing should be applied to all these lacerations and left in place for a period of 1 or 2 days.

Suturing Through Hair

Much has been stated about shaving hair and the deleterious effect of hair on a clean wound. As has been discussed in the section "Contaminated Wounds—Preparation," shaving is associated with an increased rate of infection when compared with the rate in similar wounds which are not shaved. We recommend suturing through areas such as the eyebrow, and after completion of the repair the entangled hair is pulled through the sutures and away from the wound. Using this method, one study reports no problem with infection (72). We recommend shaving only to facilitate visualization of the wound edges for suturing. Eyebrows and eyelashes take months to grow back and should *never* be shaved or removed to close a laceration. The scalp often needs to be shaved, but we would not advocate shaving wide areas around a scalp wound or other areas of the body where there is significant hair growth unless such growth interferes with the closure.

Abrasions

The debridement of abrasions has already been discussed in a previous section ("Traumatic Wounds—Debridement"). Abrasions are commonly seen in areas such as the face, forehead, and extensor surfaces of major joints such as the knees and elbows. After thorough debridement has resulted in a clean surface, the abrasion can be treated like a burn and covered

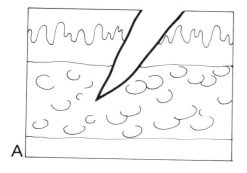

A

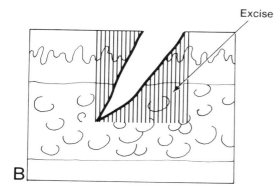

Excise

B

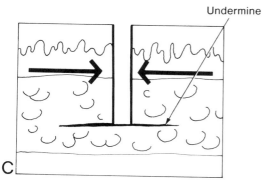

Undermine

C

Figure 9.48.   Repair of a tangential laceration. See text for discussion.

with either Xeroform® or Scarlet Red,® which will serve to seal over the abrasion with an antibacterial ointment gauze dressing. This dressing is permitted to loosen spontaneously as the abrasion heals. Sterile dry gauze dressings are then applied over the ointment gauze dressing and are changed daily as they absorb exudate from the wound which comes through the porous surface dressings. A pressure bandage is advocated over certain areas where swelling is expected to occur, such as the forehead. The area should be cleansed with a mild soap each day to remove exudate. In facial abrasions, one can leave these areas open and apply an antibacterial ointment over them. These abrasions should be cleansed four times a day to keep any exudate from accumulating.

Animal Bites

There continues to be much controversy surrounding the treatment of animal bites; some physicians advocate primary closure after irrigation, while others feel that a delayed closure should be performed in all cases (6, 14). The following regime is advocated by the authors. The area should be cleansed and debrided. Ascertain if there may be joint penetration. If it is decided that joint penetration is not likely, the wound should be irrigated thoroughly with saline. One millimeter of skin and subcutaneous tissue should be excised around the edges of the bite along the walls of the puncture wound. This resected tissue contains most of the bacterial contaminants. Following this, an ellipitical wound will result and one may close the site. This can be done in areas over joints and in all other areas of the body, including the face. In wounds which appear clean and superficial, irrigation without excision of the edges may be all that is neede, and this is followed by closure with either skin tape or sutures.

Deep subcutaneous sutures should be avoided in these wounds. These wounds must be carefully checked during follow-up for any signs of infection. If there is joint penetration, suggestion of deep structures being involved, or a severely contaminated wound, then irrigation, debridement, and a delayed primary closure should be performed. The patient should be placed on oral antibiotics. Cephalosporins are an excellent choice for most animal bites. *Staphylococcus aureus* remains the most common cause of infection in most bites. Other common agents include *Streptococcus pyogenes* and *Pasteurella multocida* (particularly in cat bites).

Human Bites

Human bites can be divided into those involving the face and those involving the hand. Controversy remains as to whether these wounds should be closed primarily; however, due to the profuse vascularity of the face, infections have not been a problem in our experience. We recommend that bites over the head or the face should be cleansed, debrided, thoroughly irrigated, and closed loosely. These patients should be placed on oral penicillin for treatment of infections from human mouth flora.

Bites of the hand are due to either a direct bite or a punch with the metacarpophalangeal region striking the opponent's teeth. These latter "bites" are associated with a much higher incidence of infection. These wounds should be debrided and thoroughly irrigated, and the patient should be placed on oral penicillin without wound closure. If there is joint penetration or if there is any sign of infection in a patient seen more than 24 hours after the bite, the patient should be admitted. Delayed closure of wound is done 4 days later or longer if still not clean. Primary closure of human bites to the hand have been advocated by some; however, no harm is produced by a delayed closure, while significant harm may be produced with a primary closure. Therefore, we advocate a primary delayed closure at 4 days or more for human bites of the hand.

In bites over other areas of the body, the decision of whether to close the wound primarily or do a delayed closure is contingent upon the location of the wound and the depth. In areas such as the penis, we advocate loose approximation after thorough irrigation and placement of the patient on antibiotics. In regions where the skin is very close to bone and periosteum may have been penetrated; i.e., the pretibial region or ulnar border of the forearm or olecranon, delayed closure should be the procedure after thorough debridement and irrigation of the wound. The antibiotic of choice for the treatment of human bites is penicillin. Under no circumstances should subcutaneous sutures be placed in a human bite unless the bite is excised.

Avulsions Of The Skin

There are a number of different types of avulsive injuries. When the skin is completely avulsed and is presented to the emergency physician, the underlying fat of the avulsed skin should be removed; the skin is then trimmed replaced as a free graft (52).

Incomplete lacerations often involve the deep layer of the dermis.

INCOMPLETE LACERATIONS

Windshield injury, in which the epidermis and papillary layer of the skin are sharply cut but the deep papillary layer is intact, producing a partial thickness avulsion of the skin, should be treated by excision of the very loose epidermal pieces of skin and either a Xeroform® or Scarlet Red® dressing placed over the wounds and a pressure bandage applied. These injuries are commonly seen on the forehead. An alternate way of treating these injuries is to apply an ointment dressing and a compression bandage for a few days; however, this method produces more scar since it involves leaving the pieces of skin in place, which are so small and "avascular" that they do not survive (72).

A curvilinear laceration, especially where there is a semicircular wound producing a trap-door type of flap, is a very difficult wound to manage, particularly when it occurs on the face. As the wound heals, contraction results and a large amount of scar tissue develops (37). A beveled wound should have its edges excised to full-thickness skin so that a 90 degree angle is produced between the incision and the skin surface. In this fashion a

minimum amount of raw surface presents for healing by scar tissue, and the stage is set for optimal healing (37) (Fig. 9.48). Undermining in these beveled flap lacerations on the face presents a problem due to the compromise in lymphatic and venous drainage, which leads to elevation and congestion of the flap as it heals. For this reason these lacerations must be treated with a compressive dressing (37). If the laceration is small or is in a "loose skin" area, complete excision and linear closure in the relaxed skin tension lines will give the best results.

COMPLETE AVULSIONS

There are five methods of treating avulsion injuries:

1. Debridement alone (abrasion).
2. Debridement and excision of soft tissue and repair primarily or secondarily.
3. Debridement and excision of avulsion flap and use of this flap as a free graft after defatting the undersurface.
4. Debridement and use of a split-thickness skin graft to cover the defect.
5. Debridement and covering the defect with a pedicle flap.

A question is always raised as to whether a flap with a small pedicle base can survive. A safe rule of thumb for extremities is that when the ratio of the width of the base of the pedicle to the length of the pedicle is 1:2 or more, the flap will usually survive. In the face, a base-to-pedicle length ratio of 1:5 or 1:6 is considered safe due to the heightened vascularity. If the pedicle appears tenuous (with the exception of the face), the safest approach is to remove it and replace it as a free graft after defatting the undersurface as suggested in #3 above. This maximizes the survivability of the pedicle.

Gunshot Wounds

Not all gunshot wounds appear to need debridement (35, 48, 73). With strict asepsis, placing the injured extremity in a splint with elevation may avoid infection in most gunshot wounds without debridement (35, 73). Debridement is unnecessary for wounds caused by bullets whose muzzle energy is less than 400 foot pounds. Devitalized and contaminated tissue is more hazardous with higher velocity wounds or shotgun wounds (73). When debridement is necessary, one should plan the incision so that it is done along the length of the tract and so that all devitalized tissue can be debrided. After debridement, the wound should be closed as a delayed closure. In some high velocity wounds in which marked tissue destruction has occurred, a graft may be needed after adequate debridement.

Escharotomy For Burns

Full-thickness burned skin has a leathery consistency and resists stretch. Edema develops beneath the burn and a tourniquet-like effect occurs on an extremity or the chest (26), resulting in circulatory embarrassment and necrosis. If respiratory embarrassment due to limited respiratory excursion is caused by a constricting eschar on the anterior thorax, then an escharotomy is imperative. The technique is as follows: a lateral incision is made in the anterior axillary line and extends from 2 cm below the clavicle to the ninth or tenth ribs, and the top and bottom incisions are joined transversely forming a square (8, 26, 45, 63) (Fig. 9.49). Hemorrhage from the incision is not usually a problem in these patients. Some may have an occasional bleeding vessel which needs ligation (8).

In circumferential burns of a limb, there may be a tourniquet-like effect on the extremity with subsequent circulatory embarrassment. During arterial tamponade, progressive loss of sensation and a impaired joint proprioception are reliable early clinical signs of vascular insufficiency. Changes in digital blood flow can be monitored with the use of a Doppler flowmeter. If it seems likely that the patient has circulatory embarrassment, then escharotomy through the burned skin restores circulation. The incision is made in the following manner: With the limb in the supine position, escharotomies are made midmedially and laterally (Fig. 9.50). The incisions should be carried into the deep fascia to provide for adequate decompres-

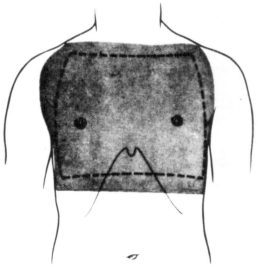

Figure 9.49. The site for escharotomy to relieve a constricting eschar of the anterior thorax. (Reprinted with permission of Aspen Systems, Inc. Edlich, R.F., Emergency department treatment, triage and transfer protocols for the burn patient. J.A.C.E.P. 7:153, 1978.)

sion (8) only for burns extending through the dermis. Most burns extend only to the dermis and can be adequately decompressed by extending the incision only to the subcutaneous layer. In making these incisions, one must be careful to avoid the radial nerve at the wrist volarly and the superficial peroneal nerve at the fibular neck. The incision should extend from the proximal extent of the burn to its distal margin and a short distance into normal skin. Midlateral and midmedial incisions are carried over the involved joints (26). Following decompression of the burn, rapid improvement in the color of the limb and return of distal pulses occur. The conscious patient often notes rapid disappearance in numbness and may experience brief, excruciating pain due to the sudden increase in blood flow. Following decompression, adequate pressure dressings should be applied to the affected limb. Some authors feel that the extremity should be covered with a light *plaster of paris* shell and elevated (9, 31, 76). We do not feel that a pressure dressing nor a plaster splint should be applied after es-

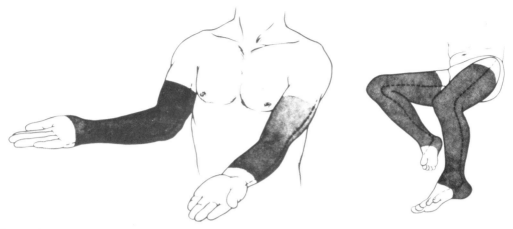

Figure 9.50.   The midmedial and midlateral escharotomies for burns of arms and legs. The burned skin is shown in the dark area. (Reprinted with permission of Aspen Systems, Inc. Edlich, R.F., Emergency department treatment, triage and transfer protocols for the burn patient. J.A.C.E.P. 7:155, 1978.)

charotomy. Instead, a burn dressing should be applied and the limb elevated.

Laterally, in the proximal and middle phalanges, the volar neurovascular bundles are straddled by two sheaths of fascia. The volar fascial sheath is called "Grayson's ligament," the fibers of which join the flexor tendon. The dorsal ligament is called "Cleland's ligament." The fibers of "Cleland's ligament" are oriented obliquely and secure the skin to the phalynx. This ligament must be incised by a lateral incision in order to decompress the vascular compartment and this is done by extending the skin incision deep into the subcutaneous tissue of the finger and undermining dorsally and volarly (69a) (Fig. 9.51).

REPAIR OF WOUNDS—SPECIAL REPAIRS

Lacerations Of The Eyelid

Eyelid lacerations can be classified as extramarginal, not involving the lid border, or intramarginal. Extramarginal lacerations can be superficial or deep. Intramarginal lacerations can be divided into those which are canalicular, usually avulsions, and those which are extracanalicular (59). Simple suturing of the edges is adequate for superficial extramarginal lacerations. When the laceration is horizontal, a simple layer-by-layer closure provides good results; however, when the laceration is vertical, contraction may occur, necessitating a Z-plasty at a later time. If less than one third of the length of the lid is missing, minimal debridement and approximation will give good results (59). *For deep extramarginal lacerations of the upper lid, the levator palpebrae and the tarso-orbital fascia must be approximated to avoid ptosis.* Repair of the orbicularis oculis muscle is also a must. For these reasons, we recommend referral of all deep extramarginal lacerations which involve a large portion of the lid.

When the margin of the lid is involved and the canaliculi are not, the margin should be perfectly approximated to avoid notching or buckling of the lid margin as shown in Figure 9.52 (52). In most cases, 4% cocaine and epinephrine (1:2000) can be instilled in the conjunctiva for adequate anesthesia of the inner portion of the lid (59). Most of these lacerations are not painful (72). Therefore, pain after an orbital or lid laceration usually indicates that a foreign body is present or there is a hematoma within the orbit and this must be evaluated. When an intramarginal laceration involves the canaliculus, a complex

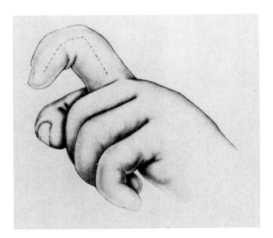

Figure 9.51. Medial skin incision from the metacarpophalangeal joint to the lateral edge of the nail to decompress a circumferentially burned finger. (Reprinted with permission of Aspen Systems, Inc. Edlich, R.F., Emergency department treatment, triage and transfer protocols for the burn patient. J.A.C.E.P. 7:156, 1978.)

repair must be performed, as shown in Figure 9.53. This repair requires meticulous care and can be associated with injury to the lacrimal duct apparatus and should be performed by a specialist.

Lacerations of the eyebrow regions should be approximated in the usual manner, depending on the wound. The eyebrows should not be shaved as shaving increases infection (see "Contaminated Wounds—Preparation"), and the eyebrow is slow to regrow. If the laceration is deep and involves the orbicularis oculi, this muscle should be approximated before closure of the skin.

Nasal Lacerations

The repair of nasal lacerations differs, depending on the area of the nose involved and the extent of the laceration. Anesthesia is provided by an infraorbital nerve block or a nose block as indicated in the chapter on regional anesthesia. Topical analgesia of the nasal mucosa is achieved with cocaine-soaked cotton pledgets. When dealing with small lacerations of the nose, a local infiltration of Xylocaine® containing epinephrine can be used. Lacerations limited to the outer aspect of the nose

(which are not through the nasal vestibule) can be repaired as simple lacerations in the routine fashion. Scars placed across areas in which there is a hollowing of the skin, such as the side of the nose, along the nasolabial junction, inferior to the lower lid and below the eye, tend to shorten and obliterate the hollow and restrict normal motion of the skin as the skin adheres to underlying fascia. Cartilage should never be sutured and should be only minimally debrided when indicated, followed by closure of the mucosa, skin, and subcutaneous tissue which will approximate the cartilage. When involved in a laceration, cartilaginous structures should be replaced in their normal anatomical position and the wound closed. Wounds of the nose should be closed with very limited or no excision of vascularly embarrassed tissue (72). This is a key point in repairing nasal lacerations as there is very little "excess" tissue on the nose which can be used. The subcutaneous tissue of the distal nose requires no approximation since the distance from the skin to the cartilaginous surface is very small and there is very little subcutaneous tissue in the interspace. When dealing with extensive lacerations, the nasal structures should be placed in an anatomical position with the wound edges approximated as closely as possible, and then sutured. Revisions can be made later, should they be required.

When the *nasal vestibule* is involved in a through-and-through laceration of the ala nasi or tip of the nose, only 3 or 4 fine Vicryl® or catgut sutures are needed to loosely approximate the nasal lining. The authors prefer to use 5-0 or 6-0 suture material in this repair. Following the approximation of the edges, a pack of ½ inch gauze impregnated with an antibacterial is placed in the vestibule in order to support the repair and promote hemostasis (72). The skin should then be repaired in the routine fashion, being careful not to incorporate the cartilaginous structures within the suture.

In *septal* injuries, the minimal number of sutures necessary to approximate the wound edges should be used. The important consideration in septal injuries is to provide adequate drainage to avoid the

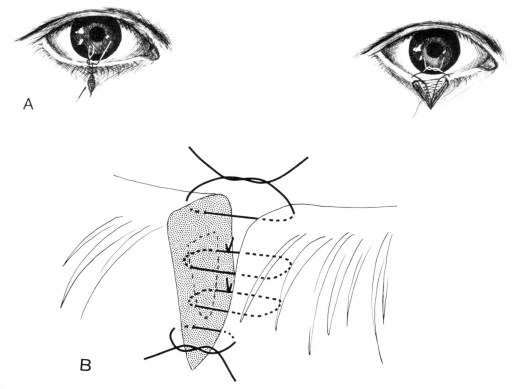

Figure 9.52.   Repair of an eyelid laceration involving the margin of the lid. The tarsal plate is approximated with fine absorbable suture material. Following this, the skin and subcutaneous tissue are approximated with 6-0 or 7-0 nylon. See text for discussion.

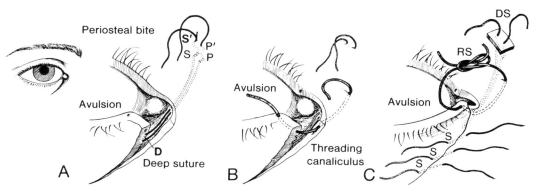

Figure 9.53.   Avulsion of the medial aspect of the lower lid. While this repair should be performed by a plastic surgeon or ophthalmologist, the technique should be familiar to the emergency physician. *A.* A mattress suture is inserted beneath the canaliculus and secures the avulsion flap securely as shown. The points marked "S" and "P" indicate periosteum having been incorporated within the suture to provide a strong anchoring stitch. *B.* The canaliculus is then threaded. Note that a suture needle is passed into the nasal aspect of the cut canaliculus and passes out of the skin on the lateral border of the nose. Heavy chromic catgut suture is used for this procedure. *C.* The avulsion is then repaired. The thread through the canaliculus should be tied very loosely to form a loop as shown. (Reprinted with permission of Surgery, Gynecology and Obstetrics. Minsky, H., Surgical repair of recent lid lacerations. 75:455, 1942.)

development of a septal hematoma or abscess. Following repair of the septum, an anterior nasal pack should be placed using ½ inch gauze impregnated with an antibacterial agent. The pack should be removed in 2 days and the wound inspected for any accumulation of hematoma or the development of infection. Another anterior pack is placed if indicated by continuing discharge from the wound.

In patients with *nasal bone* or *cartilage fractures*, the fragments are realigned and supported with an intranasal packing as well as an external splint (see Chapter 8: Otolaryngology, Ophthalmology, Dental Procedures). The alar and lateral cartilages are inspected, minimally debrided if shredded, and repositioned anatomically. The lacerations of the nasal mucosa are repaired first, followed by repair of the skin. One must always inspect the septal mucosa in patients with either a nasal bone fracture or a contusion injury to the nose. A *septal hematoma* is diagnosed when a soft and fluctuant bulge of the septal mucosa into the inferior meatus is seen. Septal hematomas are the same color as the septal mucosa and are not ecchymotic. Many of these will become infected with *Staphylococcus aureus* and the ensuing abscess will necrose the cartilage and result in a nasal deformity or perforation (54). Incision and drainage should be performed in order to relieve the hematoma. Incise just posterior to the mucocutaneous junction after anesthetizing with 4% cocaine. The technique is as follows (54):

1. Begin the incision as high as possible on the septum and carry it down to the floor of the nose, as shown in Figure 9.54.
2. A horizontal incision is then made along the floor of the nasal septum forming an L-shaped flap. If the horizontal incision is not made, the initial vertical incision will close and result in little or no drainage. Some authors remove a piece of the septal membrane at the junction of the limbs of the L to assure adequate drainage.
3. A drain is then inserted, antimicrobial therapy is begun, and the patient is

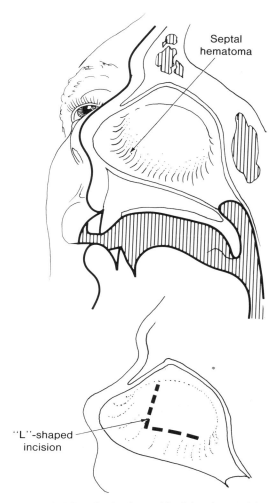

Figure 9.54. An L-shaped incision is used to drain a septal hematoma. The incision should be begun as high as possible on the septum and carried down to the floor of the nose. A horizontal connecting incision is then made along the floor of the nose, forming an "L." See text for discussion.

seen daily to evacuate any clots which may form (54).

If an avulsion of the skin is present at the tip of the nose, a full-thickness skin graft may be needed (Fig. 9.55). The donor graft usually selected is derived from behind the ear. An external splint is applied to these complex lacerations using Xeroform® ointment gauze, followed by a cot-

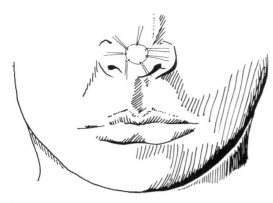

Figure 9.55. Avulsion of the tip of the nose can be treated by a full-thickness graft taken from behind the ear and applied to the tip of the nose. The graft should be secured using fine 6-0 nylon sutures and a cotton ball dressing applied over the graft. One must be certain to remove all fat from the skin graft before application.

ton ball dressing and an anterior intranasal pack for support (37).

Lip And Oral Mucosa Lacerations

Deep lacerations of the lip should be repaired in a two-layer closure. The deep musculature should be approximated with either 5-0 plain catgut or Vicryl®, followed by a surface closure of the skin and subcutaneous tissue (Fig. 9.56A) (52). One must carefully approximate the edges of the vermilion border to avoid a deformity. This border should be approximated first, before placement of any other skin sutures (Fig. 9.56B). In linear lacerations which extend vertically along the mucosal border of the lower lip to the gingival margin, the laceration should be closed with a Z-plasty primarily in the emergency center, as shown in Figure 9.56C, to prevent contracture which will result in a permanent deformity. If the wound is contaminated, a Z-plasty should not be performed in the emergency center.

Gingival Lacerations

Gingival lacerations in which the gingiva is avulsed away from the teeth, exposing the root, are seen particularly in automobile accidents where the passenger strikes his mouth against the dashboard or steering wheel. The gingiva should be sutured back into place in a manner as shown in Figure 9.57. When passed between the teeth, the needle should be passed 2 to 3 mm below the edge of the gingival margin so as to easily pass in the gap between the teeth. The suture is looped around the teeth which are used to support the gingiva in its normal position, similar to a pole holding up a plant. The knot should be cut short and should be on the inner side of the teeth so as not to irritate the inner aspect of the lip.

Ear Lacerations

The anatomy of the ear is shown in Figure 9.58. Lacerations involving the pinna can be repaired as any other soft tissue injury. Lacerations of the helix, tragus, or external meatus are discussed below.

The blood supply to the ear is excellent and incomplete avulsions heal well. Infections are a hazard, as a chondritis may develop with even small lacerations; thus, minor lacerations should be cleansed and repaired meticulously. If cartilage is missing, approximation of the skin and maintenance of the anatomical configuration are important for good results (Fig. 9.58) (72).

In repairing extensive lacerations of the ear, one should trim the cartilage to the level of the skin and then the wound should be closed by approximating the skin edges (Fig. 9.59). The perichondrium may be incorporated in the skin suture, as closure of this supports the skin closure and cartilaginous approximation. The cartilage should not be sutured. The skin in the helix of the ear is adherent to the cartilage and approximation of subcutaneous tissue (which is minimal in this area) is not indicated.

The dressing is the most important part of the repair of an ear laceration. The dressing must be well-molded to conform to the anatomical configuration of the ear in order to provide adequate support and prevent hematoma formation. Mineral oil-

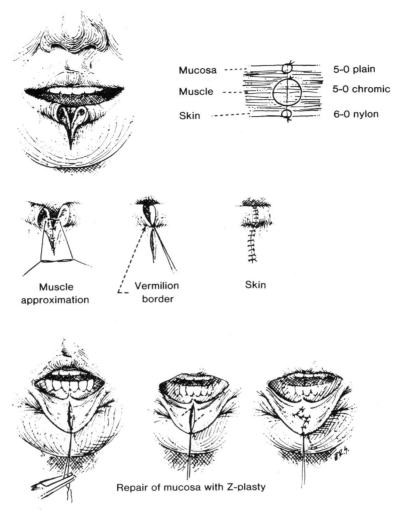

Figure 9.56. Repair of the lower lip involved in a through-and-through laceration should be by 3-layer closure, approximating the mucosa with 5-0 plain gut, muscle with 5-0 chromic, and skin with 6-0 nylon. The vermilion border must be approximated carefully. A Z-plasty is used in the repair of a linear laceration involving the inner aspect of the lower lip to avoid contraction of the scar. (Reprinted with permission of Illinois Medical Journal. Curtin, J., Basic plastic surgical principles in repair of facial lacerations. 129:658, 1966.)

soaked cotton balls packed into the natural crevices of the auricle provide an excellent "cast," because due to the oil, the cotton balls retain their initial mold. A single layer of Xeroform® gauze is used to cover the sutures before application of the cotton balls. This two-layered dressing is then held in place with a bulky head dressing composed of gauze pads, providing support behind the ear as well as in front of it

(72). This dressing should remain in place for 24 to 48 hours.

When a hematoma of the auricle is present, it should be incised and drained as shown in Figure 9.60 (37). After the application of a Xeroform® gauze dressing, saline-soaked cotton balls followed by a fluffy gauze pressure bandage encircling the head serve to protect the ear from further hematoma formation. As the cot-

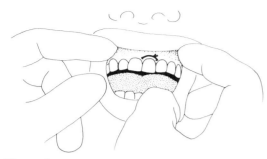

Figure 9.57. When the gingiva is avulsed away from a tooth, it can be sutured by using the tooth as an anchoring point around which to hold the gingiva in place with the suture. The suture is passed 2 to 3 mm away from the edge of the gingival margin to pass in the gap between the teeth. It is then wrapped around the posterior aspect and brought out anteriorly. One will find that a more comfortable result is achieved by bringing the knot out posteriorly behind the teeth to avoid constant rubbing against the inner aspect of the lip.

external meatus is tightly adherent to the cartilage and a cotton wick impregnated with an antibacterial otic solution will suffice to provide support as the laceration heals. Sutures are generally not indicated in this area. One must be careful to check the tympanic membrane; if there are any signs of penetration, the patient must be referred for evaluation of injury to the ossicles.

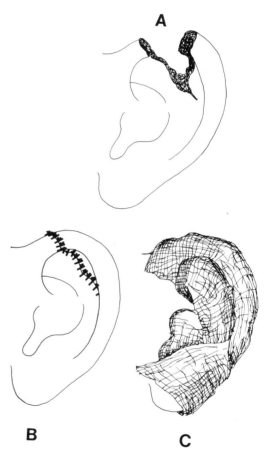

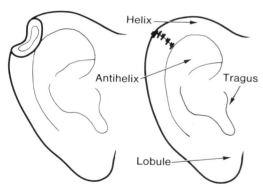

Figure 9.58. Repair of laceration involving a small segment of missing cartilage over the helix. See text for discussion.

ton balls dry, the cotton retains its shape and forms a well-molded firm cast over the ear. This dressing should remain in place for 24 to 48 hours. Serial drainage is usually necessary in these hematomas. Antibiotics are generally prescribed for a perichondrial hematoma in order to prevent a perichondritis from developing.

Lacerations may extend into the external meatus, usually as a result of a foreign object striking the ear. The skin in the

B **C**

Figure 9.59. The repair of extensive lacerations of the ear. The edges of the cartilage should be trimmed and the skin edges approximated. A Xeroform® gauze dressing is then applied over the ear, followed by a bulky gauze dressing which maintains pressure over the ear to promote healing without hematoma formation. Two folded 4 × 4s should be placed behind the ear to provide a more secure dressing when wrapping the ear.

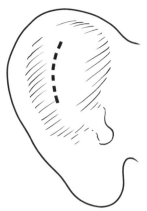

Figure 9.60. Drainage of a hematoma of the auricle. After the hematoma is drained, a Xeroform gauze dressing is applied over the incision and saline-soaked cotton balls are then packed over the Xeroform® dressing in order to form a "cast" on the ear. This is then covered with a fluffy gauze pressure bandage encircling the head.

Fingertip Injuries

A number of reports exist in the literature on the various ways to manage fingertip injuries. Five ways currently exist and are discussed below:

1. Primary closure
2. Healing by secondary intention
3. Local advancement flap
4. Skin graft
5. Pedicle flap

Primary closure, when possible, is the treatment of choice (38). When primary closure of a fingertip amputation will result in shortening and tenderness of the digit, alternative methods must be used. Skin grafts tend to contract and pose problems with regard to loss of normal sensation over the grafted skin. In 67% of cases, induration and fissuring occur at the site of the graft and there is a decrease in sensation at the site (38).

Healing by secondary intention is a conservative approach advocated by many authors and advised here (4, 21, 32, 38, 44). When the avulsion exceeds 10 mm in the adult, some prefer the use of other procedures indicated below. Remarkably good results are achieved in children including regrowth of amputated nails and phalanges with healing by secondary intention (21). The fingertip is dressed with Xeroform® gauze and Telfa®, followed by a fine mesh gauze dressing. The hand is then elevated for 24 hours, and the dressing is kept dry. The patient is placed on oral penicillinase-resistant antibiotics in the emergency center. The patient returns in 48 hours and the dressing is removed. The patient subsequently soaks his hand in warm water for 15 minutes 4 times a day for 1 week, and the wound is permitted to completely epithelialize (21, 32). In a child, even with bone exposure, the wound heals without the development of osteomyelitis (21). Occasionally the stump may be painful, and at times troublesome remnants of the fingernail persist. It may take 1 month for healing to occur (21). Most adults treated conservatively are able to return to work within a few days (32). Indurated scars occur in 48% of patients treated conservatively and reduced sensation is seen in only 13% of patients (38).

When a transverse amputation results in the bone of the distal phalanx being exposed, a number of alternative methods of closure exist. In the Kutler method of repair, a *local advancement flap* is transferred as a triangular flap from the proximal volar side of a finger amputation to the center of the wound and yields good results (33). It is important to round off the bone by removing a small amount of phalanx with a rongeur to prevent tension on the flap (33). This method is illustrated in Figures 9.43 and 9.61.

Skin grafts are commonly used to cover amputations of the distal phalanx, and some authors feel they are the treatment of choice (12). Skin grafts may be either split thickness incorporating only a portion of the dermis or full thickness. Split-thickness grafts have a tendency to shrink 70%, which draws normally tactile skin over most of the defect (12). Contraction of the graft is minimal when a thicker graft is used (7). In the emergency center, a full-thickness graft is more commonly used. When applying a skin graft, one must be certain there is no protruding bone. The bone must be at least flush with the am-

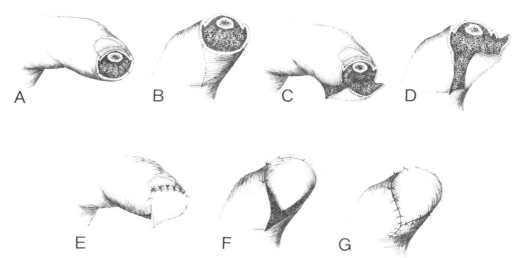

Figure 9.61. An advancement flap or Kutler procedure. *A.* Amputation of the distal tip of the finger with bone exposed. *B.* A small piece of the tip is excised. A V-shaped incision is then made on the volar surface of the finger with the point of the *"V"* just distal to the distal interphalangeal joint. *C.* The V-shaped flap is then pulled distally. *D.* The base of the flap should not be undermined and should remain in contact with the septi which nourish the flap. *E.* The flap is then trimmed slightly and carried distally to the nail margin. *F.* Fine sutures are used to secure the distal pole of the flap to the nailbed and skin folds. *G.* The lateral edges are then sutured, resulting in a Y-shaped repaired wound.

putated tissue and preferably recessed in order for the graft to be accepted. As the graft shrinks, it pulls surrounding skin over the bone. The volar surface of the forearm and the wrist are excellent sites for grafting donor skin (Fig. 9.62). Hemostasis is mandatory to insure an adequate take of the graft. After the graft is applied over the defect, it should be sutured in place with 5-0 or 6-0 nylon, and the ends of each suture tied over a bolus of moist cotton, thus providing a stent dressing. A small piece of Xeroform® gauze dressing should be placed over the grafted skin, between it and the cotton balls. The donor site can generally be closed primarily by undermining the skin edges. Continuous elevation of the finger for the first 5 days is extremely important.

A cross-finger *pedicle flap* is used in some amputations and provides a good result with regard to tactile sensation and return to normal function (44). This procedure is not one which is performed in the emergency center and is not discussed here.

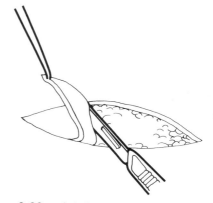

Figure 9.62. A full-thickness graft is excised as an ellipse, leaving behind as much of the fat as possible. Grafts are commonly obtained from the volar surface of the forearm or wrist.

A review of 151 partial and total amputations of a fingertip showed that the best results were achieved with early primary closure and the use of the local advancement flap with the avoidance of skin grafts (50).

In summary, treatment must be individualized for each patient depending on occupation, age, and health. In the child, most fingertip injuries can be treated conservatively with healing by secondary intention with excellent results. In the adult, conservative therapy should also be used and remains our treatment of choice whenever possible. An advancement flap as is illustrated in Figures 9.43 and 9.61 yields excellent results in patients with distal or middle phalangeal amputations. One must be careful to leave an adequate attachment of the flap to its base and to resect an adequate amount of bone so that the flap may be advanced without tension.

Nailbed Injuries

Based on the evaluation of the repairs of over 3,000 nailbed injuries, certain principles can be summarized regarding this common injury (4):

1. There should be very minimal debridement.
2. Remove the nail and accurately appose and repair the lacerated nailbed and root with 6-0 absorbable gut or other absorbable suture. If the root is not replaced, the pouch deep to the proximal skin fold is obliterated within a few days. If the root cannot be replaced easily, follow the procedure in the legend to Figure 9.67.
3. Skin folds surrounding the nail margins must be preserved. Adhesions between skin folds, nailbed, and root are prevented by preserving these spaces with a nonadherent gauze packing, such as Xeroform®, molded to the contour of the skin folds.

Immediate primary reconstruction of the nailbed and root is the treatment of choice. Before a discussion of the methods of repairing the various injuries of the nailbed, the anatomy and generation of the nail must be understood. The nail matrix is formed from three sites, the nailbed, the roof matrix at the eponychial region (Fig. 9.63), and the root matrix. The most important areas to be preserved for the generation of a normal nail are the roof and root matrix. In a child, if the nailbed is destroyed, eventually a normal nail will

regrow; however, if the nail root and roof matrix are destroyed, an entirely normal nail will never grow back. The various methods of repairing different injuries are shown in Figures 9.64 through 9.67.

Complications which arise from improper treatment include the following:

1. Split nail. A split nail occurs when the root is improperly approximated, resulting in a wide scar which produces splitting.
2. Adhesions. Adhesions of the skin fold to the nail root occur when a laceration involves both the skin fold and

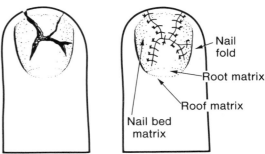

Figure 9.63. Repair of a complex nailbed injury. Often these patients present with a large subungual hematoma which necessitates removal of the nail in order to repair the nailbed. After removal of the nail, the bed is approximated with fine plain gut suture. Little debridement is necessary.

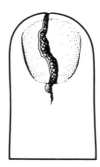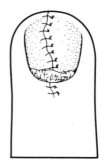

Figure 9.64. When lacerations are vertical and traverse the root of the nail as well as the distal tip, the nail must be removed and the nailbed repaired separately from the skin over the eponychial portion of the nail. To maintain the integrity of the space between the roof and root matrix, Xeroform® gauze should be packed in that space.

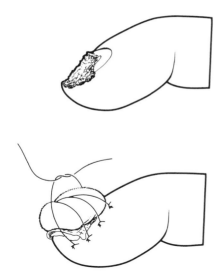

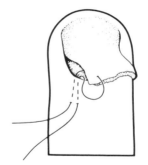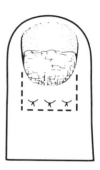

Figure 9.67. Proximal avulsion of the nailbed. When this occurs the nailbed must be reattached in its anatomical location. A suture is passed through the skin and the avulsed bed is picked up by the suture loop and secured back under the eponychia. The nailbed must not be returned to its normal location until 2 to 3 sutures are first applied, after which all are pulled, reapproximating the nailbed to its normal position, and tied. A Xeroform® dressing should be used to separate the roof and root matrix.

Figure 9.65. An avulsion of the nail involving the dorsal aspect of the distal tip. This should be treated with a simple Xeroform® dressing held in place with nylon sutures. This gauze should remain in place for 10 days.

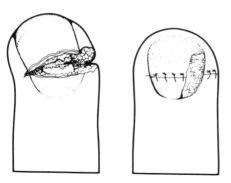

Figure 9.66. When a transverse laceration extends across the nail, the distal nail must be removed and the nailbed repaired as shown. Similarly, to the vertical laceration which extends across the eponychia of the nail the lateral nail folds should be packed with Xeroform® gauze to maintain the integrity of this space. This gauze should remain in place for a period of 10 days.

the nail matrix and they are not repaired separately, resulting in obliteration of the space. The space must be packed with nonadherent gauze packing.

Removal Of A Nail

The removal of a nail has been a controversial issue regarding when it should take place. There are no good data in the literature to support opinions regarding when to remove a nail or when not to. It would appear logical that since the base of the nail contains epithelial cells from the roof and root matrix, when possible this should be preserved. We advocate preservation of the base of the nail when a laceration extends across the nail transversely to repair the laceration. When the nail has been removed traumatically and is intact and clean, the authors feel it should be reapplied in its normal anatomical position as it provides an excellent stent over the nailbed. When open fractures occur in patients with a nail or nailbed injury, the nailbed injury should be repaired as would be routine, and the fractures treated separately. These patients should be placed on oral antibiotics, although osteomyelitis in the distal phalanx following an open fracture is quite uncommon.

When a subungual hematoma is present, this can be drained by a simple puncture of the nail with either a hot paper clip or a small drill (Fig. 9.68). A subungual he-

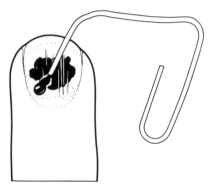

Figure 9.68. Drainage of a subungual hematoma.

matoma which is large is almost always associated with a nailbed laceration. We feel the nail should be removed, and the bed repaired. The nail is then replaced as an anatomic stent. If one does not repair the nailbed, a step off may occur with ridging of the nail when it grows back.

AFTERCARE OF NAILBED INJURIES

Sutures should remain in the nailbed for approximately 7 days. The nonadherent Xeroform® gauze dressing which is instilled in the nail folds as shown in Figures 9.61 and 9.64 should remain in place for 4 days. After the wound is sutured it should be covered with a piece of Telfa®, which will not adhere to the secretions produced by the nailbed, followed by a thick gauze dressing. The finger should be splinted and the hand elevated whenever possible. The outer dressing, excluding the Telfa, should be removed and the wound checked in 2 days. The patient must be advised that while the chances of forming a new nail are good when the injury is not severe, there is no guarantee as to what the final outcome will be.

Suture Removal

Sutures should be removed as soon as possible, as they serve as a foreign body in the wound and a nidus for infection as well as permit suture marks to form when left in place for an excessively long time. Nylon sutures can get wet for brief periods and should be dried after exposure to moisture. The technique of suture removal is shown in Figure 9.69. Using this method one avoids pulling the outside portion or the suture back through the wound and causing contamination. Sutures left in place for 3 or 4 days are unlikely to leave a permanent suture mark (52). If one removes a suture by the eighth day, the epithelial tract will regress and leave no significant mark; however, the earlier the suture is removed, the better (18). During the first 8 days, there is very little tensile strength in the wound. The closure is held by vessels crossing the wound, epithelialization, and a fibrin coagulant. In some areas of the body, such as around the joints, when sutures are removed at 8 days the wound should be supported by the use of Steri-strips (5). In the face, sutures should be removed in 3 or 4 days. In extensive facial lacerations, support is needed for longer than 3 days. Alternating sutures may be removed on day 3 and the remainder by day 5 and Steri-strips applied for added support for 5 to 7 days.

In the lower extremity, where healing is slower, sutures may remain for 14 days to assure adequate strength, especially around joints. In the upper extremity, sutures may be removed in 7 to 10 days (Table 9.9). Although sutures are removed earlier, the tensile strength of the wound does not return to normal until 21 days after closure.

Primary closure of a wound carries with

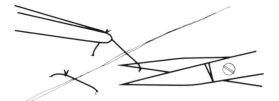

Figure 9.69. Correct method of removing a suture. The suture should be removed by cutting the end away from the knot near the skin to prevent passage of the contaminated outer portion of the stitch back through the skin. When fine sutures are used and are close to the skin, a #11 blade rather than a scissors should be used for suture removal. The tip of the blade is inserted under the suture loop, and the suture is cut.

Table 9.9. Suture Removal

Location	Time of Removal (days)
Face	3–4 (Adult)
	2–3 (Children)
Lower extremity	8–10
Upper extremity	7–10
Extensor surface of joints	10–14
Delayed closure	8–12

it the obligation to maintain optimal conditions for wound healing (55). If sutures are removed too early, the wound may be disrupted with minimal activity unless supported by Steri-strips. Separation may occur when an overwhelming force breaks the laceration open, when absorbable sutures dissolve too quickly, or when tight sutures cut through the tissue. *Dehiscence* represents the failure of the wound to gain sufficient strength to withstand stresses. When dehiscence does occur, it does so on the third to the fifth day after incision and about one half of the cases are associated with infection. *Delayed closure* should be performed on wounds which are heavily contaminated with saliva, dirt, or grease and which cannot be adequately cleansed and debrided. Closure of these wounds should be delayed to permit the wound to gain sufficient resistance against infection, at which time closure can be performed safely. In these cases the wound should be packed with fine mesh gauze and dressed with a pressure dressing, and the limb should be elevated. The wound should then be closed at 4 days. This time can be altered, depending on the area of the body. When these wounds subsequently are closed, they should be splinted and a pressure dressing applied. The sutures should remain in place for 12 days, particularly on extremity wounds (55). Delayed closure usually is not necessary on facial wounds and is not advocated. Due to the profuse vascularity of the face, wounds tend to heal well after being adequately cleansed and debrided.

Delayed wound closure can be accomplished by one of three techniques: secondary suturing after a local anesthetic is infiltrated, tying previously placed untied sutures, or pulling the wound edges together after adhesive tape is applied parallel to the wound margins. This latter method is used in closing large, gaping, linear lacerations and can be used for both delayed wound closure and primary wound closure, especially in somewhat contaminated wounds. In using this method of closure, 2 to 3 inch wide strips of adhesive tape are placed parallel to the wound margins, approximately 5 mm from the margin on both sides of the wound. A thin layer of benzoin tincture should be applied to the skin on both sides of the incision before applying the tape. The two strips of adhesive tape are laid down adjacent to the wound edges, and the longitudinal edge of the tape bordering the wound is folded one-quarter inch under each strip, thus providing a "hem" in which sutures can be placed. A running stitch is then passed through the "hems" on both sides of the wound and the wound closed in this manner. This technique combines the advantages that no anesthesia is required, no skin sutures are placed which may become infected, and no strips of tape are applied over the wound, thus permitting adequate drainage of secretions.

Elevation And Pressure Dressings

A snug pressure dressing and elevation are desirable in most instances to minimize edema formation and to prevent collection of blood and serum, hematoma formation, lymphedema, and venous congestion (5, 52). A pressure dressing also supports and protects the tissue by avoiding pull on the approximated edges (52). In certain areas such as the lips and eyelids, one may use cold compresses for 48 to 72 hours after the injury to minimize pain and swelling. In the scalp and forehead a firm pressure dressing is needed for 48 hours to prevent hematoma formation (72). A pressure dressing is extremely important, particularly in regions which are highly vascular to prevent hematoma formation which may disrupt the wound closure as well as be a source for infection. The scalp, forehead, periorbital, pretibial, and dorsal surface of the hand are common sites for hematoma formation, and pressure dressings should be applied to lacerations in these areas. In addition, wounds over the extensor surfaces of the major joints should have a pressure dressing applied to prevent hematoma formation. In children, the best way to immobilize joints is to provide a big bulky dressing over the area of laceration. A pressure dressing should be accompanied by elevation of the injured part whenever practical to accomplish the aforementioned objectives. In facial lacerations the patient should be advised to sleep upright on many pillows or in a reclining chair.

Dressings

A single layer of ointment gauze, Xeroform® or Vaseline®, can be used under the pressure dressing (5). To have an optimally aesthetic wound, prevention of dessication of the wound margins with these ointments is critical and one of the most important parts of aftercare. Where a pressure dressing is impractical (e.g., face), the wound should be cleaned daily with a mild soap and Xeroform cut to the appropriate size should be placed over the wound. After 12 to 24 hours, a mild soap should be used four times a day to cleanse the area around the wound and to remove any exudate over the Xeroform dressing. Following this, a hair blower can be used to dry the surface of the wound. The Xeroform dressing should remain in place for 7 to 14 days when dealing with a facial abrasion. All dried blood should be removed from the surface of the wound and from around the sutures, as this debris may serve as a nidus for infection (72, 75). This can be accomplished with the use of a cotton-tipped applicator. A thin layer of bacitracin ointment or similar ointment can be applied to keep the surface free of crusting. One should not use a neomycin-containing ointment since this may result in a contact dermatitis (75).

Infection

When a sutured wound becomes infected, one must relieve the constriction and provide for adequate drainage and remove the sutures which provide a nidus for infection. Always consider an undiscovered foreign body as the source of infection. The sutures should be removed in part or totally, which improves drainage and circulation and removes a foreign body. Warm packs should be applied, and the patient should be placed on penicillinase-resistant penicillins. Wounds closed by an emergency physician should always be followed, preferably by the same physician, in 48 hours. All patients should be instructed to watch for signs of infection and to return immediately if any of the signs are noted. If the incidence of infection is greater than 5%, the physician should reevaluate his technique of wound preparation and suturing and investigate possible sources of contamination during wound closures.

Suture sinuses form when a suture site becomes infected. A suture sinus is a tract leading from suture material within the wound to the skin surface which continually drains serous or purulent material. A small abscess called a *stitch abscess* often forms beneath the sinus. A suture sinus or suture abscess usually indicates that a foreign body, which may be the suture material itself, is present and has become infected in the wound. As long as the suture remains in place, the sinus will persist. These infections occur most commonly with silk and other multifilament sutures and are least often seen with monofilament synthetics. One can explore the sinus tract gently with a probe and remove the suture with a skin hook when possible; if this is not possible, one can wait a few weeks for spontaneous ejection to occur.

Scar Revision

Occasionally, the result of a repair will be poor due to the nature of the wound itself. The patient may complain of a bad cosmetic result. Scar revision is not usually performed before 6 months, to allow for scar maturation to occur, and the patient should be so advised (52, 72). In young children and in the elderly, maturation of a scar to its final appearance may take a year or more (46, 72).

Modalities such as compressive dressings and steroids injected in the intermediary may be helpful in these patients;

therefore, these patients should be referred early. Posttraumatic scars can usually be improved with surgical excision and revision since these revisions are carried out in wounds which are not traumatically induced.

ABSCESSES

Abscesses are commonly seen in the emergency center. Too often, physicians treating an abscess incise in the most "convenient" location and place the patient on oral antibiotics. Anesthesia is difficult to provide, especially when dividing the septi within the cavity of the abscess. In the treatment of abscesses, the important anatomical structures underlying the abscess must be appreciated. The location of the abscess is critical to the direction of the incision.

There are seven locations in the body where abscesses are in close proximity to major vessels. These locations are as follows:

1. Peritonsillar and retropharyngeal abscesses.
2. Abscesses located in the anterior triangle of the neck (an area enclosed by the sternocleidomastoid muscle, mandible, and anterior midline of the neck).
3. Abscesses located in the supraclavicular fossa.
4. Abscesses which lie deep in the axilla.
5. Abscesses in the antecubital space.
6. Abscesses which occur in the groin.
7. Abscesses which occur in the popliteal space.

Abscesses which occur in any of these seven locations should be aspirated with an 18 gauge needle attached to a 10 cc syringe before drainage. The aspiration is only for diagnostic confirmation. Too often, what was thought to be an abscess has been incised only to find a mycotic aneurysm and imminent exsanguination. The aspiration should not drain the abscess cavity entirely, because the purulent material serves as a marker for the hollow of the abscess cavity. The aspiration merely confirms that the material contained within the cavity is purulent and not serosanguinous or pure blood. If the latter material (mycotic aneurysm) is found, the abscess should be drained more judiciously in the operating room.

Antiseptic Preparation And Technique Of Anesthesia

The area should be surgically prepared with a topical anesthetic such as Betadine®. A regional field block anesthetic technique is used to anesthetize the abscess (1a). The injection of a ring or anesthetic material should be approximately 1 cm away from the perimeter of the erythematous border of the abscess. The entire lesion is thus anesthetized circumferentially. In providing a ring of anesthesia around the abscess, one must be certain to inject the anesthetic solution subcutaneously. A small amount of anesthetic solution is then injected into the roof of the abscess in a linear fashion along the line of the projected incision. The onset of action of the anesthetic in this location is approximately 5 minutes and is quite successful in relieving pain.

Incision

The incision should be performed along the relaxed skin tension lines to reduce scarring. When purulent material drains, a specimen for culture may be obtained at this time if desired, especially in immunosuppressed patients. A hemostat should be inserted into the abscess cavity and spread to break up the septi and loculations and to release any further pockets of purulent material. The cavity should be irrigated with normal saline before any gauze is inserted to pack the cavity. Iodoform® gauze should then be inserted into the abscess cavity with 1 cm of gauze exiting from the cavity. A sterile dressing is then applied. The Iodoform® gauze is removed in 24 to 48 hours. The Iodoform® gauze serves two purposes: it prevents the incision from sealing over and provides for adequate drainage of the abscess cavity. Following removal of the Iodoform® pack, warm wet soaks are applied to the area several times a day for a few days. The incision will heal in approximately 7 to 10 days in most cases.

In a large study, abscesses were treated with and without antibiotics (58). All the abscesses were treated with incision and drainage and all were found to heal without complications, including approximately three fourths of those cases which were treated without adjunctive antibiotics. It was concluded that the primary management of abscesses should be incision and drainage and that routine culture and antibiotic therapy were not indicated for the typical abscess in patients with normal host defenses. Abscesses which we feel should be treated with oral antibiotic therapy are those which are surrounded by lymphangitis or a large area of cellulitis. The cellulitis is determined by tenderness peripheral to the area of the abscess as well as increased warmth and redness as opposed to the nontender induration palpated around an abscess which is well-localized and which would not be benefitted by the addition of oral antibiotics. Purulent material from immunosuppressed patients should be cultured, and the patient should be placed on oral antibiotics pending the culture results (58).

Special Considerations

FELONS

A felon is an infection or abscess occurring in the pulp of the volar surface of the distal phalynx. The proper technique of draining a felon has been controversial (30). The incision which is associated with the lowest rate of complications is a simple vertical incision carried out over the center of the abscess (Fig. 9.70). The fish-mouth incision and the lateral connecting incisions which have been used in the past

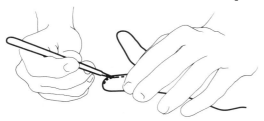

Figure 9.70. Correct incision for a felon. See text for discussion.

have been found to produce a higher incidence of fingertip anesthesia and instability (47a).

PARONYCHIA AND EPONYCHIA ABSCESSES

A paronychia, as referred to here, is an abscess under the lateral nail fold. An eponychia is an abscess under the roof matrix.

For the common paronychia, an incision is unnecessary. Instead, the tip of a #11 blade should be inserted approximately 5 mm under the surface of the nail, uplifting the cuticle (Fig. 9.71) and, thus, providing an escape for the collected suppurative material. This procedure alone provides for adequate drainage in most paronychia and eponychia.

HIDRADENITIS SUPPURATIVA

This is an infection leading to multiple abscess formation in the apocrine glands of the axilla. The matted and indurated dermis contains the apocrine glands and

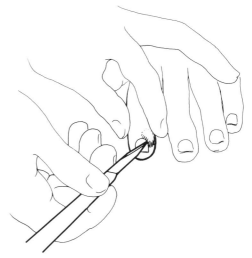

Figure 9.71. A paronychial or eponychial abscess is drained by inserting a #11 blade along the surface of the nail and uplifting the nail fold under which lies the paronychia. An incision is not necessary to drain this abscess unless it extends or is very large. The authors have found no increased incidence of recurrences with this technique. Following this warm saline soaks are used.

multiple drainage sites from these abscesses are noted. These should be incised and drained as described earlier, and a large abscess cavity should be packed in the manner described above. These patients should be referred to a general surgeon for follow-up care, as surgical excision may be needed to prevent recurrence.

PERITONSILLAR ABSCESSES

A peritonsillar abscess usually dissects into the soft palate above the tonsillar pillars, and the abscess which forms deviates the uvula to the opposite side. This abscess should be drained with a transverse incision at the site of maximal fluctuation, which is usually superior and lateral to the tonsil. To prevent pulmonary aspiration of the purulent material, a small stab should be made initially into the abscess cavity and a suction tip should be held at the site of the stab to aspirate the majority of the purulent material as it exudes from the stab. Once the majority of the suppurative material has been evacuated, the incision can be extended. These abscesses are not packed routinely, and the patient should be advised to sleep with his face down rather than on his back to provide for adequate drainage of the purulent material and avoid aspiration. This procedure is more completely discussed in Chapter 8: "Otolaryngology, Ophthalmology, Dental Procedures."

PERIODONTAL ABSCESSES

A periodontal abscess is usually seen along the border of the premolars and molars and is drained by an incision which parallels the gingival border at the site of maximal fluctuance within the oral cavity (Fig. 9.72). It is usually packed with plain gauze and the packing is removed within 24 to 48 hours. These patients are usually placed on oral penicillin to protect the surrounding sinuses from secondary infection and to treat the usual cellulitis which is seen accompanying these abscesses.

PERIRECTAL ABSCESSES

Perirectal abscesses should be drained with a radial incision which is carried into the abscess cavity and can be extended

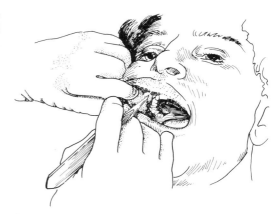

Figure 9.72. A periodontal abscess is drained by an incision made in the sulcus of the mouth where the gingiva meets the buccal mucosa. The incision should be made over the point of maximum fluctuance.

through the subcutaneous portion of the external sphincter. One has to be careful not to extend the incision through the deep portion of the sphincter as this may produce complications such as fecal incontinence when the incision heals. These abscesses are then packed with Iodoform® gauze and the patient is advised to sit in a sitz bath for 20 minutes 3 times a day for the first day and to remove the packing while in the bath. The healing is usually complete within approximately 10 days, during the course of which the patient is advised to take sitz baths twice daily. This procedure is more completely discussed in Chapter 1: "Abdominal Procedures."

PILONIDAL ABSCESS

A pilonidal abscess occurs in the midline posteriorly in the region of the coccyx. Most pilonidal abscesses contain hair (64) and, following excision and drainage, should be referred to a surgeon for definitive treatment which includes excision of the sinus. Some authors feel that definitive treatment with incision of the sinus and drainage of the abscess can be performed in the office or the hospital as a single procedure (36). Definitive treatment of repeat pilonidal abscesses during the initial visit can be done by a plastic surgeon, with total excision of the abscess and primary closure or flap closure of the defect.

FOREIGN BODY REMOVAL

Needle Embedded

A broken needle embedded in the foot is a common problem presenting to the emergency physician. This foreign body can engage the physician for hours in an attempt to remove the illusive "needle in a haystack." When it is available, fluoroscopy offers an excellent aid in removal of these foreign bodies. The patient should be transported to the fluoroscopy suite, and under sterile conditions an incision is made over the needle as judged from the anteroposterior and lateral films; the particle is localized under fluoroscopic visualization and is removed with a curved hemostat.

An alternate method has been described (51). A radiopaque marker is placed on the sole of the foot at the point of entry of the particle. A bent paper clip serves as an excellent marker placed at the entry site of the foreign body. Posterior-anterior films should be taken to show the exact size of the particle, its relation and orientation to the marker, and its configuration; a lateral projection shows its exact length. After the posterior-anterior and lateral films are taken, the marker should remain in place. The area should be prepped, draped, and anesthetized, preferably by a regional nerve block (as described in the chapter on anesthesia). Since the posterior-anterior and lateral films are obtained perpendicular to each other, with the marker in place, one can discern the exact length and orientation of the foreign body. With a #11 blade a stab incision is made at a 90 degree angle to the middle of the foreign body. Due to the width of the blade, one can insert a small hemostat in the wound with minimal probing, and the foreign body removed. The resulting stab may be covered with a single dressing after the needle is removed.

Another method is to use two 19 gauge needles placed perpendicular to each other to localize the foreign body. These are used to guide a #11 blade into position near the foreign body by intermittent exposure with a fluoroscope to pinpoint the foreign body. The patient is asked to move the extremity when needed, and the radiograph beam is turned off for each manipulation of the localizing needles. Once the foreign body is localized between the two needles, a small incision is made between the needles, and the foreign body found at the tips is removed.

Fishhook

A fishhook embedded in the subcutaneous tissue can be removed by passing the barb out through the skin as if completing its passage through the tissue. After doing this simply cut the eye of the hook and grasp the point and barb with a needle holder or pliers and withdraw the hook. One should be careful not to cut the eye from the hook until the point and barb have passed through the skin, or the embedded portion of the hook and barb may disappear beneath the skin preventing removal. In situations in which the hook is small and embedded in the face, it may be preferable to back the hook out rather than add an extra wound. When doing so, a large bore needle should be passed over the entrance tract of the barb and then inserted over the barb as the hook is being withdrawn (29a). The hook should be advanced slightly to dislodge the barb from the tissue. The hook should be pulled and twisted so that the barb is "housed" by the lumen of the large bore needle. The hook and barb then are withdrawn through the entrance wound along with the large bore needle placed over the barb as a single unit. In situations in which the hook is quite large, it may be better to pass the barb through the skin even when the face is involved, since a barb may produce a sizable irregular tear. If a fishhook is embedded in cartilage but has not passed through the skin on the opposite side, then the hook can be backed out in a manner similar to that described above using the large bore needle. If the hook has passed through the cartilage but has not passed through the other side of the skin, then the barb should be passed through the skin on the opposite side, as in the ear, clip the eye of the hook and pull the rest of the fishhook out of the skin.

The best method for removal of a fishhook is a technique popularized by Cooke (16). This method requires no anesthesia and the only material necessary is a 3 foot long piece of sewing thread or silk. The silk or thread is placed around the curve of the fishhook (Fig. 9.73A) and the other end is wrapped around the physician's hand several times in order to prevent slipping. The shank of the hook is then depressed, as shown in Figure 9.73B, until

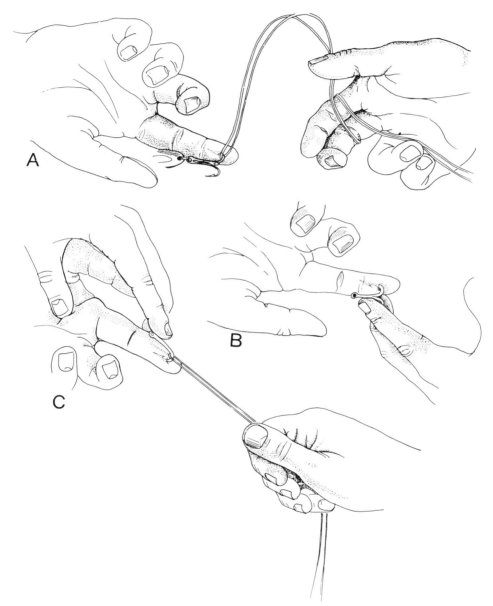

Figure 9.73. *A.* Silk suture material or a string is placed around the curve of the fishhook. *B.* The involved digit is then held firmly against a flat surface and the shank is depressed until resistance is met. *C.* While the shank is depressed and the string is held taut, a quick jerk is applied and dislodges the needle.

it meets a resistance. To provide stability, the involved digit or adjacent tissue should be held flatly against a firm surface during the procedure. The shank is then depressed and the thread is jerked in one forceful move parallel to the shank, which dislodges the hook (Fig. 9.73C). This technique is effective and produces no additional puncture wound for the patient.

References

1. Agris, J., Traumatic tattooing. J. Trauma 16:798, 1976.
1a. Albom, M., Surgical gems, J. Derm. Surg. 2:2, 1976.
2. Albert, J., Lofstrom, B., Effects of epinephrine in solutions of local anesthetic agents. Acta Anaesth. Scand. Suppl. 16:71, 1965.
3. Alexander, J.W., Kaplan, J.Z., Altemeier, W.A., Role of suture materials in the development of wound infection. Ann. Surg. 165:192, 1967.
4. Ashbell, T.S., Kleinhert, H.E., The deformed fingernail: A frequent result of failure to repair nailbed injuries. J. Trauma 7:177, 1967.
5. Backpus, L.H., DeFelice, C.A., Treatment of accidental wounds, Postgrad. Med. 27:209, 1960.
6. Baxter, C.R., Surgical management of soft tissue infections. Surg. Clin. North Am. 52:1483, 1972.
7. Bennett, J.E., Fingertip avulsions. J. Trauma 6:249, 1966.
8. Bennett, J.E., Lewis, E., Operative decompression of constricting burns. Surgery 43:949, 1958.
9. Blocker, T.G., Jr., Moyer, C.A., In Womack, N.A. (ed.) On Burns. Charles C Thomas, Springfield, IL, 1953, p. 172.
10. Borges, A.F., Alexander, J.E., Relaxed skin tension lines: Z-plasties on scars, and fusiform excision of lesions. Br. J. Plast. Surg. 15:242, 1962.
11. Borges, A.F., Alexander, J.E., Black, L.I., Z-plasty treatment of unesthetic scars. Eye, Ear, Nose and Throat Month. 44:39, 1965.
11a. Branework, P.I., American Society for Surgery of the Hand. 21st Annual meeting, Jan. 21 and 22, 1966, Chicago, IL.
11b. Branemark, P.I., Albrekisson, B., Lindstrom, J., et al., Local tissue effects of wound disinfectants. Acta Chir. Scand. Suppl. 357:166, 1966.
12. Brody, G.S., Cloutier, McL., Woolhouse, F.M., The fingertip injury: An assessment of management. Plast. Reconstr. Surg. 26:80, 1960.
13. Carpendale, M.T.F., Sereda, W., The role of the percutaneous suture in surgical wound infection. Surgery 58:672, 1965.
13a. Condie, J.D., Ferguson, D.J., Experimental wound infections: Contamination versus surgical technique. Surgery 50:367, 1961.
14. Condon, R.E., Locked vertical mattress stitch for skin closure, Surg. Gynecol. Obstet. 127:839, 1968.
15. Conolly, W.B., Hunt, T.K., Zederfeldt, B., et al., Clinical comparison of surgical wounds closed by suture and adhesive tapes. Am. J. Surg. 117:318, 1969.
16. Cooke, T., How to remove fish-hooks with a bit of string. Med. J. Australia 48:815, 1961.
17. Covino, B.G., Comparative clinical pharmacology of local anesthetic agents. Anesthesiology 35:158, 1971.
18. Crikelair, G.F., Skin suture marks. Am. J. Surg. 96:631, 1958.
19. Cruse, P.J.E., Foord, R., A five-year prospective study of 23,649 surgical wounds. Arch. Surg. 107:206, 1973.
20. Davis, J.S., Plastic Surgery. P. Blakiston's Son & Co., Philadelphia, 1919, pp. 26.
20a. Demling, R.H., Buerstatte, W.R., Perea, A., Management of hot tar burns. J. Trauma 20:242, 1980.
21. Douglas, B.S., Conservative management of guillotine amputation of the finger in children, Aust. Paediatr. J. 8:86, 1972.
22. Douglas, D.M., Tensile strength of sutures: II. Loss when implanted in living tissue. Lancet 2:499, 1949.
23. Downs, T.M., The healing of wounds. Surg. Clin. North Am. 20:1859, 1940.
24. Duke, W.R., Robson, M.C., Krizek, T.J., Civilian wounds: Their bacterial flora and rate of infection. Surg. Forum 23:518, 1972.
25. DuMortier, J.J., The resistance of healing wounds to infection. Surg. Gynecol. Obstet. 56:762, 1933.
26. Edlich, R.F., Haynes, B.W., Larkham, N., et al., Emergency department treatment, triage and transfer protocols for the burn patient, J.A.C.E.P. 7:152, 1978.
27. Edlich, R.F., Panek, P.H., Rodeheaver, G.T., et al., Physical and chemical configuration of sutures in the development of surgical infection. Ann. Surg. 177:679, 1973.
28. Edlich, R.F., Rodeheaver, G.T., Thacker, J.G., et al., Fundamentals of Wound Management in Surgery: Technical Factors in Wound Management. Chirurgecom, Inc., South Plainfield, New Jersey, 1977.
29. Elek, S.D., Conen, P.E., The virulence of Staphylococcus pyogenes for man: Study of the problems of wound infection. Br. J. Exp. Pathol. 38:573, 1957.
29a. Emerson, E.B., Fishhooks. N.Y. State J. Med. 66:2414, 1966.
30. Entin, M.A., Infections of the hand. Surg. Clin. North Am. 44:981, 1964.
31. Evans, A.J., Experience of the burns unit: A review of 520 cases. Br. Med. J. 8:547, 1956.
32. Farrell, R.G., Disher, W.A., Nesland, R.S., et al., Conservative management of fingertip amputations. J.A.C.E.P. 6:243, 1977.
33. Fisher, R.H., The Kutler method of repair of finger-tip amputations. J. Bone Joint Surg. 48:606, 1966.
34. Gant, T., A suturing refresher for family doctors. Patient Care. 13:34, 1979.
34a. Gross, C.W., Soft tissue injuries of the lip, nose, ears, and preauricular area. Otolaryngol. Clin. North Am. 2:292, 1969.
35. Hampton, O.P., The indications for debridement of gun shot (bullet) wounds of the extremities in civilian practice. J. Trauma 1:368, 1961.
36. Hanley, P.H., Acute pilonidal abscess. Surg. Gynecol. Obstet. 50:9, 1980.

37. Hoehn, R.J., Agents, mechanisms, and incidence of facial injury. Surg. Clin. North Am. 53:1479, 1973.

38. Holm, A., Zachariae, L., Fingertip lesions: An evaluation of conservative treatment versus free skin grafting. Acta Orthop. Scand. 45:382, 1974.

39. Hoover, N.W., Ivins, J.C., Wound debridement. Arch. Surg. 79:701, 1959.

40. Howes, E.L., A renaissance of suture technique needed. Ann. Surg. 48:548, 1940.

41. Huang, T.T., Lynch, J.B., Larson, D.L., et al., The use of excisional therapy in the management of snakebite. Ann. Surg. 179:598, 1974.

42. Hunt, T.K., Fundamentals of Wound Management in Surgery. Wound Healing: Disorders of Repair. Chirurgecom, Inc., South Plainfield, New Jersey, 1976.

43. Hunt, T.K., Fundamentals of Wound Management in Surgery. Wound Healing: Normal Repair. Chirurgecom, Inc., South Plainfield, New Jersey, 1976.

43a. James, R.C., MacLeod, C.J., Induction of staphylococcal infections in mice with small inocula introduced on sutures. Br. J. Exp. Pathol. 42:266, 1961.

44. Jamra, F.N.A., Khuri, S., The treatment of fingertip injuries, J. Trauma 11:749, 1970.

45. Jelenko, C., McKinley, J.C., Post-burn respiratory injury. J.A.C.E.P. 5:455, 1976.

46. Jones, L.T., An anatomical approach to problems of the eyelids and lacrimal apparatus. Arch. Ophthalmol. 66:137, 1961.

47. Ketchum, L.D., Cohen, I.K., Masters, F.W., Hypertrophic scars and keloids: A collective review. Plast. Reconstr. Surg. 53:140, 1974.

47a. Kilgore, E.S., Graham, W.P., The Hand. Lea & Febriger, Philadelphia, 1977.

48. Kim, Y.-S., A new surgical suture technique. Surg. Gynecol. Obstet. 137:669, 1973.

49. Kraissl, C.J., The selection of appropriate lines for elective surgical incisions. Plast. Reconstr. Surg. 8:1, 1951.

50. Larsen, J.S., Ulin, A.W., Tensile strength advantage of the far-and-near suture technique. Surg. Gynecol. Obstet. 131:123, 1970.

51. Leidelmeyer, R., The embedded broken-off needle. J.A.C.E.P. 5:362, 1976.

52. Lewis, J.R., Management of soft tissue injuries of the face. J. Int. Coll. Surg. 44:441, 1965.

52a. Liston, S.L., Cortez, E.A., McNabney, W.K., External ear injuries. JACEP 7:233, 1978.

53. Localio, S.A., Casale, W., Hinton, J.W., Wound healing: Experimental and statistical study. Surg. Gynecol. Obstet. 77:481, 1943.

53a. Lucid, M.L., The interlocking slip knot. Plast. Reconstr. Surg. 34:200, 1964.

54. Lynch, G., Minor surgery of the ear, nose and throat. Surg. Clin. North Am. 31:1315, 1951.

55. Lyons, C., Upchurch, S.E., The management of common superficial wounds, Surg. Clin. North Am. 31:1271, 1951.

56. Macomber, D.W., Lacerations and incisions: Technical considerations. Am. J. Surg. 26:145, 1960.

57. Madden, J.C., Edlich, R.D., Schauerhamer, R., et al., Application of principles of fluid dynamics to surgical wound irrigation. Curr. Top. Surg. Res. 3:85, 1971.

58. Meislin, H.W., Lerner, S.A., Graves, M.H., et al., Anaerobic and aerobic bacteriology and outpatient management. Ann. Intern. Med. 87:145, 1977.

59. Minsky, H., Surgical repair of recent lid lacerations. Surg. Gynecol. Obstet. 75:449, 1942.

60. Myers, M.B., Functional and angiographic vasculature in healing wounds. Am. J. Surg. 36:750, 1970.

61. Price, P.B., Stress, strain and sutures. Ann. Surg. 128:408, 1948.

62. Pryor, G.T., Local anesthesia in minor lacerations: Topical TAC vs. lidocaine infiltration. Ann. Emerg. Med. 9(11):568, 1980.

63. Quinby, W.C., Restrictive effects of thoracic burns in children. J. Trauma 12:646, 1972.

63a. Noe, J.M., Gloth, D.A., A technique for the placement of a continuous suture. Surg. Gynecol. Obstet. 150:404, 1980.

64. Raffman, R.A., A re-evaluation of the pathogenesis of pilonidal sinus. Ann. Surg. 150:895, 1959.

65. Robson, M.C., Lea, C.E., Dalton, J.B., et al., Quantitative bacteriology and delayed wound closure. S. Forum 19:501, 1968.

66. Rodeheaver, G.T., Pettry, D., Thacker, J.G., et al., Wound cleansing by high pressure irrigation. Surg. Gynecol. Obstet. 141:357, 1975.

67. Rodeheaver, G.T., Pluronic F-68: A promising new skin cleanser. Ann. Emerg. Med. 9:572, 1980.

68. Roettinger, W., Edgerton, M.T., Kurtz, L.D., et al., Role of inoculation site as a determinant of infection in soft tissue wounds. Am. J. Surg. 126:354, 1973.

69. Rubin, L.R., Langers lines and facial scars. Plast. Reconstr. Surg. 3:147, 1948.

69a. Salisbury, R.E., Taylor, J.W., Levine, N.S., Evaluation of digital escharotomy in burned hands. Plast. Reconstr. Surg. 58:440, 1976.

70. Seropian, R., Reynolds, B.M., Wound infections after preoperative depilatory versus razor preparation. Am. J. Surg. 121:251, 1971.

71. Straith, R.E., Lawson, J.M., Hipps, C.J., The subcuticular suture. Postgrad. Med. 29:164, 1961.

72. Spira, M., Gerow, F.J., Hardy, S.B., Windshield injuries of the face. J. Trauma 8:513, 1968.

72a. Spira, Hardy, S.B., Management of the injured ear. Am. J. Surg. 106:678, 1963.

73. Tejani, F., Aufses, A.H., A new technique for skin closure. Surg. Gynecol. Obstet. 142:407, 1976.

74. Van Winkle, W., Jr., Hastings, J.C., Consideration in the choice of suture materials for various tissues. Surg. Gynecol. Obstet. 135:113, 1972.

75. Walike, J.W., Suturing technique in facial soft tissue injuries. Otolaryngol. Clin. North Am. 12:415, 1979.

76. Wallace, A.B., Assessment and emergency treatment of burns. Br. Med. J. 2:1136, 1955.

77. Williams, D.F., The reactions of tissues to materials. Biomed. Engl. 6:152, 1971.

Bibliography

1. Ariyan, S., A simple stereotactic method to isolate

and remove foreign bodies. Arch. Surg. 112:857, 1977.

2. Beasley, R.W., Reconstruction of amputated fingertips. Plast. Reconstr. Surg. 44:349, 1969.

3. Bennett, J.E., Thompson, L.W., The role of aggressive surgical treatment in the severely burned patient. J. Trauma 9:776, 1969.

4. Berger, R.S., A critical look at therapy for the brown recluse spider bite. Arch. Derm. 107:298, 1973.

5. Burke, J.F., Bondoc, C.C., A method of secondary closure of heavily contaminated wounds providing "physiologic primary closure." J. Trauma 8:228, 1968.

6. Dupertuis, S.M., Musgrave, R.H., Burns of the hand.

7. Dziemian, A.J., Mendelson, J.A., Lindsey, D., Comparison of the wounding characteristics of some commonly encountered bullets. J. Trauma 1:341, 1961.

8. Edlich, R.F., Rodeheaver, G., Kuphal, J., et al., Technique of closure: Contaminated wounds. J.A.C.E.P. 2:375, 1974.

9. Fardon, D.W., Wingo, C.W., Robinson, D.W., et al., The treatment of brown spider bites. Plast. Reconstr. Surg. 40:482, 1967.

10. Forrest, J.F., An improved technique for delayed primary closure of potentially infected lesions. Surg. Gynecol. Obstet. 149:401, 1979.

11. Fryer, M.P., Brown, J.B., Bin, J.W., Repair of trauma about the orbit. J. Trauma 12:290, 1972.

12. Glass, T.G., Early debridement in pit viper bites. J.A.M.A. 235:2513, 1976.

13. Hanley, P.H., Acute pilonidal abscess. Surg. Gynecol. Obstet. 150:9, 1980.

14. Kleinert, H.E., Fingertip injuries and their management. Plast. Reconstr. Surg. 25:41, 1959.

15. Lehr, H.B., Fitts, W.T., The management of avulsion injuries of soft tissue. J. Trauma 9:261, 1969.

16. Mawr, B., The healing of wounds. Surg. Clin. North Am. 20:1859, 1940.

17. Morgan, M.M., Spencer, A.D., Hershey, F.B., Debridement of civilian gunshot wounds of soft tissue. J. Trauma 1:354, 1961.

18. Paradies, L.H., Gregory, C.F., The early treatment of close-range shotgun wounds to the extremities. J. Bone Joint Surg. 48A:425, 1966.

19. Peloso, O.A., Wilkinson, L.H., The chain stitch knot. Surg. Gynecol. Obstet. 139:599, 1974.

20. Richards, K.E., Feller, I., Grid escharotomy for debriding burns. Surg. Gynecol. Obstet. 137:843, 1973.

21. Russell, F.E., Carlson, R.W., Wainschel, J., et al.,Snake venom poisoning in the United States. J.A.M.A. 233:341, 1975.

22. Scatliff, J.H., Camnitz, P.S., Partain, C.L., Claw hammer technique for extraction of knives. J. Trauma 18:742, 1978.

23. Scott, J.E., Amputation of the finger. Br. J. Surg. 61:574, 1974.

24. Sherman, R.T., Parrish, R.A., Management of shotgun injuries: A review of 152 cases. J. Trauma 3:76, 1963.

25. Snyder, C.C., Straight, R., Glenn, J., The snake-bitten hand. Plast. Reconstr. Surg. 49:275, 1972.

26. Stevenson, T.R., Thacker, J.G., Rodeheaver, G.T., et al., Cleansing the traumatic wound by high pressure syringe irrigation. J.A.C.E.P. 5:17, 1976.

27. Tabor, G.L., Trauma to eye and orbit. J. Trauma 8:1089, 1968.

28. Tanner, J.C., Vandeput, J., Olley, J.F., The mesh skin graft. Plast. Reconstr. Surg. 34:287, 1964.

29. Trevaskis, A.E., Rempel, J., Okunski, W., et al, Sliding subcutaneous-pedicle flaps to close a circular defect. Plast. Reconstr. Surg. 46:155, 1970.

30. Wee, G.C., Shieber, W., Painless evacuation of subungual hematoma. Surg. Gynecol. Obstet. 131:531, 1970.

31. Ziperman, H.H., The management of soft tissue missile wounds in war and peace. J. Trauma 1:361, 1961.

Urological Procedures 10

BLADDER CATHETERIZATION

Many types of catheters exist which are used to catheterize the bladder including Foley catheters, coudé-tip Foley catheters, filiform, and follower catheters.

Indications

1. The relief of acute urinary retention.
2. Monitoring of urinary output in a critically ill or injured patient.
3. To obtain urine for diagnostic purposes.
4. Patients with either a neurogenic or a mechanical inability to void.

Contraindications

1. Suspicion of urethral injury. A number of signs indicate the possibility of urethral injury.
   a. Prostatic displacement on rectal examination.
   b. Perineal hematoma.
   c. Blood present at the urethral meatus.

NOTE

A number of relative contraindications exist for bladder catheterization in patients who have sustained trauma. In these patients, catheterization may be attempted; if obstruction is encountered, an alternative approach (suprapubic catheterization) should be attempted or a radiographic study of the distal urinary tract to ascertain patency of the urethra should be done. These include the patient who has sustained a severe fracture of the pelvis, particularly a straddle fracture, and trauma patients who have the desire to void but are unable.

Equipment

Most of the equipment necessary for a catheterization is contained in commercially available sets.

Drapes
Sterile lubricant
Catheter—for the average adult a 16

French* Foley catheter is used, and for the child an 8 to 10 French Foley is used.
Cotton balls
Iodinated (Betadine®) solution
Sterile disposable gloves
Syringe (10 cc) and saline for inflating balloon

MALE CATHETERIZATION

Technique

Preparatory Steps

1. Lay all of the needed materials on a sterile field.
2. Check the Foley catheter balloon for leaks.
3. Spread a sterile towel below the urethra.

Procedural Steps

1. Immobilize the penis with the non-dominant hand and retract the foreskin.
2. With the dominant hand, cleanse the glans penis with cotton balls dipped in Betadine® solution.
3. Lubricate the catheter tip.
4. Insert the catheter gently into the urethra (Fig. 10.1). An area of resistance is encountered as the catheter passes the prostate and into the membranous urethra. Gentle rotation of the catheter usually permits passage beyond this point with no difficulty. Elevating the penis and retracting it superiorly may further aid in passage of the catheter. Pass the catheter well into the bladder.

NOTE

A 16 French catheter used in the average adult is selected because a larger catheter may obstruct urethral exudates from draining properly and lead to urethritis. In some patients in which catheterization may be difficult, a larger catheter may be used and not uncommonly can be passed, even though a smaller one cannot, because

---

* One French is equal to 1 mm circumference.

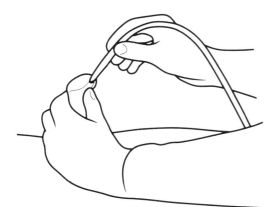

Figure 10.1. A Foley catheter is inserted into the urethra by the right hand as the penis is held firmly in position with the left hand. See text for details.

it is stiffer. A mandarin guide can be inserted inside the catheter and bent into the desired shape. The catheter is then inserted as though it were a urethral sound with digital pressure over the perineal region (Fig. 10.2) to aid in advancing the catheter through the posterior urethra.

5. Inflate the catheter balloon with 5 ml of saline.
6. Pull the catheter gently forward and connect it to a sterile closed drainage system.
7. Secure the catheter to the penis with two strips of tape opposite one another, extending from the sides of the catheter to the penis (6A). An encircling strip of tape is then placed around the catheter at the point where the catheter enters the penis. This prevents forward and backward displacement of the catheter into and out of the urethra; this displacement introduces bacterial contaminants and causes cystitis. Figure 10.3 shows a method for securing a catheter to the penis.

FEMALE CATHETERIZATION

Technique

Preparatory Steps

1. The female should be placed in the dorsolithotomy position.

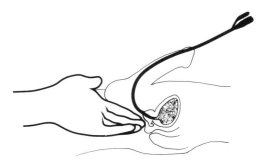

Figure 10.2. A mandarin guide may be inserted inside the Foley catheter and bent into the desired shape. This stiffens the catheter and the catheter may then be inserted as a urethral sound with perineal digital pressure applied which aids in advancing the catheter through the posterior urethra. (The mandarin guide is not shown in the diagram above.)

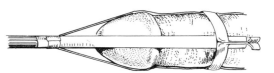

Figure 10.3. A method for securing a catheter to the penis.

2. The left hand is used to spread the labia apart to reveal the urethral orifice, above the introitus and just inferior to the clitoris.
3. The urethral meatus is identified and cleansed with cotton balls dipped in Betadine® solution, using a single wipe directed from anterior to posterior. The cotton balls are then discarded.

Procedural Steps

1. Lubricate the tip of the catheter, and with the thumb and the index finger hold the catheter 1 to 2 inches from the tip and insert it into the meatal orifice.
2. After the bladder has been entered as indicated by urine flow through the catheter, the balloon is inflated with 5 ml of saline.

CAUTION!

If the catheter inadvertently enters the vagina, a new catheter must be used to prevent vaginal contaminants from entering the bladder and causing cystitis.

3. The catheter is then securely taped to the patient's thigh.
4. After inserting the Foley catheter, the hands must be washed as these catheters are a major source of nosocomial infections. Also wash the hands after any urine sample is removed from the drainage bag or catheter (6b).

Complications

1. Urethritis. Urethritis is a common complication following catheterization, particularly in a patient with strictures or prostatic enlargement.
2. Epididymitis. This is an uncommon problem following catheterization; however, it may be encountered in a patient who has cystitis or urethritis before catheterization.
3. Bacteremia.
4. Trauma to the urethra, leading to urethral strictures.
5. Conversion of a partial urethral tear to a complete one in a traumatized patient.
6. Hemorrhage from urethral trauma during catheter insertion.
7. Creation of a false passage by inserting the catheter alongside the urethra.
8. Cystitis and pyelonephritis. Infectious complications may be unavoidable with prolonged catheterizations. Many complications may be avoided by the use of sterile technique during insertion in the emergency center. The urinary drainage should remain as a closed system with removal of urine from the bag or sterilely from connecting tubing with a needle and syringe (2a, 4a). The urine in the collecting bag should *never* be elevated and permitted to drain retrograde into the bladder.

SUPRAPUBIC CATHETERIZATION AND ASPIRATION

Suprapubic catheterization is an easy and reliable method of both obtaining urine for diagnostic procedures and draining the urinary bladder in patients in whom Foley catheterization cannot be performed. Urine may be obtained from the bladder for diagnostic purposes by simple needle aspiration, particularly in the pediatric age-group.

Indications

1. For diagnostic purposes in the pediatric age-group, when a clean catch urine is unobtainable or contamination exists.
2. To relieve urinary obstruction when one is unable to pass a urethral catheter in a patient with acute urinary retention.

Contraindications

1. A bladder which is small or nonpalpable.
2. Scars from previous lower abdominal surgery.

Suprapubic Aspiration

Equipment

22 gauge 1½ inch needle for children or a 20 gauge needle for adults
10 ml syringe
Prep solution
Anesthetic with 1% Xylocaine® with epinephrine
25 gauge needle
3 ml syringe.

Technique

Percuss the abdomen to determine the level of the bladder. Suprapubic aspiration of the bladder should not be done unless the bladder is at least partially filled with urine. This may be determined by palpation, percussion, or by the physician pressing with his fingers above the pubic symphysis and checking if this gives the patient the desire to void. The suprapubic region should be prepped and shaved. A needle (as indicated above) should be attached to the syringe and inserted in the midline approximately 2 cm above the symphysis of the pubis. The needle should be directed at an angle of approximately 45 to 60 degrees to the skin and aimed caudally. A "pop" can be felt when the bladder is entered. The urine is then aspirated and sent for analysis.

Suprapubic Catheterization
Equipment

In addition to the equipment listed above—Commercially prepared suprapubic catheters or a 14 gauge Intracath® can be used.
Closed drainage bag.

Technique (2, 3, 5, 6)

1. Percuss the abdomen to determine the level of the bladder as indicated above under suprapubic aspiration.

NOTE

One should not attempt to catheterize the bladder if it is not at least partially filled with urine.

2. Shave and prep the lower abdomen.
3. Using either a 14 gauge Intracath® or a commercially available suprapubic catheter, insert the needle attached to a syringe approximately 2 cm above the pubis in the midline at an angle of approximately 45 degrees to the skin and direct the needle caudad until the bladder is entered.
4. Introduce the catheter through the needle into the bladder (Fig. 10.4).
5. Withdraw the needle and suture the catheter to the skin of the abdomen and connect it to a sterile collecting system.

Complications

1. Leakage around the catheter (3, 6).
2. Kinking of the catheter or suprapubic tube (3).
3. Hematuria induced by the catheter or tube irritating the bladder.
4. Bowel puncture (6).

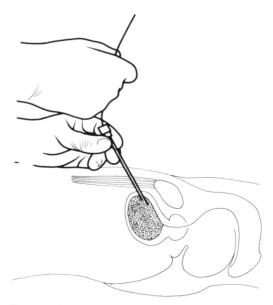

Figure 10.4. The technique of suprapubic catheterization. See text for discussion.

5. Puncture of a large vessel (6).
6. Anterior abdominal wall abscess following suprapubic aspiration (6). In the cases reported, the needle was inserted into dehydrated patients in the midline about 1 cm above the suprapubic skin crease and perpendicular to the anterior abdominal wall. The needle was advanced 2.5 cm and the syringe plunger withdrawn, and intestinal contents were aspirated.
7. The tip of the plastic catheter may be voided through the urethra (3).

NOTE

Some authors state that suprapubic tube cystostomy can be performed in patients with a ruptured bladder (2). Most feel, however, that it should not be done in patients with small or shrunken bladders or in patients with infected urine (5). When one does suspect a bladder rupture, instill about 250 ml of opaque contrast media through a patent urethra and into the bladder to perform a cystogram. Be certain rupture has not occurred (1).

CATHETERIZATION OF THE INFANT

The urethra of the female infant is C-shaped (7). The incidence of bacteremia following catheterization is remarkably high (8), approaching 30% of cases. A disposable, polyethylene, urine-collecting bag is commercially available; this bag is conical-shaped and fits well between the legs of male and of female infants (4). The collecting bag has adhesive on the sides, which stick well to the baby. This bag can be applied and removed from the child with little discomfort (4).

URETHRAL SOUNDING

Urethral sounding may be necessary in a patient who has prostatic obstruction and urinary retention and in whom one is unable to bypass the obstruction with a Foley catheter. A sound is a firm "j-shaped" instrument which is used to facilitate passage into the bladder.

Indications

Patients with prostatic obstruction in whom one is unable to insert a Foley catheter.

Equipment

Urethral sounds in assortment of sizes, 18 French and larger.

Technique

1. The penis should be held in a manner similar to that used for urethral catheterization.
2. The glans should be cleansed with cotton balls impregnated with Betadine® solution.
3. Select the size of the sound desired. One should never use a smaller sound than an 18 French in the adult male. When an 18 French sound or larger cannot be passed through the urethra, then a filiform and follower catheter should be used as this is a safer technique in bypassing an obstruction.
4. Lubricate the sound.
5. Instill a topical anesthetic through the penis and use a penile clamp to aid in retaining the anesthetic gel for several minutes before the procedure.
6. While the penis is stabilized with the left hand, the tip of the sound is advanced into the meatus with the sound held parallel to the patient's abdomen. The sound is introduced through the meatus of the penis with the handle of the sound positioned over the left iliac crest to facilitate passage (Fig. 10.5A).
7. Advance the sound into the urethra as the penis is drawn over the instrument (Fig. 10.5B). Resistance is often encountered by the sound at the bulbomembranous junction. The sound is maneuvered gently to the horizontal position to facilitate advancement through the external sphincter and vesicle neck. Digital pressure may assist in passage at this point (Fig. 10.5C). As the sound is passed toward the prostate, the handle should be depressed so the instrument can be advanced smoothly (Fig. 10.5D). In this manner the tip of the sound easily follows the curve of the posterior urethra. No force should ever be used in passing the sound or the urethra may be injured. One may aid in the passage of the sound by applying downward pressure over the root of the penis as it passes the posterior urethra to relax the penile suspensory ligaments.

CATHETERIZATION WITH A FILIFORM AND FOLLOWER

In a patient with severe urethral strictures, a filiform and follower catheter or sound may have to be inserted through the urethral meatus. The filiforms come in various sizes, as do the follower catheters. The follower catheter has a special tip which should be screwed into the filiform after the latter is passed into the bladder.

Equipment

Several filiforms, sizes 4, 5, and 6 French, with follower catheters, some with

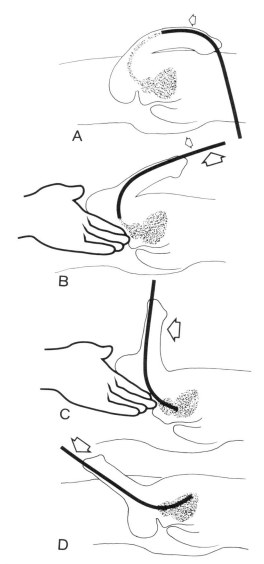

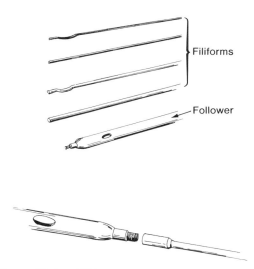

Figure 10.6. Filiforms come in many sizes. A follower catheter may be screwed into the base of a filiform catheter which has been previously inserted into the bladder.

Figure 10.5. Urethral sounding technique. *A.* While the penis is held with the left hand, the tip of the urethral sound is inserted into the meatus. The handle of the sound should be held over the left iliac crest to facilitate passage. *B.* The sound is advanced into the urethra by drawing the penis up over the instrument. The sound is maneuvered to the midline vertical position and advanced to the level of the urethral bulb. *C.* Resistance is encountered by the sound at the bulbomembranous junction. The sound is maneuvered gently to facilitate passage of the point. Digital pressure often assists in passing

curves and some without. The follower screws onto the filiform catheter as shown in Figure 10.6. Once the filiform is inserted into the bladder, the follower catheter can easily be advanced. If resistance is encountered, a sound may be attached to the filiform and passed through the penis prior to passage of the catheter.

Technique

1. Prep and drape the penis as for catheterization. The steps indicated below should be done under strict aseptic technique.
2. Pass one filiform until an obstruction is encountered. Do not attempt to force the filiform past the obstruction (Fig. 10.7A).
3. With the first filiform left in place, pass subsequent filiforms into the urethral meatus until obstruction is encountered. One of the subsequent

the sound. *D.* The handle of the sound is depressed slowly. The tip of the sound is advanced more easily over the curve of the posterior urethra. The sound is then advanced through the bladder neck.

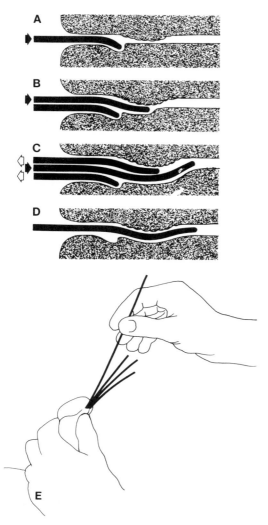

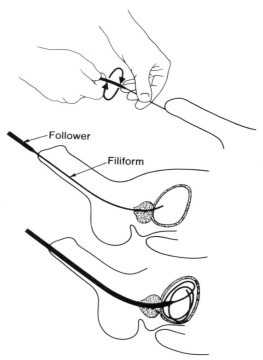

Figure 10.8. The follower catheter is screwed onto the filiform, and the catheter is advanced into the bladder. The filiform functions as a guide for the advancement of the follower catheter. The filiform remains coiled within the bladder during the time of drainage.

Figure 10.7. The insertion of urethral filiforms. Multiple filiforms are often required to bypass a stricture. Several filiforms are inserted, which obliterate the *closed* passages. The filiforms are inserted only to the point where obstruction is met (A and B). More filiforms are then inserted until the strictured segment is bypassed (C). The filiform which enters the bladder is then stabilized and the remaining filiforms are removed (D and E).

filiforms will bypass the point of obstruction on the first passage and enter the bladder (Fig. 10.7B and C).

4. Remove all superfluous filiform catheters, leaving the filiform which has entered the bladder in place (Fig. 10.7D).

5. A follower catheter is then connected to the filiform and this can be passed into the bladder (Fig. 10.8).

If one cannot pass the follower, then a LaForte sound can then be connected to the filiform, and the filiform and sound are passed together into the penis, using the same technique as for passing the sound as indicated above. The index finger placed in the rectum can be used to guide the sound into place.

References

1. Charron, J. W., Brault, J.-P., Recognition and early management of injuries to the urinary tract. J. Trauma 4:702, 1964.

2. Clark, S.S., Prudencio, R.F., Lower urinary tract injuries associated with pelvic fractures. Surg. Clin. North Am. 52:183, 1972.

2a. Finkelberg, Z., Kunin, C.M., Clinical evaluation of closed urinary drainage systems. J.A.M.A. 207:1657, 1969.

3. Hale, R.W., McCorriston, C.C., Suprapubic cystotomy with a polyethylene tube. Am. J. Obstet. Gynecol. 105:1181, 1969.

4. Hill, E.J., New method for collecting urine samples in infants. Plast. Reconstr. Surg. 22:567, 1958.

4a. Kunin, C.M., McCormack, R.C., Prevention of catheter-induced urinary tract infections by sterile closed drainage. N. Engl. J. Med. 274:1155, 1966.

5. Nystrom, K., Bjerle, P., Lindqvist, B., Suprapubic catheterization of the urinary bladder as a diagnostic procedure. Scand. J. Urol. Nephrol. 7:160, 1973.

6. Polnay, L., Fraser, A.M., Lewis, J.M., Complication of suprapubic bladder aspiration. Arch. Dis. Child. 50:80, 1975.

6a. Reinarz, J.A., Nosocomial Infections. Ciba Clinical Symposia. Vol. 30, p. 6, 1978.

6b. Steere, A., Mallison, G.F., Handwashing practice for the prevention of nosocomial infections. Ann. Intern. Med. 83:683, 1975.

7. Storts, B.P., Equipment for catheterization of female infants. Pediatrics 23:149, 1959.

8. Sullivan, N.M., Sutter, V.L., Mims, M.M., et al., Clinical aspects of bacteremia after manipulation of the genitourinary tract. J. Infect. Dis. 127:49, 1973.

Vascular Procedures

11

BASIC PRINCIPLES IN INTRAVENOUS CANNULATION

The establishment of a "lifeline" is one of the essential procedures at which an emergency physician must be as skilled as any expert practitioner. In the ensuing discussion a didactic presentation of the various types of intravenous catheters, sites of insertion and complications will be presented.

Intravenous cannulation is a means of access to the venous circulation and is useful for the administration of fluids or drugs as well as for obtaining samples of blood for laboratory evaluation. One can insert a cannula into either the peripheral system or the central system. Catheters may be inserted centrally either through a long peripheral line or through a separate site in one of the larger central veins.

Intravenous Cannulas—General Features and Complications

There are three types of cannulas available for use: hollow needles ("butterfly-type"), over-the-needle catheters (plastic catheters inserted over a hollow needle, e.g., Angiocath®), and through-the-needle catheters (indwelling plastic catheters inserted through a hollow needle (Intracath®). Plastic catheters are more commonly used for intravenous therapy than are hollow needles, since these catheters can be better secured and are less easily displaced than "butterfly catheters." Butterfly catheters are more commonly used in infants and children.

Over-the-needle catheters are available in Teflon and polyethylene and in sizes ranging from 14 to 20 gauge. The needle and catheter are inserted together; then the needle is removed, leaving the catheter in the vein. This technique prevents catheter embolism and puncture of the back wall of the vein. Through-the-needle catheters are made of the same materials. The needle must be larger than the catheter, necessitating a large needle which may make insertion difficult. Catheter embolism is a risk with through-the-needle catheters.

STIFFNESS AND THROMBOGENICITY

When comparing catheters, two properties must be mentioned: stiffness and thrombogenicity. The *stiffer* the catheter, the higher is the incidence of intimal trauma and subsequent phlebitis (24). In addition, perforation of the vein during either insertion or subsequent displacement is another hazard of a stiff catheter. The Medi-Cath Silastic catheter (over-the-needle catheter) is flexible and virtually eliminates the risk of vessel perforation and decreases the risk of intimal damage (24). *Plastic catheters initiate thrombus formation.* A fibrin layer is seen over the site of contact of the plastic with the vessel. This fibrin, in general, is not thrombogenic; the clot begins at areas of intimal contact and injury and propagates circumferentially along the catheter (24). Hoshal et al. (76) demonstrated that fibrin sleeves are present around both polyethylene and Teflon subclavian catheters. In a study by Formanek et al. (60), Teflon catheters were about twice as thrombogenic as were polyethylene or siliconized polyethylene arterial catheters.

INFUSION RATES

The amount of fluid or blood one may infuse per unit time is directly related to the diameter of the catheter and its length. Obviously, the greater the diameter the faster one can infuse a solution. The reverse is true when one considers length: the shorter the length of a catheter, the faster one can infuse a solution. Reports indicate that the time required for 500 cc of whole blood to be infused through an 18 gauge 1½ inch catheter is 15 minutes (131). When the catheter size is increased to a 12 gauge, it requires only 4 minutes. One should select as short and as large a bore catheter as possible for most urgent uses. Blood should be passed only through a catheter which is 18 gauge or larger, preferably a 14 or 16 gauge. For cannulation of a peripheral vein, a needle and catheter length of 5 cm is adequate. In central vein cannulations, a length of 8 cm is preferred.

CATHETER SHEARING

Other problems with catheters include catheter shearing. Catheter shearing occurs with the use of through-the-needle catheters when the catheter is pulled back after being advanced through the needle. The sharp point of the needle may shear off a piece of catheter, which may remain in the skin or may act as an embolus. This is eliminated by the use of over-the-needle catheters (Argyle Medicut Cannula® and Deseret EZ Cath®). Shearing also has been reduced by adding a device which retards catheter withdrawal in a through-the-needle unit (24).

AIR EMBOLISM

The possibility of air embolism is reduced by using a closed vacuum system (Medi-Cath, Intrafusor, Intracath using a closed technique). If a catheter is left open, air embolism is possible with any catheter design.

PHLEBITIS AND CELLULITIS

Contamination of the catheter is reduced by preventing contact with the skin as the catheter is threaded into the vein (through-the-needle catheters) or by preventing exposure of the catheter in a closed system. Intimal trauma is a source of phlebitis and is decreased by use of a soft, pliable catheter (Medi-Cath) (24).

Phlebitis may be difficult to prevent. One should remove a catheter at 48 hours to prevent phlebitis (36, 77). Catheter infection may be as high as 50% at 3 days and increases with time (21). The more prolonged the cannulation, the greater is the risk of sepsis; thus, it is important that the emergency nurse place the data of catheter insertion (gauge of needle, date of insertion) on the tubing for subsequent reference (138). Sometimes there are no clinical signs of inflammation present at the catheter site despite the presence of infection (18). Venous microabscesses have been shown to develop in septic phlebitis (16). In catheter-associated sepsis where the catheter was in place for 5 days, the chief organism cultured was *Staphylococcus aureus* (18). Survival after catheter-induced sepsis is influenced by the time of removal of the catheter (18). It has been shown that colonization of the plastic cannula occurs within 48 hours, phlebitis in 48 to 96 hours, and septicemia in greater than 96 hours (18).

Prevention and Treatment

One should date the catheter upon insertion. A dressing should be placed with an antibacterial ointment over the cannula, and the puncture site should be treated as any wound (138). In one study it was shown that phlebitis could be prevented by the use of 1 mg% of hydrocortisone cream over the insertion site (108). The use of topical antibiotics prolongs the time one may use an intravenous cutdown site to 4 days and may decrease infection and the number of pathogens cultured in all intravenous catheter sites. Phlebitis, however, is unaffected by the use of topical antibiotics (159). Seventy percent of intravenous cannulas associated with sepsis were placed in the emergency department and remained in place for greater than 4 days; thus, removal of plastic intravenous cannulas at 48 hours is advised (16).

SEPSIS

The majority of catheter-associated infections are due to skin flora entering the wound due to insertion of a cannula using nonsterile technique (78, 98). The primary disadvantage of the percutaneous technique of catheterization is the possibility of contaminating the catheter. Catheter contamination is primarily a function of breakdown in sterile technique, which, in turn, is a function of the experience of the operator. In patients who developed sepsis from intravenous catheters, it was found in one study in which house physicians placed only 10% of the intravenous catheters that these cannulas resulted in 90% of the infections (18). Infection at the catheter site and subsequent septic phlebitis are characterized by tenderness at the puncture site and proximal, erythema which takes a linear course along the tract of the vein and lymphadenitis with proximal adenopathy. In more advanced cases the tenderness may be noted along the length of the vein for large distances from the puncture site.

The clot that forms around the cannula tip may trap organisms and lead to sepsis (98). Septic emboli occur twice as often with intravenous catheters as compared to intravenous drug abuse. Aspiration of the vein, culture, and a Gram stain of any purulent material is helpful in identifying the organism (18).

Prevention and Treatment

Use of sterile technique is mandatory. Heat, elevation, and antibiotics should be started when septic phlebitis develops in an extremity. Oxacillin and gentamicin for staphylococcus and gram-negative organisms is advised for the first 24 hours; if no response is noted, excision of the vein and drainage of any abscess is indicated (13).

THROMBOSIS AND PULMONARY THROMBOEMBOLISM (PT)

In a double-blind controlled study of 151 patients, the addition of 1000 units of beef-lung heparin to each litre of intravenous fluid reduced the frequency of thrombophlebitis at the infusion site (42). This will not increase the prothrombin time when "keep-open" rates are used for intravenous infusion; however, if administered quickly it will prolong coagulation. In 34 patients, 5% dextrose in water containing heparin (1 u/ml) was infused for a total of 2243 hours (mean 66 hours/patient) with local inflammation necessitating a change in catheter location occurring on only three occasions. In 30 patients receiving the same solution but without heparin, infused for a total of 2659 hours (mean 88 hours/patient), 20 changes in catheter location were required.

Prevention and Treatment

It is recommended that for catheters which must remain in place for prolonged periods of time, heparin (1 u/ml) should be given.

CATHETER FRAGMENT EMBOLISM

Intravascular embolization of polyethylene catheter fragments is a significant problem, the majority caused by intravenous indwelling catheters (58).

Prevention and Treatment

One must be careful in the use of through-the-needle catheters. If one is to remove the catheter after an unsuccessful attempt, the catheter and needle should be removed together as a single unit. Sixty-nine nonsurgical retrievals of embolized fragments have been reported and a number of techniques have been used (58). The most commonly used technique is a loop snare, in which a guide wire-like device, folded in half at its midsection, is inserted through a catheter to snare the fragment. Hooked catheters, helical baskets and Fogarty catheters also have been used for retrieval of an embolized fragment (58).

HEMATOMA FORMATION

Hematoma formation is due to either unsuccessful cannulation in which pressure was not applied over the site for an adequate period of time or puncture of both the anterior and posterior walls of the vein with the needle. One should use an oblique angle when advancing the needle into a vein to minimize puncturing the posterior wall of the vein. When hematoma occurs, the needle should be removed and pressure applied over the site. Alternately, the needle may be left in the vein and a more proximal site selected, after which the original needle is removed and pressure is applied. This method permits one to use the same arm after an unsuccessful attempt without having to go to the opposite extremity.

INFILTRATION

This occurs when the cannula is not in the vein. When this occurs, one should remove the cannula and apply a pressure over the site. Alternately the needle can be left in place and a proximal site used, after which the first needle is removed.

INJURY TO NEARBY NERVES

The median nerve at the elbow may be injured with cannulation of a medial antecubital vein. Other nerve injuries are reported but are quite uncommon. The superficial radial nerve, a sensory nerve, may be injured by cannulation of the superficial radial vein. One can avoid injury to the median nerve by avoiding deep penetration when attempting to enter the vein.

Peripheral Intravenous Techniques

Various techniques are common to all the procedures whether in the upper or lower extremity veins; the differences are only with the type of catheter used. Veins in the legs should not be used except under urgent circumstances as the risk of provoking thromboembolic complications is significant.

PERIPHERAL VEINS OF THE UPPER EXTREMITY

The dorsum of the hand is a good site to find a vein for cannulation as there are a number of veins arising from the digital veins, which are interconnected forming a dorsal plexus. There are several sites along the forearm which can be used, probably the best of which is the branch of the cephalic vein called the superficial radial vein. This vein courses laterally and joins the median cephalic vein to form the cephalic vein proper in the antecubital space (Fig. 11.1). Four sites can be searched for in the patient in whom it is difficult to locate a vein. These include the ulnar veins, superficial radial vein, median basilic vein and median cephalic vein. These veins are large and relatively constant. They are shown in Figure 11.1. In the obese patient in whom veins may not be visible,

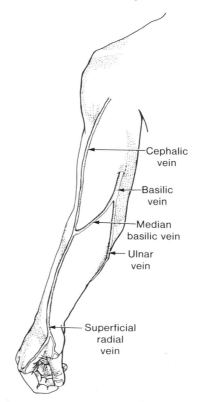

Figure 11.1. Peripheral veins of the upper extremity.

these veins are not always palpable and one may enter them "blindly." Their constant position makes them useful to the emergency physician seeking a peripheral intravenous route. When passing a long Intracath into the central system, it is best to use the median basilic vein (Fig. 11.2) as the cephalic vein courses deep in the interval between the pectoralis major and deltoid muscles and undergoes a sharp angulation after which it joins the axillary vein. It is often difficult to pass the catheter around this angulation.

A cannula may be inserted blindly into the basilic vein. When other peripheral routes fail, this procedure has a 80% success rate (160). At the antecubital fossa, 1 to 2 cm proximal to the crease, palpate the brachial artery. Enter the skin at a 45 degree angle, and just medial and slightly deep to the artery is the basilic vein which can be cannulated at this site. One may use a 16 gauge Angiocath® or smaller.

PERIPHERAL VEINS OF THE LOWER EXTREMITY

In the lower extremity, the long saphenous vein and the femoral vein are the two vessels most commonly cannulated. The long saphenous vein receives branches from the dorsal venous plexus of the foot and courses anteriorly to the medial malleolus where it lies very superficial and continues in the groove between the upper medial aspect of the tibia and the gastrocnemius. From here it passes posteriorly behind the medial femoral condyle, courses proximally to pierce the femoral fascia at the saphenous opening and enters the femoral vein approximately 1½ inches below the inguinal ligament.

Equipment

Skin preparation
Alcohol swabs
Betadine® solution
4 x 4s
Intravenous cannula
Select a plastic cannula, which can be either an over-the-needle cannula (Angiocath) or a through-the-needle cannula (Intracath) of appropriate

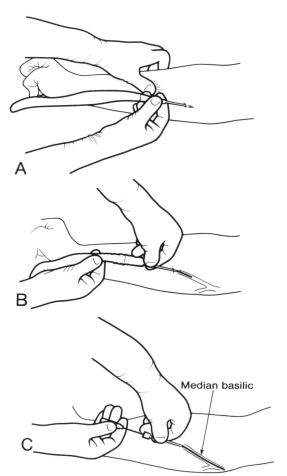

Figure 11.2. When passing a long Intracath® into the central system from a peripheral site, it is best to use the median basilic vein in the upper extremity. *A.* Insert the Intracath® through a skin puncture site after applying traction with the thumb of the left hand to retract the skin. *B.* Thread the Intracath® into the vein after the vein is entered and blood is noted to return into the lumen of the catheter. The plastic housing on the outside of the catheter keeps the catheter sterile during the process of threading the catheter into the vein. *C.* The plastic sheath then is removed and the catheter is secured into the needle hub.

size. Butterfly needles are useful, particularly in children.
Intravenous solution and tubing
Tourniquet

Blood pressure cuff (optional)
Dressing
    Antibacterial ointment
    Paper tape
    Sterile gauze of appropriate size
    Armboard
Xylocaine 1%
    25 gauge needle, 18 gauge needle and
    3 cc syringe.

Technique

The discussion of the technique refers to the upper extremity, but it is applicable to the lower extremity also.

1. Select the site. In the average patient the best site is the cephalic vein approximately 10 cm proximal to the wrist in the adult. In the infant, scalp veins are commonly used. In selecting an optimal site, four points should be observed:
   a. Use a distal site in the extremity rather than a more proximal site. If unable to enter the vein at this distal site, one may ascend to a more proximal site. If a proximal vein is used first and perforation through the venous wall occurs, distal locations along that vein can no longer be used.
   b. The nondominant hand should ideally be used; however, in an emergency situation, the extremity with the largest veins is used.
   c. One should avoid veins over joint surfaces.
   d. The optimal site in which to enter a vein is where two feeding veins join forming a Y. The junction of the three arms of the Y is a stable part of the vein, permitting entrance without lateral motion of the vein as the needle penetrates its wall which is commonly a problem.

   If unable to find a vein. A tourniquet can be applied to the extremity to distend the veins. Warm soaked towels can be applied to the extremity held in a dependent position. An alternative method of bringing a vein out is to apply a blood pressure cuff on the extremity and inflate to above systolic pressure for about 5 minutes. The cuff should then be deflated to below systolic pressure but above diastolic, and the patient is advised to open and close his fist while the arm is held in a dependent position. This may bring out a hidden vein.

2. Apply a tourniquet around the patient's arm and apply restraints with infants.

3. Prepare the skin. The skin should first be prepped with alcohol swabs. Venipuncture is less painful and more bacteriostatic once the alcohol has dried (122). The same area should then be prepped with Betadine® solution.

4. Infiltrate with 1% lidocaine. The site of infiltration should be distal to the site at which one intends to enter the vein so that there is a few millimeters distance between the skin entry site and the venipuncture site to decrease the risk of bacterial contamination at the venipuncture. The pain resulting from the injection of lidocaine intradermally through a 25 gauge needle is trivial, particularly when compared with the pain from the cutaneous insertion of a large bore cannula (48, 122).

5. Puncture vein. *Butterfly needle.* Enter the vein with a smooth motion by placing the needle flat alongside the skin. A return of blood into the tubing will be noted. Advance the needle carefully, following the course of the vein.
   Over-the-needle cannula (Angiocath). A cannula of appropriate size must be selected. An 18 gauge or larger cannula is needed for blood infusions. While maintaining traction on the skin (Fig. 11.3), enter the vein with a sudden motion at a 15 degree angle with the bevel up at site a few millimeters distal to the site of entry into the vein. Advance the needle and cannula as a unit until the vein is punctured. Once there is free backflow of blood, advance the cannula

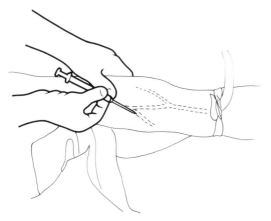

Figure 11.3. To insert a needle or catheter into a vein, hold the needle at a 15 degree angle to the skin with the bevel pointing upward at a site a few millimeters distal to the site of preferred entry into the vein. Apply traction to the skin with the thumb of the left hand to stabilize the vein and then puncture the vein along its side.

and needle a few millimeters into the vein. Slide the catheter over the needle into the vein. If difficulty is encountered, a rotating motion of the catheter back and forth will sometimes aid in entering the smaller puncture site produced by the needle. Withdraw the needle and connect the intravenous tubing. Direct pressure over the venipuncture site will control bleeding from the cannula while connecting the tubing.

Through-the-needle cannula (Intracath). The needle will be larger than the cannula and, if blood is to be infused, a size 16 gauge or larger catheter must be used. While maintaining traction on the skin, enter the vein at a 15 degree angle. Advance the needle into the vein a few millimeters. The flow of blood into the cannula confirms entry into the vein. Advance the catheter through the needle. Engage the hub of the cannula into the hub of the needle. Withdraw the wire stylet from the catheter hub and connect intravenous tubing.

CAUTION!

Do not withdraw the catheter back through the needle at any time as this may result in shearing of a piece of the catheter and a catheter embolism. If the catheter must be withdrawn during the procedure, withdraw the catheter and needle simultaneously as a single unit.

CAUTION!

If swelling or a hematoma develops, stop the procedure and remove the cannula with any of the above techniques. Apply local pressure to the site and locate an alternate site. If one does not want to pull out the cannula to control bleeding, pressure can be applied to the site leaving the needle in place and placing the tourniquet and another cannula at a more distal site along the vein. Once a vein is cannulated, remove the first needle and apply pressure over the site.

6. Apply antibiotic ointment and dressing at the puncture site.
7. Secure the line with adhesive tape or paper tape; with an upper extremity vein, use an armboard to immobilize the wrist or elbow. A butterfly catheter should be secured as shown in Figure 11.4.

Heparin Lock. This cannulation is simply a butterfly needle inserted into a vein without a continuous fluid infusion maintaining the patency of the needle lumen. The cannulation proceeds in the same fashion as for a "butterfly" needle. This cannula is maintained by using 10 units of heparin per milliliter of saline 1 to 2 ml flushed through the "butterfly" to keep the needle lumen patent. Higher concentrations increase the partial thromboplastin time (122). Three times per day and after each use, flush the line with 1 ml of the heparin flush solution. The heparin lock can be used for 4 days with minimal risk for infection (57). The heparin lock is especially useful for patients receiving intermittent intravenous drugs, e.g. antibiotics.

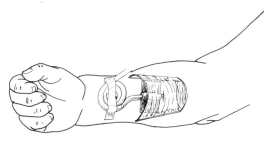

Figure 11.4. Method for securing a butterfly needle in place in a small child. A routine plastic medicine cup is cut in half and used to cover the catheter and puncture site. This protects the site from a dislodging force.

PERIPHERAL VEINS OF THE HEAD AND NECK

The *external jugular vein*, formed behind the angle of the mandible by the joining of the posterior facial vein and the posterior auricular vein, is the site most commonly used in the neck. The vein passes downward across the surface of the sternocleidomastoid muscle. At a level just above the middle of the clavicle, the vein pierces the deep fascia of the neck to end in the subclavian vein. There are several valves which may be encountered in passing a catheter through this vein. One valve lies at the entrance into the subclavian vein and another approximately 4 cm above the clavicle.

Technique

1. Place the patient in a Trendelenburg position to fill the external jugular vein; the patient's head is turned toward the opposite side.
2. Prepare the skin in the manner described on page 345.
3. Select the cannula type and size.
4. Puncture the skin at a site proximal to the site of entry into the vein.
5. Align the cannula parallel to the direction of the vein with the bevel pointing upward. The optimal site of entry into the vein is at a point midway between the angle of the jaw and the midclavicular line (Fig. 11.5).
6. Obstruct the outflow of the vein prox-

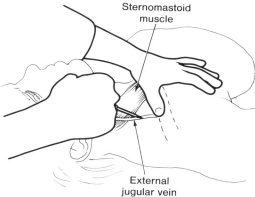

Figure 11.5. Optimal site of entry into the external jugular vein. The vein is distended by applying pressure over it with the thumb placed just above the clavicle. A Valsalva maneuver or the Trendelenburg position may aid in distending the vein.

imally to distend it by lightly placing a finger above the clavicle and pressing over the midclavicular region, as shown in Figure 11.5.

7. Cannulation of the vein should be performed rapidly during inspiration when the valves are open.
8. Cover the cannula orifice at all times to prevent air embolism.
9. Cordis® catheter may be inserted into this vessel by the modified Seldinger technique (see "Pacemaker Technique").

Central Intravenous Techniques

PERCUTANEOUS CENTRAL VENOUS ACCESS

Percutaneous central venous access by the cephalic or basilic veins with a through the needle 91 cm cannula will not be described here. The authors feel that in the emergency setting, when central venous access is needed, it must be rapid and reliable. Central venous access by a peripheral arm vein resulted in 25 to 40% unsuccessful cannulation of the central circulation (79b, 82a, 153a). Many of the unsuccessful cannulations went into the internal jugular vein; this risk may be reduced by turning the head of the patient so that his chin rests on the ipsilateral shoulder during cannulation (28a).

INFRACLAVICULAR SUBCLAVIAN VEIN CANNULATION

The subclavian is a large vein located in the root of the neck, sometimes reaching a diameter of 2 cm or more (43). The axillary vein becomes the subclavian vein as it crosses the first rib. The subclavian vein joins the internal jugular vein behind the sternoclavicular joint to form the innominate vein (43, 111). Just medial to this point, the subclavian vein lies immediately posterior to the medial third of the clavicle. It is separated from the subclavian artery by the anterior scalene muscle (the artery lies posterior to this muscle). The brachial plexus courses posterior and superior to the subclavian artery. The pleura of the lung lies behind the vein as it approaches the midline. The vein courses in close proximity to the undersurface of the medial one third of the clavicle, and it is this relationship which makes cannulation of the vein at this point possible (111). Other important structures related to the course of the vein are the vagus and phrenic nerves which course medially in front of the subclavian artery. The trachea and esophagus lie medial to the vein. No vital structures are crossed in entering the vein at the medial one third of the clavicle between the subclavian vein and the skin. The structures coursing at this point include the pectoralis major, subclavius muscle, and the costaclavicular liagment.

Indications

1. Emergency intravenous route in seriously ill or injured patient.
2. Hyperalimentation.
3. Vasopressor administration.
4. Central venous pressure (CVP) measurement and monitoring.
5. Rapid administration of large volumes of fluid (44).
6. Insertion of a transvenous pacemaker (44).
7. Passage of a Swan-Ganz catheter (55, 102).

8. Intravenous access in patients without peripheral veins (55).
9. Infusion of hypertonic or irritant solutions (48, 108).

Contraindications

1. Do not perform a subclavian puncture in a patient who is agitated and uncooperative, as there is an increased incidence of serious complications (150).
2. Distorted landmarks due to obesity (33), trauma to shoulder girdle, fibrotic changes, deformity of the chest wall, previous surgery or fracture of the clavicle.
3. Radiation therapy in the region (108, 111).
4. Vasculitis and coagulopathies (108).

Equipment

Skin preparation
Anesthetic preparation
Sterile field
Towels
14 gauge Bard Intracath® (8 or 12 inch) (62)
Intravenous solution and tubing
3-way stopcock (for CVP monitoring)
Extension intravenous tubing
Adhesive tape
Antibiotic ointment
Dressing
Tuberculin syringe

Technique

Preparatory Steps

1. Position patient. Place patient in 10 to 20 degrees of Trendelenburg (62, 123, 132, 149). When this is not feasible, one can elevate the patient's feet to transfer blood from the lower extremity into the central circulation (120). If the patient is able, a forced expiration against a closed glottis (Valsalva maneuver) held for a brief time will distend the veins in the neck.
   Place a pad under the patient's shoulders. This lifts up the shoulders and widens the space between the first rib and clavicle. In addition, it prevents the humerus from interfering with cannulation (111, 132).

Locate site of entrance and turn patient's head to opposite side (111, 123, 149). The right side is preferred to avoid the thoracic duct (43, 111). Turning the head does not alter the clavicle-vein relationship (108).

2. Prep and drape the patient (120, 132). The drapes should be placed in the shape of a V so that the suprasternal notch is easily visible and palpable (62, 111).

3. Attach needle to the tuberculin syringe. Detach the Intracath from the needle of the Bard Intracath and attach the needle to a tuberculin syringe. One needs a syringe to aspirate blood to ascertain that the vein has been entered (37). A tuberculin syringe is preferred by the authors because of the low pressure generated when aspirating to determine entrance into the vein. In many patients, higher pressures generated by larger syringes will cause collapse of the subclavian vein, particularly in the presence of hypovolemia, resulting in inability to ascertain whether the vein has been entered.

Procedural Steps

1. Locate point of insertion. A number of articles have been published indicating the "optimal" site of entrance (37, 82, 123, 132, 149). The left subclavian vein passes posterior to the clavicle near the junction of the inner and second quarters of that bone in most patients (108). The subclavian vein is more medial on the left side than on the right side, where it runs along the medial one third (149).
The site of entrance can be located by any of the following methods:
   a. The point just lateral to the midclavicular line along the inferior surface of the clavicle (149).
   b. 1 cm below the junction of the middle and medial thirds of the clavicle (37, 82).
   c. At the inferior surface of the clavicle at the point where the lateral head of the sternocleidomastoid muscle inserts.
   d. (Authors' preferred method) Palpate along the inferior surface of the clavicle and, about one third to one half the length of the clavicle from the sternoclavicular joint, one will feel a tubercle on the clavicle which corresponds to the site of entrance (132). The advantages of using the tubercle in identifying the point of insertion of the needle is that it is a definite landmark and does not involve approximating distances as does the use of the midclavicular line, junction of the middle and medial thirds of the clavicle, or other methods indicated above. One of the authors (RS) has had a remarkably high success rate when inexperienced personnel performed the procedure for the first time (131).

NOTE

One can measure the length of catheter that is needed by estimating the distance between the manubrial-sternal junction and the point of insertion. This can be done by placing the catheter over the path which it will traverse. If the catheter is too long, complications such as ventricular dysrhythmias may occur.

2. Anesthetize. Using 1% lidocaine, anesthetize the skin at the site of entrance and infiltrate around the clavicular periosteum (111).

3. Insert the needle and syringe. Place the fingertip of the index finger into the suprasternal notch as a point of reference (6, 111, 132). With the bevel pointing inferiorly, puncture the skin at the site located above. "Walk" the needle inferiorly and under the clavicle until the subclavius muscle is entered.
Aspirate the syringe and advance the needle toward the midpoint of the suprasternal notch, holding the needle and syringe parallel to the frontal plane (the back of the patient) (111). Hug the undersurface of the clavicle.

NOTE

In elderly patients the direction of the subclavian often is more inferior so one may have to aim toward the inferior margin of the suprasternal notch if the initial attempt is unsuccessful (120).

NOTE

If the first rib is struck, remove the needle and reinsert farther laterally (37).

NOTE

During cutaneous insertion a skin plug may pass into the needle due to its large bore, resulting in a dermoid cyst or plugging of the needle and inability to aspirate blood on entry into the vein. The skin plug can be removed by removing the needle after penetrating only the skin and "squirting" the plug out by forcefully expelling air through the needle. The needle then can be passed through the same puncture site, and the procedure continued.

CAUTION!

A pulsatile resistance, if noted, indicates the subclavian artery. If this should be felt, withdraw the needle and reinsert.

Alternate Method

A method published by Asimacopoulos and Bagley (7) is useful in locating the vein in the obese, uncooperative, or poorly positioned patient in whom the needle cannot be sufficiently depressed to pass under the clavicle into the vein, resulting in the needle coursing inferior to the vein. To avoid this problem the authors smoothly bend the standard #14 Intracath® needle over its entire length to form an arc of about 30 degrees (30 degrees from the point of the needle to a horizontal line extended at a tangent to the midpoint of the arc). The needle then is placed at a 45 degree angle to the skin at the point of insertion under the clavicle and as the needle follows its 30 degree arc, the vein is entered.

If blood is not aspirated on the initial attempt and the needle has been advanced to the hub, aspirate as you withdraw and the vein often is entered.

4. Grasp the needle firmly and remove the syringe. Grasp the needle between the thumb and long finger of the left hand or with a hemostat and remove the syringe.

NOTE

When the syringe is difficult to remove, hold the needle with a hemostat and then remove the syringe. This prevents moving the needle from its position in the vein. Place the index finger of the left hand over the orifice of the needle hub immediately upon removing the syringe to prevent an air embolism.

5. Advance the catheter (Fig. 11.6). Insert the catheter through the needle

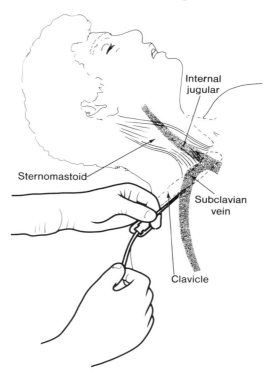

Figure 11.6. Subclavian vein catheterization by the infraclavicular approach. See text for discussion.

into the vein and remove the stylet. This should be done while the patient is holding his breath to avoid entrance of air into the vein and air embolism.

If the catheter does not advance, rotate the needle and continue to attempt advancing it. If it still does not advance, hold the needle closer to the skin. If one is able to withdraw blood from the needle but the catheter will not advance, the following may be tried:

a. Rotate the needle and angle it so that it enters the vein more acutely (hold closer to skin with needle more vertical and closer to the ear of the patient)

b. Bend the tip of the catheter and then introduce it with the bent tip pointing inferiorly.

c. Pass a guide wire through the needle with a flexible tip and then the catheter over the wire (Seldinger technique). If the catheter does not advance, remove the catheter and needle as a *single unit*.

CAUTION!

Withdrawing the catheter through the needle alone may result in a catheter embolism (6, 120, 123, 132). Always withdraw the needle and catheter together and never the catheter alone. The catheter should be advanced until it sits in the hub of the needle.

Aspirate for blood.

NOTE

If blood is not returned, the catheter is either outside the lumen of the vein, kinked, blocked by a thrombus, or lodged against the posterior wall of the vein (111). If this should occur, partially withdraw the catheter and needle while maintaining negative pressure on the syringe. If blood still is not returned, then remove the catheter (111). Remember that if the negative pressure is too strong on the syringe, one will collapse the vein and no blood will return even when the catheter is in proper place (123). This is the main reason a tuberculin syringe is recommended by the authors.

6. Attach the intravenous tubing and withdraw the needle securing it within the needle guard. After attaching the guard to the needle, lower the intravenous bottle below the level of the chest; blood should return in the tubing if the catheter is within the vein (132).

CAUTION!

Be certain to place the catheter carefully in the guard. If the catheter is mispositioned in the guard, the catheter may be severed or torn.

Aftercare

1. Suture and dress. Suture the catheter in place with 4-0 suture (Fig. 11.7). Apply tincture of benzoin around the site and antibacterial ointment to the puncture site; cover the area with a 4 × 4 dressing and tape with 3 inch adhesive taping.

NOTE

In studies in which the catheter was left in place for weeks, no infection was noted over a 2-week period when the dressing was changed every 2 days, the skin was cleansed with iodine, and Neosporin® ointment was applied to the site before a sterile dressing was placed (149). The intravenous tubing should be changed every 2 or 3 days (149). The most important precautions are to completely close the intravenous system from the bottle to the patient by taping all connections and to provide meticulous catheter care (106).

2. Check catheter position. With a CVP manometer attached to a three-way stopcock, the manometer is filled with intravenous fluid from a bottle by turning the three-way stopcock

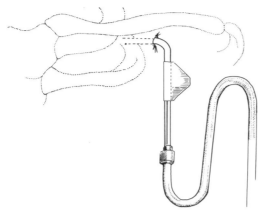

Figure 11.7. Secure the subclavian catheter in place with a suture placed around the catheter close to the puncture site. This will minimize back and forth motion between the catheter and skin which may carry skin contaminants from the puncture site into the vein. The intravenous tubing then is shaped into an "S" curve and secured into position with adhesive tape. The purpose of the double loop or S-shaped curve is that if a pulling force is applied to the intravenous tubing it will be transmitted to the first loop, thus protecting the second loop from transmitting the force to the catheter and causing dislodgement.

"off" to the patient. The tubing should be filled to approximately the 10 cm level. Following this, the three-way stopcock is turned so that it is open between the patient and the manometer. With inspiration the fluid level should fall below 2.5 cm (in the normal patient) and with each expiration it should rise again if the catheter is patent and located in the superior vena cava (111). In up to 20% of noncentral catheter placement, normal respiratory variation occurred (82a). Also, a Valsalva maneuver will raise the fluid level in the manometer.

In all cases, chest radiographs should be taken to ascertain that the catheter tip is in the superior vena cava and to check for a pneumothorax; intravenous fluids have flowed freely even when catheters were in poor positions. One must obtain a chest radiograph even if all attempts to cannulate the subclavian were unsuccessful.

Complications

Forty-four percent of complications occur when the procedure is performed as an emergency (75). Those physicians who have placed more than 50 subclavian vein cannulations have an insignificant complication rate when compared with those who have placed less than 50 and had a complication rate of 5 to 10% (20). Thus, although the list of complications below is long, the complications become uncommon as one performs the procedure more often.

1. **Pneumothorax** (6, 55, 79, 102, 152). This is one of the most common complications from subclavian vein catheterization. Pleural laceration with air leak occurs with a lung laceration. In one study it occurred in 5 of 98 catheterizations (33). Positive-pressure ventilation in a patient with a pneumothorax secondary to subclavian vein catheterization increases the chance of a tension pneumothorax within 48 hours (33, 79). Three cases have been reported; 2 of the 3 patients with tension pneumothorax due to subclavian vein cannulation died from the pneumothorax (129).

Prevention and treatment. This can be prevented by avoiding multiple attempts at cannulation. If one is unsuccessful after three attempts, another site should be selected. If the patient is receiving mechanical ventilation, he should be placed on bag ventilation, if possible, before performance of the procedure. The risk of pneumothorax is greater in children, in whom the pleural reflexion is higher than in the adult. In addition, in the thin emphysematous patient the risk is markedly increased due to the increased size of the lung in the anterior-posterior diameter (123). One probably should attempt another approach in such a patient; we recommend the internal jugular route.

2. **Air Embolism** (55, 102). Air can enter the vein through an opening due to disconnection of the intravenous infusion tubing (55) or during the initial puncture (55). During initial puncture of the subclavian vein the index finger must be placed over the hub of the needle when the syringe is withdrawn to prevent air entry into the

vein. A markedly increased incidence of air embolism occurs with hypovolemia (79). In subclavian punctures performed in dogs, only those with hypovolemia developed air embolism (25). One can prevent this complication by positioning the patient in the Trendelenburg position and maintaining a closed system at all times. Approximately 100 ml of air per second can pass through a 14 gauge needle (25). Patients with hyperalimentation lines, cachexia, and/or hypovolemia are at a high risk for air embolism, even after the subclavian catheter has been removed (121)! This can be prevented by covering the wound and tract with Vaseline® gauze (121) after removal of the catheter.

Air can pass from the right side of the heart to the left through a patent foramen ovale, resulting in coronary, cerebral, or renal infarcts. In arterial air embolism, air in the retinal vessels on ophthalmoscopic examination is termed *Liebermeister's sign*. A sharply defined area of pallor on the patient's tongue, marbling of the skin (especially over the superior parts of the body), and air bubbles on incision of skin (termed *air-bleeding*) (46b) are associated clinical signs of arterial air embolism.

Symptoms and signs of cyanosis, tachypnea, hypotension, and a millwheel murmur (sounding like a washing machine) over the precordium, due to the air and water mixing, are indicative of venous air embolism (46c, 55). Death due to air in the pulmonary outflow tract may ensue shortly (46c). When symptoms of air embolism develop, immediately place the patient in the Trendelenburg position with the patient's left side down so air will enter the right ventricle from the pulmonary outflow tract and is "churned" into small bubbles in the right ventricle which then pass through the pulmonary circulation (46c). Give the patient oxygen (55). Lastly, aspirate blood quickly from a central venous catheter which permits aspiration of the air from the ventricle (74a, 197, 135).

3. *Catheter Embolism* (55, 102). This complication may be due to traction on the bevel tip of the catheter while inserting the needle (55) or, occasionally, may be due to excessive motion of the patient (55). To prevent this complication, during unsuccessful cannulation, the needle and catheter must be removed together as a single unit to avoid shearing the catheter (55). If this complication does occur, the catheter fragments must be removed to prevent the common complications of catheter embolism (56, 74, 145) which include: myocardial thrombi, recurrent septicemia, endocarditis, coronary artery thrombosis, and cardiac perforation with pericardial tamponade (45).

The treatment of this complication may be by many methods. An infraclavicular incision along the path of the catheter may occasionally be successful in retrieving it if it is lodged in the subcutaneous tissue (55). Subclavian venography may demonstrate the catheter, and one then may remove the catheter with wire loops, baskets, hooked catheters, or endoscopic forceps (47, 99, 100, 139). If the above techniques are unsuccessful, a supraclavicular approach to remove the cannula may be used (55).

NOTE

A medial supraclavicular incision is made; the clavicular head of the sternocleidomastoid is divided, freezing the medial clavicle. The clavicle then is divided at the junction of the medial and middle thirds. Elevation of the ends of the bone and retrieval of the catheter fragment using vascular clamps is then possible. If angiographic studies localize the catheter fragment in the superior vena cava or the pulmonary outflow tract, then a right thoracotomy to remove the catheter is necessary to prevent pulmonary hypertension, pulmonary infarction, or endocarditis.

4. *Infection* (55, 102, 137). There is an increased incidence of infection with catheter-induced sepsis in catheters remaining for more than 48 hours (15, 151).

Osteomyelitis due to pseudomonas (92) and *Staphylococcus aureus* have both been reported involving the clavicle. *Septic arthritis* of the sternoclavicular joint secondary to pseudomonas also has been reported (92).

5. *Hemothorax* (55, 137). Hemothorax may occur as a result of penetration of the vein wall by the catheter tip (102). A pleural rent with secondary bleeding also may cause this complication. Excessive motion during insertion can cause laceration of the internal mammary artery near its origin, resulting in a hemothorax (150). Lethal exsanguination has been reported following subclavian vein penetration (55). If the catheter tip has penetrated the vein wall, bleeding may not necessarily occur. Administration of blood through such a cannula may simulate a hemothorax. Indigo carmen dye may be injected into the subclavian catheter and the presence of the indigo dye in a thoracostomy bottle is indicative of this complication (102). This test is useful in the patient who is injured and has a hemothorax, but one is not certain of its association with the subclavian catheter.

6. *Hydrothorax* (4, 22, 102, 129, 152). Perforation of the catheter tip through the subclavian vein and into the thorax may cause a hydrothorax. Prevent this complication by demonstrating free backflow of blood immediately after placing the catheter (4, 33). One cannot tell on radiograph if the cannula is extraluminal since the catheter may advance along the vein from an intraluminal position then to become extraluminal (4). In addition, with intrapleural insertion, one may see respiratory variation of the CVP which may be misleading. To prevent this complication, in part, do not insert a subclavian in a patient with suspected injury to the subclavian vein (55).

7. *Hydromediastinum* (102, 137). Perforation of the catheter tip through the innominate vein may lead to a hydromediastinum. Injection of radiopaque dye through the cannula will confirm this complication (46). The onset of symptoms may be delayed for 30 hours after cannulation. Treatment is to aspirate the mediastinum (by suctioning what one can) if cardiopulmonary embarrassment occurs and withdraw the catheter.

8. *Hydropericardium* (1, 55, 75, 131). Perforation of the catheter tip through the right atrium into the pericardial space causes hydropericardium (46, 146) and pericardial tamponade. During cardiac tamponade one may see only a moderately increased CVP but massively increased neck veins 24 to 48 hours post-insertion. Injection of radiopaque dye through the cannula will confirm this entity (46). Catheters initially in normal position may move (75) to an abnormal position such as the pericardial space, so be certain that normal respiratory movement occurs with each CVP reading. The treatment is to withdraw all fluid from the pericardial space through the cannula, and then remove the catheter and treat tamponade if still present. To prevent this complication, the catheter should not be placed in the right atrium but in the superior vena cava (46, 146).

9. *Venous Thrombosis* (55, 102, 126, 153). A late complication of central vein cannulation is venous thrombosis. In a prospective study, three types were found in 90% of cases: sleeve thrombus which accounted for 80% of cases, mural thrombus in 13%, and major venous thrombosis in 7%, with pulmonary emboli occurring in 3 cases (3). Thrombosis in this instance was not prevented by anticoagulation (15, 151). There is a high association between thrombosis and suppuration at the catheter site (153). Superior vena cava thrombosis secondary to central vein cannulation has been reported (153).

10. *Pulmonary Emboli* (3, 53). See above.

11. *Subclavian Artery Puncture* (36, 67). There are no serious complications associated with this puncture according to some authors (33); however, hemothorax, (67, 93), arteriovenous fistula, false aneurysms, and compressive hematomas have been reported as a result of inadvertent subclavian artery puncture (54, 93). One should repair any subclavian arterial puncture that causes a hemothorax; for most subclavian artery punctures, observation is all that is needed (93).

12. *Internal Mammary Laceration* (91, 150). The internal mammary artery may be lacerated, resulting in an upper mediastinal mass due to the hematoma formation. One must obtain a chest radiograph to

diagnose this condition, even in those situations in which all attempts to cannulate the subclavian vein were unsuccessful (91).

13. **Diaphragmatic Paralysis.** Diaphragmatic paralysis from phrenic nerve injury may result from attempts at subclavian vein cannulation. A raised hemidiaphragm is seen with paralysis and lack of diaphragmatic motion confirmed by fluoroscopy. This complication can be prevented by directing the needle as anteriorly as possible (52) when entering the vein.

14. **Puncture of the Cuff of the Endotracheal Tube (ET Tube).** This presents as a sudden persistent air leak (27) in patients with an ET tube. Sudden extubation of the patient with motion also may occur.

15. **Faulty Positioning of the Catheter Tip.** The subclavian catheter may proceed retrograde into the internal jugular vein, which may result in swelling of the neck (33). If this occurs, the line can still be used for infusion of fluids but cannot be used to register a CVP. This complication can be prevented by turning the patient's head to the ipsilateral side when advancing the cannula, thereby increasing the acuteness of the subclavian-internal jugular vein angle.

16. **Brachius Plexus Injury.**

17 **Knotting and Kinking.** This complication may present as difficulty in withdrawing the catheter (22). One can prevent this by not using too long a catheter, which then coils around itself in the atria.

18. **Arrhythmias** (102). Atrial or ventricular arrhythmias may result with intracardiac positioning of the catheter. These arrhythmias are usually resistant to standard antiarrhythmics and can be stopped promptly by withdrawal of the catheter.

19. **Ascites.** Abnormal communication between the chest wall and the abdominal cavity with concomitant intrapleural administration of fluid results in this complication. Lack of recognition of this abnormal communication led to the administration of 12 liters of fluid "intra-abdominally" in 1 case (4).

20. **Hematoma at Puncture Site.** Raise the head of the bed to reduce pressure in the hematoma after the procedure is completed. A pressure dressing aids in the management of this complication.

21. **Chylothorax.** Avoid the left side when feasible in central vein cannulation where the thoracic duct may be accessible. Extrinsic compression can be used (148) to treat this complication. A pleural drain should be used and losses of medium chain triglycerides measured and replaced if needed.

22. **Dermoid Cysts.** Dermoid cysts can occur from skin plugs "squirted" subcutaneously (63b) and, therefore, the practice of removing the skin plug by squirting it into the subcutaneous tissue is not encouraged. When a skin plug is a problem, it can be expelled by withdrawing the needle and "squirting" out the plug, then reinserting the needle into the same puncture site.

Supraclavicular Subclavian Vein Cannulation

An alternate approach to central venous cannulation is the supraclavicular subclavian method. The advocates of this method state that it avoids the major complication of the infraclavicular approach—pneumothorax (63, 87, 157). This approach is primarily indicated when one cannot perform subclavian vein cannulation by the infraclavicular route.

There are numerous advantages to this approach: 1) Instead of cannulating the subclavian per se, the junction of the subclavian and internal jugular which is a larger "target" is used (87). 2) The needle is directed toward the mediastinum, thus avoiding the pleura (63, 87). 3) It is less painful since the needle does not "walk" down the periosteum of the clavicle (63, 157). 4) The distance between the skin and the vein is shorter than in subclavian vein cannulation (63). 5) The variability of the space between the first rib and the clavicle is avoided by this technique (63, 157). 6) A much greater success rate is achieved by inserting the catheter in the proper position due to the more direct course taken by the catheter into the superior vena cava. In some studies there were no instances of catheter malposition, as is common with the infraclavicular approach and other central approaches (63, 157). 7) The procedure can be performed on the patient in the *upright position*, if necessary, for persons with severe orthopnea.

Technique

Preparatory Steps

1. Position the patient. Place the patient in the Trendelenburg position which minimizes the risk of air embolism and causes venous distension. This position is not mandatory to the performance of the procedure, which can be performed in the upright position. Turn the patient's head to the opposite side.
2. Prepare and drape the supraclavicular region.
3. Identify the site of entrance (Fig. 11.8). The site of entry is at the junc-

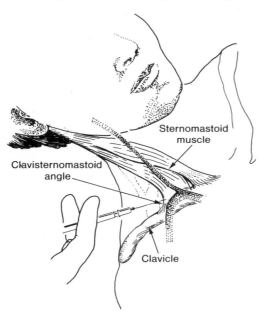

Figure 11.8. Supraclavicular subclavian approach. The site of entry is at the junction of the lateral aspect of the clavicular head of the sternocleidomastoid muscle with the superior border of the clavicle, called the clavisternomastoid angle. The needle should be directed at a 5 degree angle from the coronal plane, at 50 degrees from the sagittal plane, and at 40 degrees from the transverse plane. See alternate method in text.

tion of the lateral aspect of the clavicular head of the sternocleidomastoid muscle with the superior border of the clavicle, called the clavisternomastoid angle (63, 87, 157). The identification of this angle is the key to the procedure. In the obese patient identification is made easier by having the patient tense the sternocleidomastoid muscle by raising his/her head against the resistance of the physician's hand placed on the forehead.

NOTE

The right side is preferred for two reasons: 1) There is danger of injury to the thoracic duct on the left (63) and 2) the right subclavian has a straighter course in relation to the innominate and superior vena cava and may result in more successful catheterization when compared to the left side (157).

4. Anesthetize the site of entrance.

Procedural Steps

1. Puncture the site indicated above with a standard #14 gauge Bardic-Intracath needle attached to a tuberculin syringe.
2. Advance the needle. While applying negative pressure to the syringe, advance the needle, directing it posteriorly at a 5 degree angle from the coronal plane, at 50 degrees from the sagittal plane, and at 40 degrees from the transverse plane (63, 87). An alternate and preferred technique is to pass the needle 10 to 15 degrees below the coronal plane and 45 degrees lateral to the sagittal aiming at the retromanubrial area.* The needle is expected to enter the junction of the internal jugular and subclavian veins after advancing it 2 to 3 cm in the average adult. After the vein is entered, advance the needle a few millimeters farther.

---

* Coronal plane separates anterior from posterior, sagittal plane separates right from left, and transverse plane separates superior from inferior.

3. Detach the syringe and advance the catheter. The syringe is detached from the needle and the hub is covered by the gloved thumb to prevent air entry. The catheter then is inserted through the needle and connected to intravenous tubing and an infusion is started.
4. Secure the needle into the needle guard and suture the catheter in place.

Complications

Complications are uncommon with this procedure (33).

1. Phrenic nerve paralysis
2. Hemothorax (78a)
3. Pneumothorax
4. Hydrothorax
5. AV fistula
6. Brachial plexus injury
7. Air embolism (78a)
8. Pulmonary artery laceration. This occurs from penetration into the superior pulmonary vessels during passage of the needle.

INTERNAL JUGULAR VEIN CANNULATION

Due to the incidence of complications with the subclavian approach, the internal jugular vein is the site preferred by many authors for access to the central circulation (44, 51, 78b, 125).

The internal jugular vein emerges from the base of the skull posterior to the internal carotid artery. During its course through the neck, it lies lateral and then anterolateral to the carotid artery and is covered superficially throughout its length by the sternomastoid muscle (51). With the head turned to the opposite side, the internal jugular vein, in the lower part of the neck, lies just lateral to a line joining the medial portion of the clavicular head of the sternomastoid to the mastoid process. The vein is subject to almost no anomalies or positional variations.

The vein has two valves immediately above the inferior bulb (a bulge formed by the junction of the subclavian and internal jugular veins). The vein can be cannulated quickly despite profound shock or even obesity. Catheterization of the right side is preferred since the internal jugular, the innominate, and the superior vena cava form a nearly straight line into the right atrium. In addition, in the adult the right internal jugular vein is larger and when distended it may reach a diameter of 2.5 cm. Finally, the apex of the pleura is higher on the left than on the right (44, 65, 125).

DeFalque has listed the advantages and disadvantages of internal jugular venous cannulation over the subclavian route as follows (44):

Advantages

1. Lower risk of pleural puncture.
2. If a hematoma forms in the neck, it is visible and easily compressible.
3. It has a superficial and constant position. It is particularly useful in the elderly or the obese patient. In the patient with a short, thick neck, the infraclavicular subclavian route is preferred.
4. Malpositioning of the catheter is rare with internal jugular vein cannulation but can be as high as 25% by the subclavian route.

Disadvantages

1. Failure rate is higher with internal jugular than with subclavian route.
2. Internal jugular vein may collapse in the hypovolemic patient. This is alleviated by placing the patient in the Trendelenburg position.
3. It is more uncomfortable for the patient than is the subclavian route and may dislodge or kink due to neck motion.

Indications

Same as for infraclavicular subclavian cannulation.

Equipment

Same as for infraclavicular subclavian cannulation.

Technique

Two approaches are used in entering the internal jugular vein, the anterior approach and the posterior approach. Both are described below.

Preparatory Steps

1. Position the patient. Fifteen to 20 degrees of Trendelenburg is recommended (26, 125). Turn the patient's head to the contralateral side (25, 44, 125).

NOTE

In infants and small children in whom the head is relatively large and the neck short, it is best to have the neck well extended by placing the body on a pillow or a folded towel beneath the shoulders. Place a roll of towel or pad under the shoulders to enhance the neck structures (26).

2. Prepare and drape the neck.
3. Locate the site of entrance.
   Anterior approach. Locate the triangle formed by the sternal and clavicular heads of the sternocleidomastoid muscle superiorly and the clavicle inferiorly. The point f insertion is at the apex of this triangle (Fig. 11.9).
   Posterior approach (Fig. 11.10). The site of insertion with this approach is along the posterior border of the sternocleidomastoid muscle just cephalad to where the external jugular vein crosses that border (26). Alternately, when the external jugular vein cannot be visualized the needle is introduced under the sternocleidomastoid muscle at the junction of the medial and lower thirds of the posterior margin (44, 114).
4. Anesthetize the site.

Procedural Steps

1. *Anterior approach* (Fig. 11.9). With a needle connected to a tuberculin syringe, puncture the skin at the apex of the triangle as indicated above. Insert the needle at an angle of 30 to 40 degrees to the skin. Direct the needle lateral and caudad toward the ipsilat-

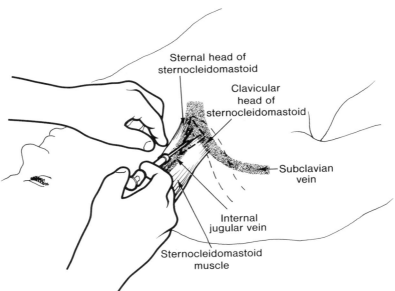

Figure 11.9. Anterior approach for internal jugular vein cannulation. The point of insertion is at the apex of the triangle formed by the junction of the sternal and clavicular heads of the sternocleidomastoid muscle superiorly and the clavicle inferiorly. Insert the needle at an angle of 30 to 40 degrees to the skin and direct the needle slightly laterally and caudad toward the ipsilateral nipple. See text for discussion.

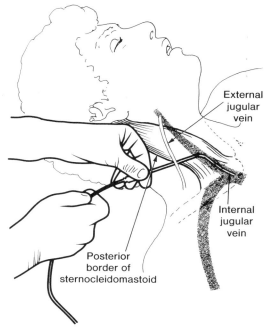

Figure 11.10. Posterior approach to cannulation of the internal jugular vein. Insert the needle along the posterior border of the sternocleidomastoid muscle just above the site where the external jugular vein crosses that border. Alternately, when one cannot see the external jugular vein, introduce the catheter at the junction of the medial and lower one third of the posterior margin of the sternocleidomastoid muscle. The vein should be entered in 5 to 7 cm. See text for discussion.

eral nipple or midclavicular line (40, 125). The vein should be entered after 1 to 2 cm as it is quite superficial in this location. If one misses the vein, direct the needle 5 to 10 degrees more laterally (44). If by 4 to 5 cm the vein is not entered, remove the needle.

As the needle is advanced, one should aspirate. If one does not enter the vein, aspirate as you withdraw.

Posterior approach. Insert the needle at the site indicated above. Advance the needle and syringe under the sternocleidomastoid, aiming at the midpoint of the suprasternal notch (44). One should enter the vein in 5 to 7 cm (26).

NOTE

Some authors advocate the use of a small gauge needle and syringe to locate the vein before cannulating with the large Intracath® needle (125). We feel this is helpful in the difficult patient whose anatomy is not discerned readily.

2. Insert the cannula (Fig. 11.10). Advance the cannula through the needle. If resistance is met, remove the catheter and needle together so that the catheter is not sheared resulting in a catheter embolism (125). The catheter should be advanced while the patient holds his breath to prevent air entrance into the vein (44). Advance the catheter until it is lodged in the hub of the needle.
3. Withdraw the needle and aspirate for blood. If blood does not return into the tuberculin syringe, this may be because of hypovolemia and vascular collapse. Withdraw the catheter a centimeter or so and aspirate again. If one still cannot aspirate blood, then assume improper positioning and remove the catheter.
4. Attach the intravenous tubing and secure the needle guard.

Aftercare

1. Lower the intravenous bottle to check that the catheter is in the vein. Blood should return into the tubing.
2. Anchor the cannula to the skin with sutures and apply antibiotic dressing.
3. Loop the plastic intravenous tubing behind and over the patient's ear and tape into position (26).

Complications

1. ***Hematoma.*** Hematoma can occur from either venous or arterial bleeding. This complication may result from inadvertent puncture of the carotid artery (44, 125). If one side of the neck develops a large hematoma, the other side should not be cannulated as a bilateral hematoma can result and compromise the patient's airway. The hematoma should be treated with a compression dressing (44).

2. *Thoracic Duct Injury.* This complication is rare. A case of chylothorax necessitating surgery has been described (84). If this occurs the resulting chylothorax should be treated with repeated thoracocentesis and replacement of lost proteins with medium chain triglycerides.

3. *Hemothorax.* Hemothorax is secondary to puncture of either the lung or a major vessel such as a subclavian artery, aorta, or carotid. Deaths as a result of hemothorax have been reported (125). Hemothorax is treated by chest tube drainage and, if secondary to arterial injury, the artery may need repair.

4. *Pneumothorax.* Pneumothorax is secondary to puncture of the lung. This is much less common with internal jugular vein cannulation than with subclavian puncture.

5. *Pneumomediastinum and Hydromediastinum.* This is more common in infants, in whom laceration of the trachea may occur (44). To prevent hydromediastinum carefully insert the catheter and check for blood reflux into the intravenous tubing on lowering the bottle. Avoid directing the needle medially in the infant.

6. *Air Embolism.* This is especially common in hypovolemic patients (135). One always should make certain that the connections in the intravenous tubing are tight. The index finger must be placed over the hub of the needle when the syringe is withdrawn. For therapy see "Air Embolism" in the section "Infraclavicular Subclavian Technique."

7. *Phlebitis.*

8. *Infection.* Catheter tips cultured for organisms were found to have an 11% incidence of organisms which were pathogenic; however, only 1 patient in 70 developed clinical infection (96).

9. *Catheter Embolism.* See subclavian discussion.

10. *Myocardial Puncture.* See subclavian discussion.

11. *Nerve Damage.* No significant neurologic damage is reported in the literature (44). Only Horner's syndrome, probably due to puncture of the stellate ganglion, has been noted (125).

FEMORAL VEIN CANNULATION

Indications

Rapid placement of a large bore intravenous route, especially during external cardiac compression when motion of the neck and subclavian region necessitates cessation of cardiac compression for central venous cannulation.

Drawing blood when unable to locate vein elsewhere.

Radiographic procedure.

Emergency intravenous route when unable to find access elsewhere or when there is clinical contraindication to use of an upper extremity vessel.

Rapid placement of a transvenous pacemaker.

Technique

Preparatory Steps

1. The overlying skin must be meticulously prepared as contamination is a significant problem.
2. Locate vein. Palpate the pulse of the femoral artery. The vein is located 1 cm medial to the artery (63a). In the patient with vascular collapse or cardiac arrest in whom the femoral artery pulse cannot be palpated, one can find the vein by extending a line between the anterior superior iliac spine and the pubic tubercle. Divide this distance into thirds. The artery is found at the point where the medial third joins the lateral two thirds. The vein is found 1½ cm medial to the estimated artery (63a).
3. Anesthetize with 1% lidocaine.

Procedural Steps

1. When the catheter and needle are chosen, position the needle two fingerbreadths (2 to 3 cm) below the inguinal ligament (23) and medial to the artery; direct the needle cephalad at a 45 degree angle with the skin and aim the bevel of the needle toward the umbilicus. In difficult cases, one may enter the vein perpendicular to the skin and then change the direc-

tion of the needle to 45 degrees to cannulate the vein.

2. Attach intravenous tubing.
3. Dressing. Apply dressing with anti-bacterial ointment and sterile gauze.

Complications

1. **Thrombosis and Phlebitis.** A very common problem with prolonged femoral cannulation is thrombosis, which may extend proximally into the deep veins and into the inferior vena cava (23, 66). Twenty-four patients with femoral catheterizations which remained in place 3 to 14 days were studied (151). Five patients developed caval thrombosis and 2 patients had pulmonary emboli. Four of the patients developed suppurative thrombophlebitis and sepsis. Patients who developed serious complications had the catheter in place for 13 days, while those without complications had the catheter in place for 6 or less days.

In the *prevention and treatment* of these complications, one should remember to remove the femoral cannula as early as possible. One must use strict aseptic technique and the fluid infusion sets should be changed every 48 hours (14, 29). The use of heparin in a bottle as indicated in the section "Complications Common to All Techniques" is advocated for patients undergoing prolonged cannulation of central veins, especially the femoral.

2. **Hematoma.** This is a common problem (8). In *preventing and treating* this complication, one should apply a good pressure dressing over an unsuccessful cannulation site. When the vein is entered and the cannula removed, pressure should be applied for a full 5 minutes. Avoid the use of the femoral vein in patients with coagulopathies (97).

3. **Septic Arthritis of the Hip** (8, 23, 97). This results from piercing the hip capsule which lies under the vein. The development of anterior thigh edema and decreased extension and internal rotation of the hip joint should suggest this complication. The most common organism is *Staphylococcus aureus* (8).

The *prevention and treatment* of this complication involves avoidance of piercing the posterior wall of the femoral vein and avoidance of contact with bone. Strict aseptic technique is encouraged so that if the capsule is penetrated, septic arthritis does not result (8).

4. **Femoral Nerve Damage** (8, 23). The femoral nerve courses lateral to the femoral artery. In the obese patient in whom landmarks are difficult to define and arterial pulsation is difficult to identify, one may cause damage to the femoral nerve by inadvertently aiming the needle too far laterally.

5. **Penetration of a Viscus in an Unrecognized Femoral Hernia** (23).

6. **Psoas Abscess** (8, 23). A psoas abscess may result from introduction of skin bacteria into the psoas fascia which lies beneath the femoral artery and vein.

Saphenous Vein Cutdown at the Ankle

The saphenous vein in the ankle is probably the ideal vein for cannulation. It is the only vessel of importance in this location and its constant location just anterior to the medial malleolus permits ready access. Its elasticity permits the vein to be dissected easily through a short incision without rupture. The disadvantages of this site are the greater risk of phlebitis, the difficulty in rapidly infusing fluids via this route due to the valves in the leg veins, and the low flow rates through these relatively small caliber veins (127).

In addition to the ankle, other sites can be used for cannulation (Fig. 11.11). The saphenous vein in the groin is especially useful when one needs to place a large-bore line, such as intravenous tubing, for voluminous fluid and blood administration in a patient with a traumatic cardiopulmonary arrest. In addition, the saphenous vein in the groin is easily accessible and can be cannulated rapidly in infants and children. The basilic vein located in the medial antecubital fossa is another site which can be cannulated. Catheters can be inserted through this route for central monitoring. This site is the most com-

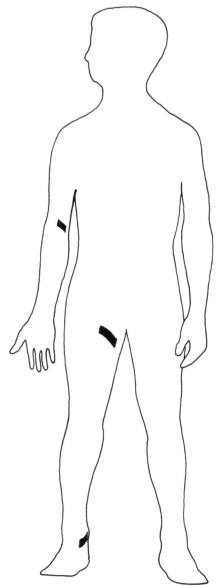

Figure 11.11. Antecubital, groin, and ankle cutdowns are perhaps the most commonly performed.

monly used cutdown site in the upper extremity. The cephalic vein located on the lateral aspect of the antecubital fossae is another available site; however, it is infrequently used because of the difficulty in passing a catheter (if a CVP line is needed) past the sharp angulation as this vein enters the axillary vein. Also, there is the possibility of injury to the lateral cutaneous nerve at the cutdown site. According to some authors (41), in the upper extremity the cutdown site of first choice is the median basilic because of its superficial location and large caliber; the brachial vein is the second choice, and the median cephalic is the third choice (Fig. 11.1).

Indications

1. Poor peripheral sites for intravenous cannulation, e.g., obese patients and drug addicts, in whom a central line cannot be placed.
2. Hypovolemic shock in which rapid volume replacement through a large-bore cannula is needed.
3. Placement of a central venous pressure monitor or Swan-Ganz catheter, in patients in whom a central line is not preferred.
4. Pacemaker insertion.
5. Cardiac arrest in infants and small children, in whom access to a central line is unsuccessful.

Contraindications

1. Injury to vessels proximal to the site of cutdown.
2. Unstable fractures proximal to the site of the cutdown which may increase the risk of phlebitis due to swelling proximally.

Equipment

One scalpel with a #10 and 11 blade
One curved Kelley hemostat
One small mosquito hemostat
Fine-toothed forceps
Scissors, iris and sharp cutting
Anesthetic prep
Skin prep
Drapes and towel clips
At least two sizes of polyethylene tubing
One sterile intravenous extension tubing
Sterile sponges, 4 × 4
Syringes, 5 cc
Self-retaining retractors
Small rake
Needle holder
Silk 3-0 and 4-0 suture
Injectable saline

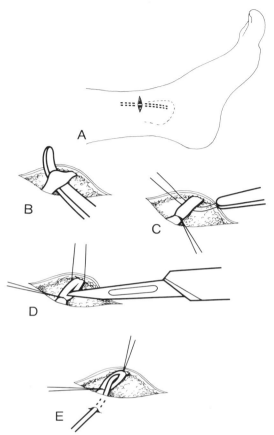

Figure 11.12. Procedure for a cutdown over the saphenous vein at the ankle. See text for discussion.

Intravenous tubing and solution
Dressings with antibiotic ointment

Technique

The technique discussed here is for the saphenous vein at the ankle. The same principles are applicable to other sites and the differences between this site and the others will be discussed separately.

Preparatory Steps.

1. Select site and position the patient.
2. Prepare and drape.
3. Infiltrate with local anesthetic if necessary.

Procedural Steps.

1. Incise the skin and subcutaneous tissue (Fig. 11.12A). Make a transverse incision over the vein, 1.5 to 2.5 cm in length (depending on size of patient) and extending from anterior to the medial malleolus to the anterior tendons (extensor hallucis longus) just superior to the malleolus.
2. Isolate the vein (Fig. 11.12B). With a curved hemostat pass from the medial malleolus deeply along the fibrous layer over the tibia exiting next to the tibialis anterior tendon, one will "scoop" the tissue containing the vein. Dissect bluntly in this tissue and the vein is rapidly found. *Alternate method.* The vein may be localized easily in a thin patient by blunt dissection just beneath the subcutaneous tissue rather than "scooping up" the tissue as indicated above and then dissecting out the vessel.
3. Isolate the vein between two ligatures passed beneath the vein and separated by 1 to 2 cm from each other (Fig. 11.12C).
4. Select a cannula approximately one size larger than the vein appears.
5. Make a sharp incision into the vein (Fig. 11.12D). This incision can be a linear or a transverse incision made after passing a closed hemostat beneath it. When using a transverse incision, it should extend approximately one half the diameter of the vessel. This venotomy should be between the two sutures. This can be done with either a #11 blade or an iris scissors. Bleeding is controlled by lifting up on the proximal ligature.
6. Insert the cannula into the vein. A vein introducer (small plastic insert) can be inserted into the venotomy site to aid in cannulation. With the bevel facing the posterior wall of the vein, relax the proximal ligature and gently advance the cannula. Stabilize the vein with gentle traction on the distal suture.
   Alternate method. An alternate technique is to pass the cannula through a separate stab wound distal to the site of the incision for the

cutdown (Fig. 11.12E). A 14 gauge needle or larger is passed through the skin from inside the incision to the skin distal to the cutdown site so as not to introduce bacteria from the skin. The cannula is passed through the needle after which the needle is removed. The cannula then is inserted into the vein as discussed above. This decreases the incidence of infection at the incision site and at the vein, since the cannula does not pass through the incision, acting effectively as a "drain within an abscess cavity." This is our preferred approach; however, one may not be able to do this technique in an emergency situation when time is of the essence.

7. Check position. Aspirate to confirm that one is in the vein and not in a false passage in the wall of the vein. Following this, inject a few milliliters of sterile saline so as to prevent clot formation at the tip and assure free flow.
8. Attach the cannula to the intravenous solution.
9. Secure the proximal ligature around the cannula now within the vein and ligate distally.
10. Close the wound.

Aftercare

1. Suture cannula to the skin, using nylon or silk suture.
2. Apply antibiotic ointment over the incision site and site of cannula exit and dress with 4 × 4 gauze. Tape securely and immobilize the ankle in a splint.

Saphenous Vein Cutdown at the Groin

Through a saphenous vein cutdown at the groin, one can infuse 500 cc of whole blood within 5 minutes (118) with a large-bore cannula. The authors feel this is the best route for massive trauma patients in whom large volumes of fluid are needed over a short period of time. In such a situation, a sterile intravenous extension tubing with the tip cut off at a 45 degree angle is used as the cannula. In a dire emergency, one can perform a cutdown at this site within 60 seconds (118). Catheters at this site should, however, be removed within 24 hours to avoid phlebitis as this is not a sterile area.

Technique

1. In the pulseless patient the incision begins at the point where the scrotal fold (labial fold) joins the medial thigh. The incision is carried laterally in a transverse direction approximately 6 cm. If one can feel the femoral artery pulse, the incision is carried to a point just lateral to the pulse. The vein lies just medial to the artery (Fig. 11.13).
2. Dissect through Scarpa's fascia and the greater saphenous vein lies just beneath this fascial layer (Fig. 11.13). If the anterior thigh were divided into thirds, the vein lies at the junction of the inner and middle thirds.

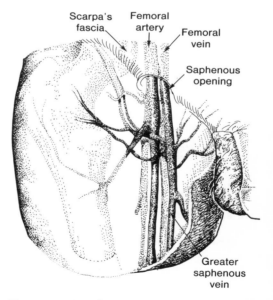

Figure 11.13. Saphenous vein cutdown at the groin. Note Scarpa's fascia. With one sweep of a #10 blade, the physician can go through the skin and subcutaneous tissue to Scarpa's fascia. Following this, one can quickly identify the greater saphenous vein which is seen piercing the fascia, superiorly.

3. After the vein is isolated, a venotomy is made and intravenous extension tubing is passed.

Basilic Vein Cutdown

This cutdown is performed with the patient's elbow extended and the forearm supinated. It is traditionally taught that in this cutdown a 2.5 cm incision is made two fingerbreadths superior to the medial epicondyle with the center of the incision being over the brachial pulse. When this pulse is not palpable, the transverse incision should be centered between the biceps and triceps muscles at the junction of the distal one fourth and proximal three fourths of the arm. The vein courses just over the triceps muscle. The vein will be found superficial to the neuromuscular bundle between the biceps and the triceps on the medial side of the arm. The vein will lie just medial and deep to the brachial artery and median nerve. Proceed as in the saphenous cutdown.

Complications

1. *Thromboembolism and Phlebitis.* This complication can occur from prolonged catheterization, infection from the cutdown site extending into the vein, or irritation from the cannula against the vein wall. It is more common with lower extremity cutdowns than with upper extremity sites (118).

2. *Infection.* In a double-blind study using Neosporin® (not recommended here), bacteria were cultured from the wound in 18% as compared with 78% in a placebo group. Some patients who developed phlebitis subsequently had sterile wounds, and some benign-appearing wounds grew pathogenic bacteria (78, 113). One should use aseptic technique and, if possible, bring the cannula out through a separate stab wound.

3. *Injury to Associated Arteries and Nerves.* The median nerve lies in close proximity to the basilic vein and can be injured. The saphenous nerve courses adjacent to the saphenous vein at the ankle. The lateral antecubital nerve courses close to the cephalic vein at the elbow. There are cases in which the artery is mistaken

for a vein. To avoid this, feel for arterial pulsation in the vessel. This may be a problem, especially in a child or in a patient in shock in whom pulsations may not be evident.

4. *Catheter Embolism.* Discussed in the section on subclavian cannulation.

5. *Air Embolism.* Discussed in the section on subclavian cannulation.

6. *Perforation of Vein Proximal to Puncture Site, Resulting in Fluid Infusion into the Subcutaneous Tissue Proximally.* This occurs from puncture of the vein wall with a sharp cannula or previous attempts at intravenous insertion proximally or as a result of traumatic injury.

Intravenous Cannulation of the Infant

Several sites of cannulation are available on the infant, both peripheral and central. However, due to the relatively infrequent need of a large intravenous cannula in an infant, experience with these approaches is limited; therefore, the physician often is somewhat fearful when central cannulation becomes necessary. To avoid redundancy we have concentrated on those procedures which are useful in establishing an intravenous route, and both peripheral and central approaches are discussed. The reader should be familiar with the techniques for intravenous cannulation, such as subclavian and internal jugular veins, in adults as only the pertinent dissimilarities or striking similarities will be discussed in this section on intravenous cannulation in the infant. Since cutdowns are used in emergency medicine in difficult infant intravenous cannulations, these also are discussed here.

Several primary sites exist where veins have a constant position in the infant (156) and can be used for peripheral, central, or cutdown venous cannulations. These include the long saphenous vein at the ankle (anterior to the medial malleolus) and the cephalic vein at the wrist over the lateral surface of the distal end of the radius. Secondary sites are on the back of the hand and in the antecubital fossa (basilic and median antecubital veins). The external jugular vein in the neck and the long saphenous vein at the medial knee and in the groin also are places where access to the circulation can be attained in the infant.

Perhaps the most commonly used veins in small infants are the scalp veins, as they are readily accessible. When one dresses these venous sites with antibiotic ointment, there is a decreased incidence of colonization and the infection rate decreases from 36% to 3.7% (19). Infection associated with scalp vein cannulation is infrequent even when the cannula remains in place for 3 or 4 days (39). Scalp veins have a lower incidence of phlebitis than do other veins and can be used repeatedly (39).

Use as large a catheter as possible. Generally a vein will take a catheter 1 size larger than it appears (156). This is especially true when one is dealing with a cutdown. A 2 French catheter will not permit even saline to flow well without an infusion pump (156). A 3 French allows saline to pass but not blood, while a 4 French is a good all-purpose catheter (156). This is the smallest size recommended for most cutdowns performed on infants. The long saphenous in the full-term neonate generally takes a 4 French catheter easily.

PERIPHERAL INTRAVENOUS LINES IN THE INFANT

One should select a site, usually a scalp vein or a vein on the dorsum of the hand initially. The technique using a butterfly is discussed below. For intravenous cannulation, use a small gauge Angiocath®; the technique is similar to that in the adult.

1. In starting an intravenous line in a child with small veins, it is important to connect the butterfly needle to the intravenous tubing first. Fill the tubing with the intravenous solution.
2. Apply a tourniquet to the forearm or a rubber band to the scalp.
3. Secure the arm and hand to an armboard when one of these veins is used. With scalp veins, the covering used over the site (Fig. 11.4) should protect the needle or cannula from dislodging.

4. Flush a small amount of solution into the site by pressing on the end of the tubing after the needle has penetrated the skin. This creates a negative pressure in the system and assures prompt blood return once the vein is entered.
5. Cannulate the vein at a 15 degree angle and once the vein is entered do not advance the needle further. The exception to this is when a large vein is cannulated and advancement can be performed under direct vision without the hazard of going through the vein.
6. Begin the intravenous infusion.
7. Secure the line in place, wrapping several loops of the tubing (attached to the butterfly needle) adjacent to the site.
8. Cut a small plastic disposable medication cup (15 cc) in half vertically. Cover the site with the half-cup forming a "hood" over the puncture site to protect the needle from displacement (see Figure 11.4).

INTERNAL JUGULAR VEIN CANNULATION IN THE INFANT

English et al. reported a success rate of 91% in cannulation of the internal jugular vein in a group of 85 infants and children (51). In another study, 100 children underwent cannulation between the ages of 2 weeks and 9 years without any complications (72). The reader is referred to the adult section for a full discussion of the procedure.

Technique

Preparatory Steps.

1. Position the infant. Place the child in 15 to 20 degrees of Trendelenburg, with the head held firmly over the edge of the table (88, 125). Turn the infant's head to the opposite side and have an assistant hold it, hyperextending the neck to tense the sternocleiodmastoid muscle (72, 88, 125).
2. Prep and drape as routine (72, 125).
3. Select a catheter. Various authors have recommended different sizes; however, generally either a 16 gauge

Abbott® or Desert® venocath (72) or a 17 gauge Intracath® (88) is used.

Procedural Steps (same as in adults).

1. Insert needle attached to a tuberculin syringe at the site.
    Anterior approach (Fig. 11.14). The apex of the triangle formed by the two heads (sternal and clavicular) of the sternocleidomastoid is the site of insertion. The needle is directed at a 45 degree angle to the skin caudally and is aimed toward the ipsilateral nipple (125) (Fig. 11.9).
    Posterior approach (Fig. 11.14). The site of entrance is at the junction of the middle and lower thirds of the posterior border of the sternocleiodmastoid muscle (88). Advance the catheter to the midpoint of the supra-

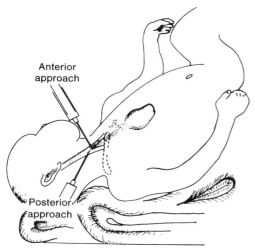

Anterior approach

Posterior approach

Figure 11.14. Catheterization of the internal jugular vein by the anterior and the posterior approach in the infant. With the anterior approach, the apex of the triangle formed by the two heads of the sternocleidomastoid is the site of insertion. The needle is directed at a 45 degree angle to the skin caudally. In the posterior approach, the site of entrance is at the junction of the middle and lower thirds of the sternocleidomastoid muscle. The needle should be held at a 30 degree angle to the skin. (Reprinted with permission of Surgery, Gynecology and Obstetrics. Craux, M.M., Percutaneous cannulation of the internal jugular vein in infants and children 148:593, 1979.)

sternal notch (72, 88). The needle should be held at a 30 degree angle to the skin (72).

NOTE

Some authors prefer to use a 22 or 23 gauge needle attached to a 5 ml syringe to locate the vein before introducing the cannula above (72).

2. Aspirate and advance. With the anterior approach, one usually enters the vein in 1 to 2 cm (88, 125); if not, aspirate during withdrawal.
3. Remove the syringe and insert the catheter. Place the thumb or index finger over the hub of the needle as you remove the syringe so as not to permit air entry. Thread the catheter into the superior vena cava. Aspirate after the catheter is in place to check position and withdraw the needle and catheter out of the puncture site once the catheter is securely locked into the hub of the needle.

CAUTION!

The same precautions apply in infant cannulations as with the adult. Should it be necessary to remove the catheter, remove the needle and catheter as a single unit and never withdraw the catheter through the needle since this may result in shearing and catheter embolism.

4. Connect the intravenous solution and lower the infusion bottle to check for return of blood into the tubing indicating the proper location in the vein (88, 125).

Aftercare

1. Tape and secure. Radiographs should be obtained to check proper location in the superior vena cava. If one has difficulty seeing the catheter tip, 5 ml of contrast material can be injected to visualize the position (88). An antibiotic ointment and the dressing should be changed three times a week, and the intravenous tubing once a day.

SUBCLAVIAN VEIN CANNULATION IN THE INFANT

There seems to be an inordinate amount of fear associated with introducing a catheter into the subclavian vein of a child. We feel this is inappropriate when such a procedure may be lifesaving in an emergency situation. In 103 subclavian catheterizations in infants between 6 months and 2 years of age, few complications were noted when the procedure was performed properly (69).

The reader is referred to the adult section for a full discussion of subclavian catheterization.

Technique

Preparatory Steps.

1. Position the infant. Place the child in 15 to 20 degrees of Trendelenburg (69). Restrain the infant with the head turned to the opposite side.
2. Prep and drape in routine fashion.
3. Select catheter. While a 16 or 17 gauge catheter can be used in larger children, in the smaller infant we prefer a 19 gauge 1½ inch Bardic® or Deseret® type catheter. This size fits well between the infant's clavicle and first rib (69).

Procedural Steps.

1. Insert the needle attached to a tuberculin syringe into the site. The site of insertion is somewhat different than that advocated for the adult. In addition, the direction in which the needle should be passed is slightly different due to the more horizontal position of the clavicle in the infant than in the adult. The site is the *midclavicular region*, and the needle should be directed in a straight line between the *first rib* and the clavicle. The vein is entered directing the needle 1 to 1½ cm above the suprasternal notch (57a, 113, 69).
2. Aspirate and advance.
3. Remove the syringe and insert the catheter. Place thumb or index finger over the orifice of the needle. It is often necessary to manipulate the catheter into the superior vena cava

in contrast to the adult where the catheter goes in easily (69). This manipulation of the catheter is by backward and forward motion as well as slight rotation as the catheter tends to proceed into the opposite subclavian or internal jugular vein when being passed. This displacement, in the authors' experience, has been more common in the infant than in the adult. If the catheter bends, then withdraw the needle and catheter together as a *single unit*.

4. Check position. Lower the intravenous bottle to check proper position of catheter in the vein.
5. Secure and dress in the routine fashion.

CATHETERIZATION OF THE STRAIGHT SINUS IN THE INFANT

This procedure was introduced by Kunz (89) and is used only in a dire emergency. It is not advocated as a routine procedure, although in Kunz' article there was a very low incidence of complications. We cannot find reports testing the procedure elsewhere in the literature. It can be used for emergency transfusions of blood or fluids.

Technique

1. The infant is placed on one side with his back toward the operator and, an assistant immobilizes his head and body similar to the position in which one placed an infant when performing a lumbar puncture.
2. The center of the posterior fontanelle is palpated, and the skin is prepped.
3. A 2.5 cm, short bevel, 20 to 22 gauge needle (Angiocath®) is introduced 3 to 4 mm. The point is directed toward the uppermost part of the forehead in the sagittal plane.
4. Aspirate blood from the straight sinus. For transfusions, place the needle 1 to 1.5 cm below the skin in the straight sinus.
5. One must inject blood very carefully with as little pressure as possible and frequent checking of proper needle placement. Since the catheter gauge is very small, blood must be injected

slowly rather than administered by drip as one would with a 16 gauge catheter.

SAPHENOUS VEIN CUTDOWN AT THE ANKLE IN THE INFANT

For a detailed discussion of this procedure refer to the adult section on cutdowns. While the procedure described here is for the saphenous vein at the ankle (most commonly used site), the same procedure can be used in other accessible veins including the basilic and cephalic.

Technique

Preparatory Steps.

1. Select a catheter. A 4 French catheter is used for most full-term newborns. One should have other catheters available, and a catheter selected which is 1 size larger than appearance of the vein.
2. Immobilize the leg and foot on an armboard.
3. Prep and drape in the routine fashion.

Procedural Steps.

1. Incise skin and subcutaneous tissue. Make a transverse incision 0.5 cm long directly over the site of the vein (156), which lies just superior and anterior to the medial malleolus.
2. Dissect the vessel. With a mosquito forceps, open the wound widely. Wipe the blood out of the field with a swab held in the forceps. With a *scooping motion,* using a closed curved hemostat inserted directly anterior to the medial malleolus, the entire tissue beneath the skin incision is lifted upward onto the closed hemostat. This tissue then is dissected to find the vein (156). Make certain that the vein is not left behind and is accompanied by the saphenous nerve (156).
3. Ligate the distal end of the vein. With forceps held under the vein, two pieces of catgut are placed under the vein (distal and proximal) and the distal end is ligated (156).
4. Make a transverse incision in the vein. With a mosquito forceps under

the vein to stabilize it, a small transverse incision is made in the vein with a #11 blade or a nick with an iris scissors.
5. Insert catheter. With the bevel of the catheter directed downward (156), the catheter is inserted. To do this, the mosquito is removed from under the vein to relax the proximal end and the distal ligature placed in step 3 is tensed distally by gentle traction. The catheter is usually passed easily with this technique (156). An introducer also can be used, which is inserted into the vein to dilate the puncture site.
6. Tie proximal stitch. Tie the proximal stitch around the catheter. We prefer 4-0 chromic to silk (2) in children. The catheter should not be tied too tightly.

Aftercare

1. Immobilize the catheter with tape after securing it with a suture.

SAPHENOUS VEIN CUTDOWN IN THE INFANT GROIN

While this procedure is infrequently used in the child, it is commonly used in the adult who has sustained a traumatic arrest and is severely hypovolemic. A very large bore cannula can be introduced with ease into the saphenous vein, where it enters the femoral vein at the groin. This site is recommended in the child in a similar situation or in any circumstance in which large volumes of fluid must be administered very rapidly. In situations in which a cutdown is needed for other than such a dire circumstance, we prefer the saphenous cutdown at the ankle.

Technique

Preparatory Steps.

1. Identify the femoral pulse below the inguinal ligament (73).
2. Select the catheter. Even the neonate will admit a 16 gauge catheter at this site. In larger children, one can pass a 12 or 14 gauge catheter. When large volumes of fluid are needed in larger children, one may pass the intrave-

nous tubing itself, approximately 8 gauge.
3. Prep and drape.

Procedural Steps.

1. Make incision. An incision should be made at the upper thigh over the femoral pulse parallel to the groin crease (2). Dissect through the subcutaneous tissue and identify the saphenous vein.
   In the pulseless infant the incision should begin at the point where the scrotal (or labial) fold meets the medial thigh. The incision should extend laterally to approximately the mid position of the inguinal ligament. The saphenous vein lies just beneath the subcutaneous tissue one to two fingerbreadths lateral to the scrotal or labial fold.
2. Insert the catheter after incising the vein. Make a small nick with an iris scissors transversely into the vein and insert the catheter into the femoral vein.
3. Advance the catheter into the inferior vena cava.
4. Pass a suture ligature around the vein at the puncture site proximally and distally, tie the catheter in place proximally and then ligate the distal end of the saphenous vein. Since this is an emergency, this step is not done until now.

Aftercare

1. Suture the skin wound closed loosely with 4-0 nylon.
2. Secure the catheter in position with tape and dress the wound with an antibiotic ointment and gauze dressing.
3. The infant should be restrained if necessary.

UMBILICAL VESSEL CATHETERIZATION

Umbilical vessel catheterization is a useful procedure for establishing an intravenous line in a newborn who is in distress. Occasionally the vein is mistaken for an artery, but this is not common. The vein is thin-walled and there are two veins adjacent to one another. The artery is a single thick-walled vessel which is usually constricted. The umbilical artery is the preferred vessel (12); venous catheterization can be used also when arterial catheterization is not successful (50, 86). It is usually still possible to insert the catheter for the first time in neonates 48 to 72 hours of age (70, 86); some catheters have been passed successfully up to 10 days after birth. The orifices of the umbilical artery are easily identifiable after 72 hours of age only if the umbilical cord stump is sterile (70). Within a few minutes of birth the umbilical arteries constrict. This process is delayed with hypoxia and acidosis (86). In newborns who require umbilical artery catheterization for management of cardiorespiratory distress, successful catheterization is almost always possible in the first 15 to 30 minutes of life. The vast majority can be catheterized in the first day of life (86) with relative ease.

Catheterization can be performed by one person. Unless the infant is limp or the procedure is done as an extreme emergency, he should be restrained loosely before the procedure.

The catheter will not advance beyond 2 cm, or at 6 to 8 cm, in 10% of cases. If this does pose a problem, then one needs to proceed to the other vessel (34).

Indications

1. Administration of fluids and blood (70, 86) in a newborn infant.
2. Repeated arterial blood pH and gas determinations (134). Repeat specimens for blood gas analysis can be obtained by direct arterial puncture. With this procedure, however, peripheral vasoconstriction in the ill infant may result in inaccurate measurements (70). If the child cries during the procedure, this lowers the $PaCO_2$ (70). It is not practical to obtain repeated samples by percutaneous puncture, so sampling of arterial blood through the umbilical artery catheter is preferred (70, 86).

One should try to keep the aortic PO_2 between 55 and 70 mm of Hg. Excessively high O_2 tensions may injure the retina, resulting in retrolental fibroplasia (86). If an arterial catheter cannot be placed, then in the healthy infant central venous pH can be determined and is usually 0.02 to 0.03 pH units lower than arterial values. Central venous PCO_2 is 5 to 6 mm Hg higher than respective arterial values (86). These values do not hold for blood from the portal system. The O_2 tensions in venous blood are lower but do not correlate with arterial samples. Therefore, venous samples cannot be used to guide oxygen therapy (86).

Samples should not be obtained while the infant is straining or crying. The technique for obtaining a sample is as follows (86):

a. There should be a constant inspired O_2 level.

b. Infant should not be crying.

c. Flushing fluid should be removed from catheter so it does not contaminate the specimen. Withdraw a volume equal to three times the capacity of the catheter system (usually 0.2 ml). A 0.4 ml sample should be removed if withdrawn from the stopcock port.

d. Withdraw a sample in a heparinized syringe (see section on arterial blood gas).

e. Infuse a volume of fluid equal to the sample volume taken to maintain a constant blood volume.

3. Administration of alkali (86). The authors recommend an arterial not a venous route to administer bicarbonate, since bicarbonate is diluted by the aorta and also capillary vessels. Bicarbonate administered in a vein, especially if the catheter is in a portal vessel, decreases blood flow, and thrombosis and phlebitis may develop (86). If the catheter tip is in the inferior vena cava or atrium, alkali may irritate the sinoatrial node and cause cardiac arrhythmias.

4. Measurement of blood volume and cardiac output (86).

5. Exchange transfusion (86, 134). This procedure can be performed through an umbilical venous or arterial catheter or both. The procedure is usually performed with the venous catheter tip placed in the portal circulation. One should attempt to pass the catheter through the ductus venosus and into the inferior vena cava since citrated blood is acidotic and may produce hypokalemia and hypocalcemia. Rapid infusion of blood into the inferior vena cava can cause arrhythmias. The blood should be buffered before administration. The best way to perform exchange transfusion is with two catheters which are of the end-hole type (hole at end rather than on side of catheter); the venous catheter is used for transfusion and the arterial catheter is used to withdraw blood samples for pH and blood gas determination (86). In placing a catheter from the umbilical vein to the inferior vena cava, some authors (86) advise an end-hole catheter so that suction during exchange transfusion does not perforate the very thin-walled inferior vena cava.

Equipment

Kitterman (86) states that the ideal catheter should have the following characteristics:

1. It should be flexible and not kink as it follows the curves of the vessels.

2. It should be made of nonwettable material so clots do not form on its surface.

3. He prefers the single end-hole variety, to avoid clotting in the tip which is a problem with the side-hole catheters.

4. It should be radiopaque.

5. Its capacity should be small so that only small amounts of blood need be withdrawn before samples are taken. The best catheter at present is the Argyle umbilical artery catheter, 3.5 French for infants less than 1.5 Kg and 5 French for larger infants.

Circumcision drape with 2 × 2 inch hole in center

4 small towels
Straight iris scissors
Large sharp scissors
2 mosquito forceps
2 curved eye dressing forceps
2 umbilical cord tape ties
2 small needle-holders
Gauze sponges
Syringes (2 or 5 ml)
No. 18 needle (blunt)
Three-way stopcock
3-0 silk on atraumatic noncutting needle
Medicine glass. A heparin solution is made by adding 250 units of heparin to a 250 ml bottle of isotonic saline to fill the medicine glass.

Technique

Preparatory Steps.

1. Keep infant warm. The infant should be kept warm in an incubator (70, 134). Babies are best placed on an ambient warmer with supplemental oxygen as it is hard to maintain the oxygen tension in the incubator sufficiently high (70). Infants should be placed under a radiant heat source when not in an incubator (134).
2. Prepare the infant and catheter. The gloves should be rinsed with sterile water to remove talcum powder (86). This avoids introduction of talcum into the vessel.
   To facilitate sampling, fill the catheter with a heparinized solution with a concentration of 0.3 u/ml. This concentration prevents thrombus formation (50, 134). Gastric contents should be emptied with a pediatric feeding tube to avoid vomiting and aspiration during the procedure. When dealing with a newborn infant, the aspiration of meconium from the stomach is a serious problem leading to severe pneumonitis (134).
   Attach a three-way stopcock to the catheter filled with heparinized saline (86).
3. Prep the umbilical cord and drape. Prep the umbilical cord with povidone-iodine (Betadine®) followed by

alcohol to prevent any iodine burns (50, 70, 86, 144).
Drape with a circumcision drape with a hole cut out of center.
Sharply transect the cord 0.5 to 1 cm from the abdominal wall after antiseptic preparation (50, 70, 86, 134, 144).
Identify the vessel to be catheterized and carefully dilate the lumen (134) with the tip of a mosquito forceps.

NOTE

When blotting the cut surface, one will see a single, large, thin-walled oval vein and two smaller, thick-walled arteries which are rounded. After birth the artery constricts to the size of a pinpoint. It can be dilated by gently inserting the closed tip of a small curved iris forceps into the lumen (50, 86). The forceps can be opened to dilate the artery further (144).

The cord stump should be held upright with 2 × 2 gauze. Tie either a cord ligature or preferrably umbilical tape loosely around the base of the umbilical cord to prevent brisk arterial bleeding or venous oozing (70). Tie it loosely with a single knot (86) tight enough to prevent bleeding during the procedure. One may have to loosen the knot later to permit passage of the cannula.

Procedural Steps.

1. Insert catheter into umbilical artery or vein (Fig. 11.15). A 3.5 or 5 French catheter is threaded gently. Once within the arterial orifice, the catheter can usually be advanced easily (70).

NOTE

Obstruction can occur at two points. At 1 to 2 cm where the vessels suddenly course downward at the level of the anterior abdominal wall and at 5 to 6 cm at the level of the urinary bladder (86), where the umbilical artery may go into spasm as it

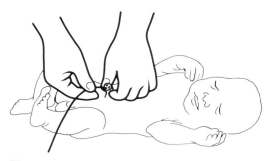

Figure 11.15. Umbilical artery catheterization. In the emergency center, this procedure is performed only in the newborn infant who requires neonatal resuscitation. See text for discussion.

Table 11.1. Distance Catheter Must be Inserted to Reach the Diaphragm

Weight (gm)	Distance (cm)
1000	8–10
1000–1500	10–11
1500–2000	10–12
2000–2500	12–13
2500+	14–15

enters the iliac vessel. The first site of obstruction often can be overcome by pulling the stump upward toward the baby's head (70, 144). The second site of obstruction may be overcome with 30 to 60 seconds of gentle steady pressure. Do not repeatedly attempt to thread the catheter past the point of obstruction. At 6 to 10 cm, blood easily can be withdrawn from the catheter (70). If unsuccessful at relieving the obstruction, do the following:

   a. Fill the tip of the catheter with 0.1 to 0.2 ml of sterile 2% lidocaine without epinephrine.

   b. Reinsert to the point of obstruction.

   c. Inject the lidocaine. Do not try to pass the catheter; wait 1 to 2 minutes for the artery to relax, then advance (86).

   d. If this fails, use the other umbilical artery.

2. Position the catheter tip. The umbilical artery catheter should be placed in the aorta (50, 134). Advance the catheter until approximately 2 cm past the point where blood is obtained (86). Here the tip is usually at the aortic bifurcation. Radiographs should be obtained in the anterior-posterior and lateral projections to check the position of the catheter (chest and abdominal films). It should be placed with the tip at T7-8. It has been found that with the tip at this

level, there is one half the complication rate than with the catheter tip at L3-4 (112).

When the umbilical vein catheter is passed, it should go through the ductus venosus and into the inferior vena cava to the level of the right atrium or (50, 86, 144), preferably, it should remain in the inferior vena cava.

NOTE

Table 11.1 will help guide the distance estimated for the size of the infant (70).

   After positioning the catheter, attach a three-way stopcock and withdraw blood and return the sample to the infant.

3. Fix the catheter and connect. With a purse string suture of fine silk, suture the catheter in position.

Tape it to the abdomen (70, 134) (Fig. 11.16).

Antibiotic ointment is placed at the junction of the catheter and the umbilical cord (134, 144).

NOTE

The catheter volume is 0.2 ml. Each time a sample is drawn, flush with 0.3 ml heparinized saline (0.3 u/ml) (70). This is not necessary with a constant infusion which flushes the catheter (70).

Connect to infusion pump. If a Harvard constant infusion pump is not available (50), then the solution infused should be at a high enough pressure to overcome arterial pressure (134), when the umbilical artery is used.

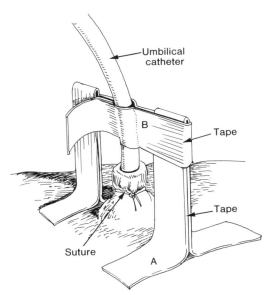

Figure 11.16. A method for securing an umbilical catheter to the abdomen was introduced by William Pearl. He folds a strip of adhesive tape back over itself in the middle as shown in *A.* Two strips of the folded tape are then secured on either side of the infant's umbilicus. *B.* While holding the catheter in place, he applies two strips of tape on either side of the catheter. This secures the catheter in place. In addition, the catheter should be secured with a suture placed around the umbilical cord as shown.

NOTE

Keep catheter free of blood to prevent formation of clots (86). Each time blood is withdrawn from the catheter, flush with enough heparinized saline (three times the capacity of the catheter) to clear the blood. Flush the catheter every hour when a constant infusion is not used. If using a continuous infusion, heparin 1 u/ml of parenteral fluid can be added.

NOTE

All infants with umbilical catheters are treated with penicillin 50,000 u/kg/day and kanamycin 5 mg/kg/day intramuscularly for the duration of catheterization plus an additional 48 hours (144).

4. To remove the catheter. Remove it slowly over 30 to 90 seconds. Tie the

purse-string suture (134, 144) which allows the vessel to constrict and minimizes bleeding.

Complications

The mortality associated with exchange transfusion through umbilical veins is less than 1% in major centers (134). Umbilical artery catheters carry an overall complication rate of 10% according to some authors (134). The utilization of umbilical venous catheters was associated with a twofold increase in the overall complication rate as compared with that of umbilical arterial catheters and a fourfold increase in pathologic changes demonstrated at necropsy (144). At autopsy, thrombi were noted in 6% of those with umbilical artery catheters and in 44% of those with umbilical venous catheters. The incidence of complications with umbilical artery catheters is related to the length of time the catheters are left in place; however, the complications associated with umbilical venous catheters are unrelated to length of time the catheters are in place (144). Although the ease of placement of venous catheters has resulted in their common use, the greater complication rate should result in reserving their use to those cases in which the arterial route has proved impossible and catheterization is needed (144).

1. *Vasospasm.* Vasospasm of the umbilical artery (134) and blanching of an extremity occur in some infants. Occasionally in infants, the leg will blanch during the procedure, and this is attributed to vasospasm (86). Leg blanching is relatively frequent with the umbilical artery cannulation (70).

2. *Loss of Pulse and Development of Gangrene.* This complication has occurred in some infants following umbilical artery catheterization (50, 86, 134, 155), leading some authors to recommend its use only in those patients in whom other routes cannot be used.

3. *Extravascular Catheter Placement.* Perforation of the colon has been reported (31). Thus radiographs are needed to exclude pneumoperitoneum and to determine catheter placement. It is rare for this to occur with catheters that have rounded

tips; thus, catheters with sharp beveled tips should not be used (86). Large bowel perforation can occur (50, 86, 134). In addition, venous catheters should be positioned in the inferior vena cava and not in the portal system through the ductus venosus.

4. *Cardiac Arrhythmias* (134). A short PR interval without Wolf-Parkinson-White Syndrome has been reported; bigeminy and prolonged sinus bradycardia also have been observed (50).

5. *Thrombosis and Phlebitis* (134). Portal thrombosis and liver necrosis can occur (134). In one study, 12.5% of patients who came to autopsy with umbilical catheters had thrombosis (155). The most commonly reported complication of umbilical vessel catheterization is thrombosis (86). The incidence of thrombosis varies from 3 to 5% at autopsy (86). These thrombi vary from small fibrin thrombi to thrombi of the renal arteries or aorta (86). Umbilical venous catheter thrombosis varies from 3 to 33% as determined by autopsy or clinical examination (53, 155). Portal vein thrombosis may occur due to injection of hypertonic solutions (86) into the portal vein. Hypertonic dextrose, bicarbonate, and trihydroxymethylaminomethane (THAM) all can cause thrombosis (86). Portal vein thrombosis occurs more commonly when the venous catheter tip is in the portal system (10, 70, 155). Necrotizing phlebitis and aortitis also have been reported (34). If the catheter is used for blood transfusion, then there also is an increased incidence of thrombosis (34). Hepatic necrosis secondary to the administration of undiluted bicarbonate can occur also (155). Sixteen percent of infants of diabetic mothers develop thrombosis with umbilical catheters (119). Neonatal hypertension secondary to renal infarct has been reported (17). Transverse myelitis and paraplegia secondary to spinal artery infarct have been reported from umbilical vessel catheterization (10). For venous catheters, no correlation exists between the length of time the catheter is in place and thrombosis (65). With umbilical artery cannulation the risk of thrombosis is present almost exclusively during the first 12 hours, with the highest risk being shortly after catheterization. To prevent thrombi, keep the catheter size small and the duration of catheterization and length of the catheter as short as possible. Avoid manipulating the catheter (134). Infuse hypertonic solutions into large vessels with a rapid flow rate (86) to reduce the risk of thrombosis in vessels like the aorta or inferior vena cava. Reduce the rate of infusion with bicarbonate to 2 mEq/kg/min (86). If a catheter is clotted and the clot cannot be removed, then a new catheter should be inserted and may be inserted into the same artery (34).

6. *Embolism.* Catheters in the umbilical vessels may cause emboli from clots formed on the catheters or from air injected through the catheter tip (86). Emboli from the umbilical artery are lodged at the tip of the lower abdominal aorta and will go to the lower extremity, with infarction occurring most commonly in the toes. If infarction occurs, the catheter should be removed. Emboli from venous catheters are lodged in the portal system. If the catheter is passed through the ductus venosus, the emboli infarct lung tissue (86, 155). Due to patent foramen ovale or patent ductus arteriosus, venous emboli may be widely disseminated throughout the systemic circulation (86).

For air embolism to occur in the arterial catheter, the air must be injected at a higher pressure than that of the systemic circulation (86). Venous air embolism can occur during inspiration, when the chest develops a more negative intrathoracic pressure, and can "suck" not only the fluid in the catheter into vessels in the chest but also air. When this complication occurs in the larger vessels, it can be fatal (86). Thus, never open the umbilical veins to atmospheric pressure. (See "Air Embolism—Infraclavicular Subclavian Vein Cannulation—Complications.")

7. *Hemorrhage.* Umbilical artery catheters in the aorta have a constant risk of hemorrhage and must be observed for this complication (50, 70, 86, 155). The catheter should be observed for disconnection which may produce exsanguination. The infant may pull or kick the catheter and to prevent this, he should be restrained. If bleeding is significant, restore volume as soon as possible (86).

8. *Infection.* The catheter is a frequent source of infection, especially in infants who have received bicarbonate via the catheter (86). Gram-negative bacteremia may occur in some infants (50). Omphalitis is not uncommon (70). The infection rate is higher with umbilical vein than with umbilical artery cannulation (12). There is no difference in the infection rate with the administration of antibiotics (155), and, therefore, some authors do not support the prophylactic administration of antibiotics. There is reportedly a lower incidence of cord colonization with pathogens in infants on systemic antibiotics (12).

To decrease the risk of infection, umbilical dressing should be changed daily and an antibiotic ointment applied. Remove the catheter as soon as possible and adhere to aseptic technique during handling (12).

SPECIAL PROCEDURES RELATED TO INTRAVENOUS CANNULATION

Central Venous Pressure Monitoring

Central venous pressure monitoring is a simple method of assessing the status of blood volume. Although it has considerable value in acutely ill patients for regulation of fluid or blood replacement, one must be aware of its shortcomings (147). Inaccurate measurements often are obtained by aberrant lodging of the venous catheter tip in addition to other problems (see "Technique"). Radiographic identification of the location of the catheter tip is essential to the elimination of some of these problems (64, 147). Patients with hypovolemia may have an elevated central venous pressure, particularly when the cause of the hypovolemia is concomitant with pulmonary contusion or other injuries which elevate the CVP. The important parameter in measuring the central venous pressure is not the isolated value per se but the *response* to a sudden fluid infusion. The response of the CVP is a more reliable indicator of the patient's volume status than the *actual* CVP. If after rapidly infusing 200 to 300 cc of crystalloid one notes no change in the CVP or a decrease in the pressure, one can safely assume the patient is volume depleted.

Indications

When a Swan-Ganz catheter is available and the skill and equipment necessary for insertion are at hand, this catheter is the preferred method to monitor central venous pressure.

1. Sepsis
2. Management of shock syndromes

More specifically, if a hypotensive patient does not respond to a volume infusion or responds but subsequently becomes hypotensive again, then central venous pressure measurements would be important. In addition, central venous pressure monitoring is useful in patients who are hypotensive but in whom volume infusion is prohibitive (e.g., patients with renal failure or congestive heart failure). In patients with probable hypovolemia one may initially attempt to observe neck vein distension carefully and obviate central venous pressure monitoring providing the neck veins are flat and easily visualized.

3. Massive hemorrhage
4. Severe blunt chest trauma
5. Evaluation of cardiac tamponade

Technique

Discussed is the technique of obtaining a central venous pressure reading after the catheter has been inserted into the superior vena cava by any of the routes discussed in the chapter.

1. Place the patient in a supine position.
2. Place the zero point of the manometer in the midaxillary line at the fourth intercostal space. The column should be held vertically. Mark this point with a skin pen so that an accurate and reproducible measurement can be subsequently obtained for comparisons (Fig. 11.17).
3. Fill the manometer with intravenous fluid by opening the three-way stopcock to the intravenous solution. Remove all air bubbles from the tubing and manometer.
4. Open the three-way stopcock to the patient so that the channel which is open is that between the patient and the fluid-filled manometer.

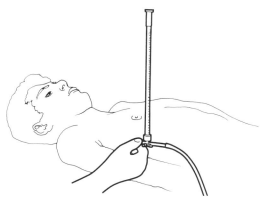

Figure 11.17. Zero point of the manometer should be placed at the midaxillary line of the fourth intercostal space. This provides for more accurate central venous pressure readings.

5. Observe for respiratory fluctuations in the column of fluid in the manometer. With a patent channel (and a properly positioned catheter tip) the fluid level should rise with expiration and fall with inspiration. There is generally a 2.5 cm variance between the inspiratory and expiratory levels. A Valsalva maneuver also will increase the fluid level in the column.
6. Measure the CVP reading and then open the line from the patient to the intravenous bottle so that a clot does not form in the catheter.

Transvenous Cardiac Pacemaker

Electrical pacing of the heart can be instituted rapidly at the bedside with the introduction of a transvenous electrode by a percutaneous route. Temporary cardiac pacemakers have been used for some time in the management of heart block and bradycardia associated with low cardiac output (128). Fluoroscopic control, while optimal, is generally not available in emergency centers and a number of authors have documented excellent results with bedside cardiac pacing (11, 80, 110, 128). In the past, prolonged unsuccessful catheter insertion was attributed to soft pliable catheters and indirect approaches to the central venous system. A number of catheters have been employed which can be divided into three types: unipolar, bipolar,

and dipolar. Although some authors report a high success rate with unipolar electrodes (128), the latter two types are the best for use in the emergency center (140) since unipolar catheters require direct endocardial contact which may be difficult to achieve. The newly introduced Elecath® semifloating bipolar pacemaker catheter has resulted in a very high percentage of successful insertions (11, 85, 128).

There are three techniques which have been described for placement of percutaneous transvenous pacemakers into the right ventricle: fluoroscopic positioning, electrocardiographic positioning, and blind positioning. Transfer of the severely ill patient to another unit may be hazardous and bedside cardiac pacing is often preferred, making electrocardiographic and blind positioning the only two methods of importance to the emergency physician and, therefore, the only two which are discussed here. Electrocardiographic positioning is the preferred technique; however, it requires that cardiac activity be present. It is especially useful for the patient who is in complete heart block with bradycardia following an anterior myocardial infarction. In patients without spontaneous cardiac action, the blind technique is used.

A number of venous routes have been advocated by various authors, each having their favorite site including the antecubital vein (128, 130), external jugular vein (140), femoral vein (32, 103, 140), and the subclavian and internal jugular vein (110, 128). While any of these approaches can be used to gain access to the right atrium and thence to the ventricle, it would appear that three sites offer the advantages of ease of access and rapidity with which the veins can be cannulated (32, 35, 85, 103, 110, 128, 130, 140). These sites, preferred by the authors, are the *right internal jugular vein, left subclavian vein,* and either *femoral vein.* The right internal jugular vein proceeds directly into the superior vena cava. The left subclavian vein is preferred to the right subclavian vein, because the natural curve of the catheter follows that of the left subclavian vein permitting entrance into the superior vena cava easier than with the right, where the catheter must make a sharper bend. When introducing the electrode using the blind technique for positioning, by far the most rapid and preferred approach is through the femoral vein (32, 103, 140). In one study involving 31 patients, the catheter could be introduced via the femoral vein in less than 30 seconds and cardiac pacing initiated in 1 to 3 minutes (103).

Indications for Pacemaker In Emergency Center

1. Asystole or bradycardia (<60/mm) with altered hemodynamic state or ventricular irritability (escape beats) which is unresponsive to atropine or isoproterenol (49, 80, 110). In the presence of myocardial infarction, isoproterenol is contraindicated for bradycardia but not for asystole.

NOTE

In patients who enter the coronary care unit with a myocardial infarction, 6 to 8% will develop the complication of heart block with 85% occurring in the first 48 hours (80).

Equipment

Monitor and ECG machine
Skin preparation
Alligator clips and connecting wire
4 towels
Towel clips
Gloves
Anesthetic prep
Elecath® catheter (packages in a kit) or any semifloating bipolar catheter. For femoral route a 100 cm long #5 bipolar catheter in which the distal 10 cm are in a "J" configuration is recommended.
Skin suture
Dressing
14 gauge Angiocath® or Cordis® catheter

Technique

Preparatory Steps

1. Select catheter. The 4F Elecath® semifloating catheter which is packaged in a kit and fits through a 14 gauge needle yields the best results with either technique and is the authors' preferred electrode catheter for cardiac pacing (85, 128, 130, 140). The catheter is 100 cm long and is bipolar with two platinum ring electrodes at the distal tip separated 1.5 cm by a balloon (130).
   For the femoral approach, the somewhat different 5 F bipolar catheter in which the distal 8 to 10 cm are in a "J" configuration is preferred (103).

2. Select site. The basilic vein in the upper extremity, cannulated through a cutdown approach, was more commonly used in the past (128) but currently is not recommended by most authors (32, 110). There is a high frequency of dislocation of the electrode tip when the extremity is raised over the patient's head. There is as much as 2.5 cm displacement of the electrode tip from the right ventricular wall with such motions as elevation of the arm (32, 110). The subclavian and internal jugular venous routes are commonly recommended (110, 128). If one is to select either of these routes, we would recommend that the right internal jugular vein be used as this is a direct route into the superior vena cava (58a). When the subclavian vein route is selected, the left is preferred since the catheter follows a natural curve and cannulation into the superior vena cava is more easily achieved when this side is used (110). The femoral vein is less commonly used than either of the above routes; however, many authors feel that it is the preferred route for emergency pacing due to the rapidity and success of the procedure as discussed above. Our preferred approach is the right internal jugular vein initially; if rapid catheterization is not achieved, we recommend the femoral vein route.

3. Position the patient. *Internal jugular or subclavian.* Place the patient in 10 to 20 degrees of Trendelenburg. Place a roll under the shoulders. Turn the patient's head to the opposite side of the entrance site.

Femoral vein. Place the patient supine.

4. Prep and drape.

Procedural Steps

1. Cannulate the vein. Cannulation of the vein is performed in the routine fashion as discussed in other sections of this chapter. Use a 14 gauge Angiocath® or a Cordis® catheter.

2. Introduce the electrode catheter and position by ECG (in the patient with cardiac activity):
Electrocardiographic positioning (11, 10, 128, 130). Attach the limb leads of the ECG to the patient in the routine fashion. Attach the precordial lead (V_1) to the distal end of the electrode catheter and record the electrical activity on the V lead as the catheter is advanced. The catheter may be attached to the precordial V lead by the use of an alligator clamp. The ECG recorded from this electrode tip localizes the position of the electrode tip (Fig. 11.18).
As the catheter is passed, one will see a recording similar to that seen normally in AVR. Advance the catheter into the right atrium, where the recording will show a large negative P wave on the precordial lead. At this point, inflate the balloon which then will "float" the catheter into other locations. Advance the catheter across the tricuspid valve into the right ventricle. If an obstruction is met, counterclockwise rotation and forward - backward motion help pass the catheter across the tricuspid valve. When the catheter tip is in the right ventricle, one will notice a wide QRS pattern of left bundle branch block.
Deflate the balloon.
Advance 3 to 5 cm until premature beats or ST elevation in the intracardiac V lead is noted. This finding indicates firm contact with the right ventricular endocardial surface. When the J-shaped catheter is used, it is pulled back against the endocardial surface.
One is now ready for pacing.

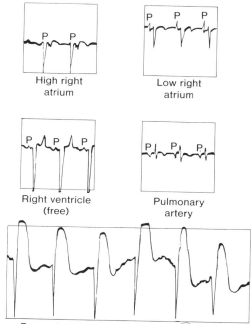

High right atrium   Low right atrium

Right ventricle (free)   Pulmonary artery

Femoral catheter lodged against RT ventricle endocardium with marked ST elevation.

Figure 11.18.   ECG tracings taken from the precordial lead attached to the pacemaker catheter at various levels in the heart.

At this point the pulse generator is connected; adequate positioning can be definitely ascertained before connecting a pulse generator if a current of injury is noted on the ECG.
Femoral approach (103). Introduce the catheter 15 cm into the vein.
Inflate the balloon.
Connect the distal terminal of the electrode to the V lead of the ECG and attach the limb leads to the patient in the routine fashion.
Float the electrode tip into the right ventricle. Entrance into the right ventricle and across the tricuspid is signalled by abrupt appearance of large negative intraventricular complexes as noted above.

3. Establish pacing. Connect the catheter to the generator.
Bipolar—distal end to the negative terminal, proximal end to the positive terminal.
Unipolar—connect subcutaneous needle to the positive ter-

minal electrode and then to the negative terminal.

Pacing generator settings:
  Demand mode
  Rate of 70/min
  2.5 to 6 mA output until pacing established

Turn generator on.

Slowly increase milliamperes output until generator shows pacing spikes followed by a wide QRS.

Decrease generator output to threshold (where pacing ceases) and then resume pacing at 2 mA above threshold.

AXIOM

Good positioning is indicated in part when pacing threshold is below 1.5 mA (32, 128). The 12 lead ECG should show a pattern during pacing. If an RBBB is demonstrated, then the electrode is positioned in the pulmonary outflow tract or in the left ventricle due to septal perforation by the electrode.

Alternate Method

An alternate method of establishing pacing is to turn the pacemaker generator to maximum output (mA) and once pacing is established to then decrease the output slowly.

Aftercare

1. Secure the catheter. Place two loops of the catheter next to the side of the puncture site, and suture catheter in place.
  Obtain anterior-posterior and lateral chest films. An overpenetrated radiograph may be helpful to visualize the electrode wire.
  The patient with a femoral catheter is asked to cough, deep breathe, or shift position to be certain the catheter is well lodged.

Alternate Technique

Blind Positioning.

Slide the catheter into the superior vena cava, via the right internal jugular vein.

Attach the external end of the pacemaker catheter to the generator.

Set the generator to maximum output (mA), and a rate of 70/min.

Turn the generator on.

Advance the catheter until ventricular pacing occurs.

Confirm position by anterior-posterior and lateral chest radiograph.

Femoral Approach (preferred) (104). The usual routes for blind passage of a pacing catheter have many well-known disadvantages. The technique indicated here for the insertion of a "flow-directed" bipolar pacing catheter through the femoral vein is optimal. A 5 French catheter is used with a balloon located between the two electrodes which are 1 cm apart and in which the distal 8 cm of the catheter is preformed into a J configuration. A stiffer wire with a balloon can be used when there is no cardiac activity, rather than a flow-directed catheter. The technique is similar to that indicated in the section on insertion through the femoral route. The inverted J-shaped tip predisposes to attainment of a stable position in the right ventricular apex.

Complications

1. ***Myocardial Perforation.*** This occurs at the free wall of the right ventricle or atrium with hemorrhagic pericarditis or pericardial tamponade as a consequence. This complication may be secondary to excessive advancement of a stiff electrode. One will note a transient pericardial rub with the catheter tip rubbing against the epicardial surface. In one case a diaphragmatic twitching was noted with perforation (11).

No therapy is generally needed other than the withdrawal of the catheter. Pericardial tamponade secondary to continued hemorrhage is unusual.

2. ***Catheter Dislodgement or Excessive Loops in the Catheter.*** Frequently there is a failure to sense or an increase in the pacing threshold. This dislodgement or looping occurs due to the catheter being inadequately anchored. This may cause arrhythmias with the paced beats having the same configuration as the ectopic beats since they are produced by the same sec-

tion of myocardium (61b, 150a). Some catheter arrhythmias produced by the dislodged catheter will be bizarre and uninterpretable, while others will occur during inspiration only (61b, 150a). Ventricular bigeminy may occur but the coupling interval may vary. Even high doses of antiarrhythmics will be ineffective (61b, 150a). Atrial arrhythmias also may occur (140, 95a). With excessive loops, each atrial systole thrusts the catheter tip against the myocardium, causing aberrant beats (140, 95a). The beats will be preceded by P waves and occasionally there may be fusion beats (140, 95a).

The treatment is to remove or reposition the catheter (61b, 150a). When redundant loops are the problem withdraw the loops carefully.

3. **Perforation of the Interventricular Septum or Ventricular Wall.** *Septum.* This results in the catheter tip being displaced into the left ventricle. There are a number of clues to this occurrence:

a. The pacer shows a change from an LBBB pattern to an RBBB pattern (141b).
b. The chest radiograph shows the catheter tip in the left ventricle (141b).
c. There is an increase in the pacing threshold.

Ventricular wall. In one study when the right ventricle was perforated without tamponade the patients had no signs of perforation (61a). It was discovered incidentally at thoracotomy. In other cases the only manifestation was failure to capture (61a).

4. **Movement of the Catheter Tip across the Tricuspid into the Hepatic Vein, Inferior Vena Cava, or Coronary Sinus and Loss of Positioning for Optimal Pacing.**

5. **Failure to Obtain Capture or Sense QRS.** This may occur as a consequence of a massive myocardial infarction, extreme electrolyte imbalance, hypoxemia, low oxygen transport, or a faulty generator. This complication is seen frequently (45% of cases) (61a), especially in cardiac arrest. It was successfully managed in one third of cases by repositioning of the catheter tip, replacement of the generator, catheter removal and replacement,

tightening of the electrode connections, or adjusting the sensitivity of the amperage (61a). In pacemaker malfunctioning, 75% of episodes occur in the first 24 hours (61a).

6. **Phlebitis.** This complication may occur at the catheter puncture site. The treatment is warm soaks and antibacterial cream applied to the site. If dressings are changed frequently, the catheter may remain in place for 1 to 2 weeks.

7. **Arrhythmias.** Ventricular fibrillation or ventricular tachycardia may occur (61a, 61b, 85a, 150a). These arrhythmias may occur during insertion, making the diagnosis easy, or may occur after insertion. There is a 6% incidence of catheter-associated arrhythmias (85a, 95a, 140), and the emergency physician should have a defibrillator immediately available.

8. **Diaphragmatic Pacing.** a. Faulty insulation; b. Myocardial perforation.

9. **Muscle Spasm.** Faulty insulation and stimulation of muscles by electrical current. Antebrachial site of pacemaker insertion could lead to muscle contractions at the same rate as the setting on the pacemaker impulse generator. To diagnose this entity, vary the pacing rate on the generator, and the muscle contractions will vary in a like manner.

Transthoracic Cardiac Pacemaker

This is not the preferred approach for placement of a pacemaker. It is used only in emergencies. Transthoracic pacemakers have been used most frequently in the emergency center in patients who have had a cardiac arrest and are in asystole. One must discontinue cardiopulmonary resuscitation during insertion of the catheter and, thus, the procedure should be done rapidly. The femoral route offers a quick access into the heart even in the patient who has sustained a cardiac arrest without having to stop cardiopulmonary resuscitation; however, the transthoracic approach is more reliable and one is more certain of accurate placement in the patient with cardiopulmonary arrest. Tintinalli and White report that in brady-asystolic arrest, ultimate outcome was unaffected by transthoracic pacing despite 40% of patients having good capture (148a).

Equipment

Anesthetic prep

Skin prep

Transthoracic pacemaker kit

6 inch #18 spinal needle with obturator

Monitor and ECG

Indications

1. Cardiac arrest in which the transvenous approach is not feasible due either to inability to pass a central catheter or to lack of skill or equipment.
2. Transvenous approach unsuccessful and emergency in a deteriorating patient (see indications for transvenous approach).

Technique

Preparatory Steps.

1. Monitor the patient.
2. Prep the left chest over the fourth intercostal space or the area around the xyphoid process (should be done quickly in the patient in cardiopulmonary arrest).
3. Anesthetize area if indicated.

Procedural Steps.

1. One may use the subxyphoid approach and this is discussed in more detail in Chapter 4: "Cardiothoracic Procedures."

   Alternately, introduce a 6 inch #18 spinal needle with obturator into the fourth intercostal space at the region of the apical impulse. Aim the needle at the tip of the right scapula.
2. Remove the obturator and attach a syringe. A brisk flow of blood indicates entrance into the ventricle.
3. Pass a bipolar electrode through the needle.
4. Attach to the pacing unit. The lead marked distal is attached to the negative pole and the proximal lead to the positive pacing unit.
5. Set the current at 1.5 mAmp and observe for ECG capture. Increase the intensity of the current until capture occurs.

Aftercare.

1. Suture the catheter in place.

Complications

1. **Pericardial Hemorrhage and Tamponade.** This results from cardiac injury or injury to the coronary arteries. This is a very serious complication, and there is no method of preventing it, due to the "blind" technique of insertion.

2. **Arrhythmias.**

Swan-Ganz Catheterization of the Pulmonary Artery

This procedure is commonplace in intensive care units. It may be useful in the emergency center when, due to circumstances beyond the physician's control, the patient may have a prolonged stay in the emergency center or a "holding unit." This catheter measures pulmonary artery pressure (PAP), pulmonary capillary wedge pressure (PCWP), right ventricular pressure (RVP), right atrial pressure (RAP), CVP, and cardiac output using a thermal dilution technique. The PCWP correlates well with left atrial pressure, when PCWP is <15 mm Hg or positive and expiratory pressure is <10 cm water. The Swan-Ganz catheter is a triple lumen tube, one at the tip for PAP and pulmonary artery blood sampling, one 30 cm further back for CVP and central venous blood sampling, and one for inflating and deflating the balloon and a thermister at the tip. The cardiac output usually is measured by a transducer after 0 to 4° C water is injected into the central venous part rapidly. The temperature of the blood as it reaches the thermister correlates with cardiac output and is computed and usually provided as a digital value on ancillary equipment. The measurement of the pulmonary artery wedge pressure and cardiac output is useful in patients who have hypotension and subclinical, chronic, or acute congestive heart failure or renal failure, and one wishes to administer large volumes of fluids, e.g., the patient who is hypovolemic following acute trauma. It is also useful in the patient who is in shock of undetermined etiology, and in monitoring the volume status and effects of therapy in patients with cardiogenic shock (5, 30, 59, 61, 136, 142, 143). For a detailed discussion of Swan-Ganz catheters, the following articles are excellent (28, 81, 142, 143).

Indications

1. Measurement of pulmonary artery wedge pressure.
2. Measurement of cardiac output.

Equipment

Skin prep
Anesthetic prep
4 towels
Towel clips
Setup for subclavian or internal jugular vein cannulation with a 16 gauge Angiocath® and guide wire
Balloon flotation catheter kit with introducer
    5, 6, or 7 French double lumen catheter or 7 French triple lumen catheter
In the adult, a 6 French catheter is used with the introducing cannula one size larger. One needs a 12 gauge needle to pass a 7 French Swan-Ganz catheter. In the Seldinger technique a smaller needle is used since a dilator is then inserted.
Monitors
    Pressure transducer
    ECG monitor
    Pressure recorder
Connecting tubing and a three-way stopcock
Heparinized saline 1000 units/100 ml
Defibrillator

Technique

Preparatory Steps.

1. Introduce a #16 Angiocath® via the right internal jugular or left subclavian vein approaches as discussed in another section of this chapter.
2. Attach the Swan-Ganz catheter via a three-way stopcock to monitor the pressure.
3. Connect the pressure monitor to the other limb of the stopcock.
4. Calibrate the recorder (technician).

Procedural Steps Modified Seldinger Technique (28, 81).

1. Slide the guide wire through the #16 Angiocath.®
2. Remove the Angiocath® and replace with the introducer and sleeve. One

may have to puncture the skin with a #11 blade to provide a hole large enough for the introducer.
3. Remove the guide wire.
4. Remove the introducer and leave the sleeve in position.
5. Occlude the hub of the sleeve with the thumb to prevent air embolism. (See "Air Embolism—Infraclavicular Subclavian Cannulation—Complications.")
6. Slide the Swan-Ganz catheter (7 French) through the introducer.
7. Advance the catheter into the right atrium. When the catheter tip reaches the superior vena cava, inflate the balloon on the syringe with 0.7 to 0.8 ml of air to take advantage of the buoyancy of the balloon and "flow-direction."
8. Advance the catheter. Inflate the balloon and pass the catheter into the pulmonary artery (Fig. 11.19). Follow the pressure tracings to determine catheter location (Fig. 11.20). Normal pressures are listed in Table 11.2.

NOTE

Pass the catheter smoothly to prevent vasospasm.

Once the catheter occludes the pulmonary artery and a wedge pressure

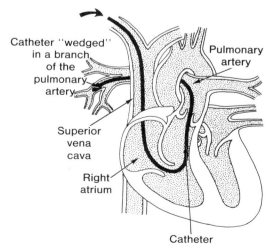

Figure 11.19. Swan-Ganz catheter wedged in a branch of the pulmonary artery.

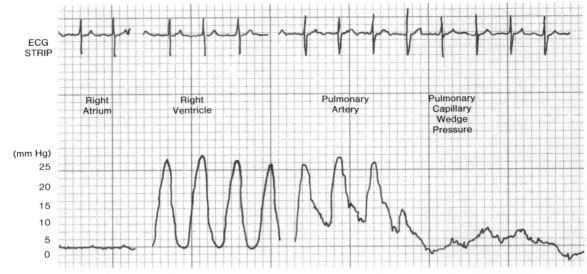

ECG STRIP

Right Atrium | Right Ventricle | Pulmonary Artery | Pulmonary Capillary Wedge Pressure

(mm Hg)
25
20
15
10
5
0

Figure 11.20. Cardiac and pulmonary artery pressures with a concomitant ECG tracing.

Table 11.2. Normal Pulmonary and Cardiac Pressures

Region	Systolic (mm Hg)	Diastolic (mm Hg)	Mean (mm Hg)
Central venous			1–6
Right atrium			1–6
Right ventricle	20–30	<5	
Pulmonary artery	20–30	<10	<20
Pulmonary capillary wedge pressure			4–12

tracing is observed, deflate the balloon (Fig. 11.19) and the pulmonary artery pressure tracing is obtained.

9. PA diastolic pressure usually approximates PA wedge pressure and often may be used to follow the clinical course of a patient, when the PA wedge pressure is no longer obtainable.

CAUTION!

Watch the ECG closely for ventricular irritability. Persistent irritability requires that the catheter be withdrawn.

CAUTION!

Inflate the balloon only when the wedge pressure is needed.

10. Check proper positioning of the catheter. With proper positioning the pulmonary artery wedge pressure is lower than the mean pulmonary artery pressure and, in most patients, is equal to the pulmonary artery diastolic pressure. Note the characteristic pressure waves obtained, indicating right atrial, ventricular, pulmonary artery and pulmonary wedge pressure cannulation (28, 81).

NOTE

To deflate the balloon, remove the syringe. Manual deflation of the balloon may cause inversion of and damage to the balloon.

11. Suture the catheter to the skin and dress the wound. Record data from the catheter and insert on the dressing catheter.
12. Attach heparin flush. The concentration used is 100 units/100 ml saline. Infuse at a rate of 2 to 3 ml/hour.
13. Always obtain a radiograph to insure the proper position.

Complications (105, 133)

1. ***Balloon Rupture.*** This is due to over-inflation or frequent deflation of the balloon, damaging the balloon wall. It is heralded by a "damped" pulmonary wedge pressure. Prevent this complication by adding only 0.8 to 1.0 ml of air to the balloon and avoid unnecessary deflation.

2. ***Septic Phlebitis*** (68, 154). To prevent this complication, use sterile technique, change the tubing every 24 to 48 hours, and remove the catheter every 4 days.

3. ***Traumatic Endocarditis.*** The catheter may injure the tricuspid or pulmonary valve or the right ventricular myocardium, resulting in thromboembolization. To prevent see "Septic Phlebitis."

4. ***Catheter Kinking or Knotting.*** This results from placing too much catheter in the ventricle, producing redundant loops. Looping in the atrium may produce atrial, then ventricular, and then atrial wave forms due to catheter tip "Flipping" into the ventricle as the catheter is withdrawn.

5. ***Arrhythmias.*** This occurs when the catheter is advanced to the right ventricle which may be irritated by the catheter tip. Periodic arrhythmias may occur during looping of catheter in the right ventricle. One should avoid positioning the catheter in the right ventricle and remove it from this location as soon as poosible.

6. ***Pulmonary Infarction*** (30, 59). This complication occurs when the balloon remains inflated too long or the uninflated catheter tip becomes wedged in a small pulmonary artery. To treat continuous wedging, aspirate blood from the catheter; if wedged firmly, blood will withdraw with difficulty. Always deflate the balloon if this is suspected. If still wedged, inject heparinized saline to help dislodge the catheter tip. If wedged continuously, withdraw catheter slowly until PA waveform appears. If this fails, check catheter placement on chest radiograph.

7. ***Damped Waveform or High Waveform.*** This complication may be due to the catheter being up against a wall of a vessel, clot at the tip of the catheter, or air bubbles in the transducer. To treat this complication, flush the catheter with a large volume of fluid after blood withdrawal from the catheter. If these procedures do not improve the waveform, obtain a radiograph to check catheter position. If air bubbles are in the transducer, flush rapidly through transducer.

8. ***Abnormally Low or Negative Pressure.*** This complication is due to improper transducer level or incorrect zeroing and calibration of the monitor. To correct, the technician should recalibrate the transducer at midchest level and register zero.

9. ***No Pressure.*** This complication is due to the transducer not being open to the catheter or the amplifier being on calibrate, zero, or off. Treatment is to recalibrate.

ARTERIAL PUNCTURE

A number of sites, including the radial, ulnar, brachial, and femoral arteries, are commonly used. The radial is perhaps the most commonly used site and is the one recommended here. The radial pulse is medial to the radial styloid where the artery courses over the distal end of the radius.

Equipment

Skin prep
Anesthetic prep
Heparin (concentration 100 u/ml)
Ice and container
Cap for syringe
Glass syringe
  (All of the above with the exception of the skin prep and anesthetic are contained in commercially available kits.)
Butterfly needle, 23 or 25 gauge preferred
  Alternative: 23 gauge ⅝ inch needle

NOTE

The butterfly needle is preferred because of its ease of handling in regard to entering the artery, especially the radial artery. For larger deeper arteries, a 22 gauge 1½ inch needle is preferred.

Technique

Preparatory Steps.

1. Prepare the selected site.
2. Coat the syringe with the heparin solution. This can be done by drawing heparin into the syringe, connecting the butterfly needle, and ejecting all of the heparin through the needle. The amount retained in the butterfly needle and tubing is enough to provide adequate heparinization.
   Alternate method (for step 2). When using a larger vessel, one can draw 1 to 2 ml of heparin into a syringe, connect a 22 gauge 1½ inch needle to it, and eject all of the heparin; the amount retained on the sides of the syringe is all that is needed to prevent the arterial blood from coagulating.

Procedural Steps.

1. Palpate the arterial pulse. Careful palpation is mandatory before needle puncture. Delineate the longitudinal course of the artery between the tips of the second and third fingers (Fig. 11.21). Using a butterfly or a straight needle, puncture the skin at a 60 degree angle at the midpoint between these two fingers. One can feel the pulse through the needle as the needle rests on top of the artery.
2. Puncture the artery. One will obtain a pulsatile flow which will raise the plunger of the syringe. A nonpulsatile

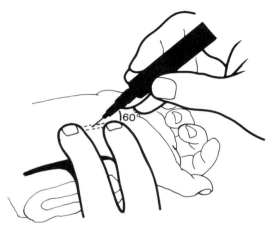

Figure 11.21. Radial artery puncture. See text for discussion.

but steady flow may occur in patients with high central venous pressures. If bone is contacted, slowly withdraw the syringe; one may still retrieve a sample on withdrawal through the back wall of the artery. It is not advisable to pierce or "spear" the artery because, occasionally, osteomyelitis or large hematomas have occurred in this fashion.

3. Remove air bubbles from the syringe. To remove air bubbles without disseminating drops of blood, apply an alcohol wipe over the needle tip and eject the bubbles onto the alcohol wipe.
4. Apply a cap to the tip of the needle or a rubber cap over the syringe (supplied in kits). Place the sample on ice and send for analysis.

Aftercare.

1. Apply pressure to the site for 5 minutes. Patients on anticoagulants must have pressure applied to the site for 10 minutes. These times should not be estimated but actually timed.

Complications

1. **Compression Neuropathy.** The median nerve at the antecubital fossa may be injured during the puncture of the brachial artery. This complication can occur with an antecubital brachial artery puncture due to bleeding and nerve compression; pain and paresthesias in the distribution of the median nerve are noted. This is more likely to occur with anticoagulated patients (75). The treatment is to discontinue anticoagulation if possible, elevate the extremity, and observe for 6 to 12 hours. Definitive treatment involves fascial decompression and hematoma removal. When nerve compression occurs in the leg, the results are poor (94).

2. **Pseudoaneurysm.** This complication can occur especially with femoral punctures. The patient presents with a "pulsating tumor," with a bruit anterior to the artery. These occur more often when the hematoma is large. Treatment is by removal of the pseudoaneurysm.

3. **Arteriovenous Fistula.** An arteriovenous fistula may form after femoral punc-

ture. This complication is another reason for advocating the use of the radial artery, as there is no accompanying major vein.

4. *Arterial Spasm.* Arterial spasm occurs after puncture and may lead to vascular compromise. This complication is fivefold more common with brachial artery puncture than with femoral (141).

5. *Hematoma Formation.* One should maintain pressure over the punctured artery for 5 minutes to avoid this complication. There is an overall 10% incidence of complications with arterial punctures (101). In patients who are anticoagulated, there is a fourfold increase in the overall complication rate.

6. *Septic Arthritis.* This is a complication following puncture of the femoral artery. The authors do not advocate penetrating to the bone in performing arterial puncture at this site.

ARTERIAL CANNULATION

Two methods of arterial cannulation are used: percutaneous cannulation, in which the radial artery is the site most commonly used, and the cutdown approach (81). Both of these are discussed below.

Indications

1. Arterial pressure monitoring.
   a. Difficulty in obtaining cuff blood pressure in a critically ill patient who is severely hypotensive.
   b. Monitoring a patient who requires potent dilators or pressors for accurate pressure management, i.e., nitroprusside.
2. Repeat arterial blood sampling.

Contraindications

1. Severe injury to the extremity.
2. Positive Allen's test.
3. Injury to the site proximal to the vessel to be cannulated.

Equipment

Percutaneous Technique.

Armboard
Folded towel
1 inch wide adhesive tape
Skin preparation
Sterile field
Local anesthetic
10 ml syringe
18 gauge Angiocath® or Medicut® cannula
Stopcock
Heparin 1 ml of 100 units/ml
30 ml vial injectable saline
Dressing
Arterial pressure transducer
Pressure tubing
Calibrated oscilloscope

Cutdown Technique.

Sterile sponges
#3 knife handle
#15 scalpel blade
Curved iris and suture scissors
Fine-toothed forceps
2 curved mosquito clamps
1 small self-retaining retractor
Needle-holder
3-0 silk ligatures
10 ml plastic syringe
Angiocath 18 gauge or Medicut® cannula
   18 gauge needle
Three-way stopcock
Heparin 1 ml, 1000 u/ml
30 ml vial injectable saline
4-0 nylon sutures for skin

Technique

The route discussed is with the radial artery.

Preparatory Steps.

1. Select site. The radial artery is preferred. Alternate sites include the brachial artery (although thrombosis may occur at this site) and dorsalis pedis. Do not use the femoral artery.
2. Perform the Allen's test (3a, 120a). Compress both the ulnar and the radial arteries at the wrist and ask the patient to squeeze his fist several times to drain venous blood from the hand. Have the patient relax the hand with no flexion or extension at the wrist and note the blanching (68a). Release the ulnar artery and observe the effect on blanching. In the hand with a patent ulnar artery, the palmar surface should return to normal color

(pink). Repeat using radial artery occlusion and note the return of pink color to the palm on release of the radial artery. If either artery is occluded, as demonstrated by delay of return or by no return of normal skin color, then do not cannulate either vessel.

3. Place the wrist in a supine position, with the arm abducted. Dorsiflex the wrist over a folded towel placed between the wrist and the armboard to make the artery more prominent. Tape the hand to the armboard to maintain the position shown in Figure 11.22.
4. Anesthetize the skin over the site.
5. Prep and drape.
6. Prepare the syringe with heparin. A 10 ml heparinized syringe is used. A stopcock should be attached to the syringe. Adequate heparin concentration used is 500 u/10 ml saline.

Procedural Steps.

1. *Percutaneous approach.* Puncture the skin first with the 18 gauge needle to produce a small skin incision and avoid a skin plug.

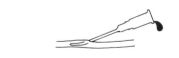

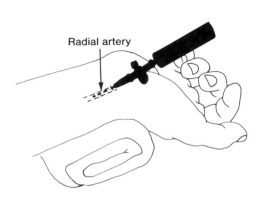

Radial artery

Figure 11.22. Radial artery cannulation. Secure the hand and wrist to the armboard with the wrist placed in extension as shown. See text for discussion.

Through the skin puncture site advance the 18 gauge Angiocath® at a 30 degree angle to the skin and parallel to the artery.
Insert the Angiocath® into the artery at a 45 degree angle to the axis of the vessel.
Cutdown approach. Make a transverse incision proximal to the flexion crease at the wrist.
Mobilize the artery, exposing 1 to 2 cm of the length of the vessel.
Ligate the distal end with a 2-0 suture.
Place an elevating clamp beneath the artery.
Using an Angiocath,® puncture the artery proximal to the elevating clamp.

2. Cannulate the artery.
Percutaneous approach (authors' preferred method). Transfix the artery between two fingers.
Puncture the artery and advance the cannula after pulsatile bloodflow is noted (Fig. 11.21).
Alternate method.
When the artery is punctured through its back wall, it is transfixed.
Arterial flow confirms entry into the artery.
Remove the needle, leaving the cannula in place.
Slowly withdraw the cannula until arterial blood is noted to "spurt out."
Advance the cannula into the artery.
Cutdown approach. Slide the needle and cannula into the artery until the tip lies in the arterial lumen.
Remove the needle and advance the cannula.

3. Attach a three-way stopcock with a heparinized syringe used to prevent thrombosis in the arterial cannula.
Flush the cannula after aspirating to confirm good blood flow.
After flushing with heparinized saline, close the stopcock to the cannula and remove the syringe from the stopcock.

Aftercare.

1. Connect the transducer.
2. Control bleeding with pressure dressing. Apply pressure over the artery at

the tip of the cannula for 5 minutes to stop bleeding. Release the tape on palms and remove towel and tape the hand to the armboard.

Complications

1. Local infection or sepsis (140a).
2. Hematoma. This is due to pressure not applied to the cannulated artery for a sufficient time.
3. Vasculitis.
4. Nerve damage.
5. Embolism. Retrograde arterial embolism can occur from retrograde flushing of the cannula, and emboli may enter the cerebral circulation (46a, 94a). This danger is greater with smaller patients. To maintain patency of the artery in children, use volumes of heparinized solution smaller than 3 ml or maintain a slow continuous flushing because thrombi may be dislodged (46a, 94a).
6. Tissue necrosis with distal ischemia (79a, 156a). This complication is due to excessive arterial trauma resulting in thrombosis. One should avoid several consecutive punctures at the same site. Certain arteries especially the brachial and femoral arteries, are more prone to ischemic complications and should be avoided. Finger ischemia occurs commonly in patients in shock and in those with poor ulnar artery flow. One must perform the Allen's test before cannulating the radial artery; if the patient is in shock, the benefits must be weighed against the potential complications.

Intramuscular Injections

The upper outer quadrant of the buttocks is the site of choice for intramuscular injection. In this quadrant the muscle is maximally thick so that one may inject deeply. This area avoids the blood vessels and nerves which are present in the inner quadrants. No other quadrant of the buttocks is acceptable (158). Zelman feels that injections in the deltoid and other muscles are less satisfactory due to the greater sensitivity of these muscles, smaller mass, and their proximity to nerves (158).

From the anatomy of the gluteal muscle and the distribution of the intramuscularly injected substances, it has been shown that injections into the lower central portion of the buttocks endanger the greater sciatic nerve, if the injection extends through the gluteus maximus. More commonly there is a temporary sciatic-like pain extending down the back of the leg; this pain is attributed to irritation of the small sciatic nerve which overlies the greater sciatic nerve in this area.

Technique

The intramuscular injection should be given with the patient in the prone position with the toes facing inward and heels outward.

After retracting the skin and subcutaneous tissue, introduce the needle. When the needle is later withdrawn, the return of these superficial tissues to their normal position breaks the direct needle track and decreases the likelihood of subcutaneous seepage of the injected material from within the muscle belly.

One must remember to aspirate the syringe to exclude entry into a blood vessel. If blood or any other fluid is obtained, the needle is withdrawn, another site is chosen, and the inoculum discarded (158).

The needle should be passed through the skin and muscle in a single movement to a depth of 3 to 4 cm; the medication is injected slowly. The material should be injected slowly to allow time for distension of the accommodating space within the muscle to decrease the pain of injection. Deep firm massage of the muscle favors spread of the medication through a wider area of tissue and more rapid absorption.

Alternate Site

An alternate site, suggested by Grey Turner (71), is the region of the outer side of the thigh over the vastus lateralis muscle. He feels this is the ideal place for intramuscular injections. The area does not contain any important nerves or large blood vessels and is a large muscle mass. The needle should be introduced at the middle of the outer side of the thigh. If the bone is reached, the needle should be slightly withdrawn before an injection is made.

An Emergency Intramuscular Site for Drug Administration

Lidocaine and other local anesthetics can be injected lingually (124). Periorally injected lidocaine has been shown to produce peak blood levels rapidly. An intravenous bolus of lidocaine is the most rapid method of achieving peak blood levels (2 minutes); however, when an intravenous site is not available, intralingual injection of lidocaine without epinephrine produces peak blood levels in 10 minutes (124). It should be stated that in such a patient, if an endotracheal tube is in place, the administration of the drug by this route is probably the second most rapid method of achieving peak levels; however, the time varies widely from 5 to 25 minutes. In another study (115) in which epinephrine or aminophylline was injected along the lateral ventral surface of the tongue, it was found that an effect was noted on the electrocardiogram and in depth and rate of respiration within 35 seconds.

References

1. Adar, R., Mozes, M., Fatal complications of central venous catheters. Br. Med. J. 3:746, 1971.
2. Adelman, S., An emergency intravenous route for the pediatric patient. J.A.C.E.P. 5:596, 1976.
3. Ahmed, N., Payne, R.F., Thrombosis after central venous cannulation. Med. J. Aust. 1:217, 1976.
3a. Allen, E.V., Thromboangiitis obliterans: Methods of diagnosis of chronic occlusive arterial lesions distal to the wrist, with illustrated cases. Am. J. Med. Sci. 178:237, 1929.
4. Allsop, J.R., Askew, A.R., Subclavian vein cannulation: A new complication. Br. Med. J. 4:262, 1975.
5. Archer, G., Cobb, L.A., Long-term pulmonary artery pressure monitoring in the management of the critically ill. Ann. Surg. 180:747, 1974.
6. Ashbaugh, D., Thomson, J.W.W., Subclavian-vein infusion. Lancet 2:1138, 1963.
7. Asimacopoulos, P.J., Bagley, F.H., McDermott, W.F., A modified technique for subclavian puncture. Surg. Gynecol. Obstet. 150:241, 1980.
8. Asnes, R.S., Arendar, G.M., Septic arthritis of the hip: A complication of femoral venipuncture. Pediatrics 38:837, 1966.
9. Aulenbacher, C.E., Hydrothorax from subclavian vein catheterization (letter). J.A.M.A. 214:372, 1970.
10. Aziz, E.M., Robertso, A.F., Paraplegia: A complication of umbilical artery catheterization. J. Pediatr. 82:1051, 1973.
11. Baird, C.L., Transvenous pacemaking: A bedside technique. Br. Heart. J. 33:191, 1971.
12. Balagtas, R.C., Bell, C.E., Edwards, L.D., et al., Risk of local and systemic infections associated with umbilical vein catheterization: A prospective study in 86 newborn patients. Pediatrics 48:359, 1971.
13. Baker, C.C., Petersen, S.R., Sheldon, G.F., Septic phlebitis: A neglected disease. Am. J. Surg. 138:97, 1979.
14. Band, J.D., Maki, D.G., Safety of changing intravenous delivery systems at longer than 24 hour intervals. Ann. Intern. Med. 91:173, 1979.
15. Bansmer, G., Keith, D., Tesluk, H., Complications following use of indwelling catheters of inferior vena cava. J.A.M.A. 167:1606, 1958.
16. Barenholtz, L., Kaminsky, N.I., Palmer, D.I., Venous intramural microabscess: A cause of protracted sepsis with intravenous cannulas. Am. J. Med. Sci. 265:335, 1973.
17. Bauer, S.B., Feldman, S.M., Gelli, S.S., et al., Neonatal hypertension: A complication of umbilical-artery catheterization. N. Engl. J. Med. 293:1032, 1975.
18. Bentley, D.W., Lepper, M.H., Septicemia related to indwelling venous catheter. J.A.M.A. 206:1749, 1968.
19. Bergentz, S.-E., Hansson, L.O., Norback, B., Surgical management of complications to arterial puncture. Ann. Surg. 164:1021, 1964.
20. Bernard, R.W., Stahl, W.M., Subclavian vein catheterizations: A prospective study: I. Noninfectious complications. Ann. Surg. 173:184, 1971.
21. Bogen, J.E., Local complications in 167 patients with indwelling venous catheters. Surg. Gynecol. Obstet. 110:112, 1960.
22. Borja, A.R., Masri, Z., Shruck, L., et al., Unusual and lethal complications of infraclavicular subclavian vein catheterization. Int. Surg. 57:42, 1972.
23. Bosch, D.T., Kengeter, J.P., Beling, C.A., Femoral venipuncture. Am. J. Surg. 79:722, 1950.
24. Bower, E.B., Choosing a catheter for central venous catheterization. Surg. Clin. North Am. 53:639, 1973.
25. Braux, E., Cardiac tamponade following penetrating mediastinal injuries. J. Trauma 19:461, 1979.
26. Brinkman, A.J., Costley, D.O., Internal jugular venipuncture. J.A.M.A. 223:182, 1973.
27. Brown, H.I., Burnard, R.J., Jensen, J., et al., Puncture of endotracheal-tube cuffs during percutaneous subclavian-vein catheterization. Anesthesiology 43:112, 1975.
28. Buchbinder, N., Ganz, W., Hemodynamic monitoring: Invasive techniques. Anesthesiology 45:146, 1976.
28a. Burgess, G.E., Marino, R.J., Penler, M.J., Effect of head position on the location of venous catheters inserted via the basilic vein. Anesthesiology 46:212, 1977.
29. Buxton, A.E., Highsmith, A.K., Garner, J.S., et

al., Contamination of intravenous infusion fluid: Effect of changing administration sets. Ann. Intern. Med. 90:764, 1979.

30. Calvin, M.P. Savage T.M., Lewis C.T., Pulmonary damage from a Swan-Ganz catheter. Br. J. Anaesth. 47:1107, 1975.

31. Castor, W.R., Spontaneous perforation of the bowel in the newborn following exchange transfusion. Can. Med. Assoc. J. 99:934, 1968.

32. Cheng, T.O., Percutaneous transfemoral venous cardiac pacing. Chest 60:73, 1971.

33. Christensen, K. H., Nerstrom, B., Baden, H., Complications of percutaneous catheterization of the subclavian vein in 129 cases. Acta Chir. Scand. 133:615, 1967.

34. Cochran, W.D., Davis, H.T., Smith, C.A., Advantages and complications of umbilical artery catheterization in the newborn. Pediatrics 42:769, 1968.

35. Corman, L.C., Levison, M.E., Sustained bacteremia and transvenous cardiac pacemakers. J.A.M.A. 233:264, 1975.

36. Corso, J.A., Agostinelli, R., Brandriss, M.W., Maintenance of venous polyethylene catheters to reduce risk of infection. J.A.M.A. 210:2075, 1969.

37. Corwin, J.H., Moseley, T., Subclavian venipuncture and central venous pressure: Technic and application. Am. Surg. 32:413, 1966.

38. Crenshaw, C.A., Prevention of infection at scalp vein sites of needle insertion during intravenous therapy. Am. J. Surg. 124:43, 1972.

39. Crossley, K., Matsen, J.M., The scalp-vein needle: A prospective study of complications. J.A.M.A. 220:985, 1972.

40. Daily, P.O., Griepp, R.B., Shumway, N.E., Percutaneous internal jugular vein cannulation. Arch. Surg. 101:534, 1970.

41. Daly, B.D.T., Berger, R.L., Antecubital approach for intravascular monitoring. Surg. Gynecol. Obstet. 135:434, 1972.

42. Daniell, H.W., Heparin in the prevention of infusion phlebitis: A double-blind controlled study. J.A.M.A. 226:1317, 1973.

43. Davidson, J.T., Ben-Hur, N., Nathen, H., Subclavian venipuncture. Lancet 2:1139, 1963.

44. DeFalque, R.J., Percutaneous catheterization of the internal jugular vein. Anesth. Analg. 53:116, 1974.

45. Doering, R.B., Stemmer, E.A., Connolly, J.E., Complications of indwelling venous catheters: With particular reference to catheter embolus. Am. J. Surg. 114:259, 1967.

46. Dosios, T.J., Magovern, G.J., Gay, T.C., et al., Cardiac tamponade complicating percutaneous catheterization of subclavian vein. Surgery 78:261, 1975.

46a.Downs, J.B., Chapman, R.L., Hawkins, J.F., et al., Prolonged radial artery catheterization. Arch. Surg. 108:671, 1974.

46b.Durant, T.M., Long, J., Oppenheimer, M.J., Pulmonary (venous) air embolism. Am. Heart J. 33:269, 1947.

46c.Durant, T.M., Oppenheimer, M.J., Webster, M.R., et al., Arterial air embolism. Am. Heart J. 38:481, 1949.

47. Edelstein, J., Atraumatic removal of a polyethylene catheter from the superior vena cava. Chest 57:381, 1970.

48. Edin, M.B., Dudley, H.A.F., The local complications of intravenous therapy. Lancet 2:365, 1959.

49. Effert, S., Skykosch, J., Emergency pacing techniques. Ann. N.Y. Acad. Sci. 167:614, 1969.

50. Egan, E.A., Eitzman, D.V., Umbilical vessel catheterization. Am. J. Dis. Child. 121:213, 1971.

51. English, I.C.W., Frew, R.M., Pigott, J.F., et al., Percutaneous catheterisation of the internal jugular vein. Anaesthesia 24:521, 1969.

52. Epstein, E.J., Quereshi, M.S.A., Wright, J.S., Diaphragmatic paralysis after supraclavicular puncture of subclavian vein (letter). Br. Med. J. 1:693, 1976.

53. Erkan, V., Blankenship, W., Stahlman, M.T., The complications of chronic umbilical vessel catheterization (abstract) Pediatr. Res. 2:317, 1968.

54. Farhat, K., Nakhjavan, F.K., Cope, C., et al., Iatrogenic arteriovenous fistula: A complication of percutaneous subclavian vein puncture. Chest 67:480, 1975.

55. Feliciano, D.V., Mattox, K.L., Graham, J.M., et al., Major complications of percutaneous subclavian vein catheters. Am. J. Surg. 138:869, 1979.

56. Fenn, J.E., Stansel, H.C., Jr., Certain hazards of the central venous catheter. Angiology 20:38, 1969.

57. Ferguson, R.L., Complications of heparin lock needles. Ann. Intern. Med. 85:583, 1976.

57a.Filston, H.C., Grant, J.P., A safer system for percutaneous subclavian venous catheterization in newborn infant. J. Pediatr. Surg. 14:564, 1979.

58. Fisher, R.G., Ferreyro, R., Evaluation of current techniques for nonsurgical removal of intravascular iatrogenic foreign bodies. Am. J. Roentgenol. 130:541, 1978.

58a.Fletcher, G.F., Insertion of a temporary transvenous pacemaker. In Cardiac Procedures, p. 329.

59. Foote, G.A., Schabel, S.I., Hodges, M., Pulmonary complications of the flow-directed balloon-tipped catheter. N. Engl. J. Med. 290:927, 1974.

60. Formanek, G., Frech, R.S., Amplatz, K., Arterial thrombus formation during clinical percutaneous catheterization. Circulation 41:833, 1970.

61. Forrester, J.S., Diamond, G., McHugh, T.J., et al., Filling pressures in the right and left sides of the heart in acute myocardial infarction: A reappraisal of central venous pressure monitoring. N. Engl. J. Med. 285:190, 1971.

61a.Fort, M.L., Sharp, J.T., Perforation of the right ventricle by pacing catheter electrode. Am. J. Cardiol. 16:610, 1965.

61b.Furman, S.D., Escher, J.W., Transvenous pacing; A seven year review. Am. Heart J. 71:408, 1966.

62. Gallitano, A.I., Kondi, E.S., Deckers, P.J., A safe approach to the subclavian vein. Surg. Gynecol. Obstet. 135:96, 1972.

63. Garcia, J.M., Mispireta, L.A., Pinho, R.V., Percutaneous supraclavicular superior vena caval cannulation. Surg. Gynecol. Obstet. 134:839, 1972.

63a.Getzen, L.C., Erich, W.P., Short-term femoral vein cannulation. Am. J. Surg. 138:875, 1979.

63b.Gibson, T., Norris, W., Skin fragments removed by injection needles. Lancet 8:983, 1958.

64. Gilday, D.L., Downs, A.R., The value of chest radiography in the localization of central venous pressure catheters. Can. Med. Assoc. J. 101:363, 1969.

65. Goetzman, B.W., Stadalnik, R.C., Bogren, H.G. et al., Thrombotic complications of umbilical artery catheters: A clinical and radiographic study. Pediatrics 56:374, 1975.

66. Goldbloom, R.B., Hillman, D.A., Santulli, T.V., Arterial thrombosis following femoral venipuncture in edematous nephrotic children. Pediatrics 40:450, 1967.

67. Goldman, L.I., Maier, W.P., Drezner, A.D., Another complication of subclavian puncture: Arterial laceration (letter). J.A.M.A. 217:78, 1971.

68. Greene, J.F., Fitzwater, J.E., Clemmer, T.P., Septic endocarditis and indwelling pulmonary artery catheters. J.A.M.A. 233:891, 1975.

68a.Greenbow, D.E., Incorrect performance of Allen's test: Ulnar artery flow presumed inadequate. Anesthesiology 37:356, 1972.

69. Groff, D., Subclavian vein catheterization in the infant. J. Pediatr. Surg. 9:171, 1974.

70. Gupta, J.M., Roberton, N.R.C., Wigglesworth, J.S., Umbilical artery catheterization in the newborn. Arch. Dis. Child. 43:382, 1968.

71. Grey Turner, G., The site for intramuscular injections. Lancet 2:819, 1920.

72. Hall, D.M., Percutaneous catheterization of the internal jugular vein in infants and children. J. Pediatr. Surg. 12:709, 1977.

73. Haller, J.D., Cerruti, M.M., Silver, W., A simple method for arterial and venous monitoring of neonates. Surg. Gynecol. Obstet. 134:489, 1972.

74. Harken, D.E., Zoll, P.M., Foreign bodies in and in relation to the thoracic blood vessels and heart: III. Indications for the removal of intracardiac foreign bodies and the behavior of the heart during manipulation. Am. Heart J. 32:1, 1946.

74a.Hart, G.B., Treatment of decompression illness and air embolism with hyperbaric oxygen. Aerospace Med. 45:1190, 1974.

75. Henzel, J.H., DeWeese, M.S., Morbid and mortal complications associated with prolonged central venous cannulation. Am. J. Surg. 121:600, 1971.

76. Hoshal, V.L., Jr., Asuse, R.G., Hoskins, P.A., Fibrin sleeve formation on indwelling subclavian central venous catheters. Arch. Surg. 102:353, 1971.

77. Indar, R., The dangers of indwelling polyethylene cannulae in deep veins. Lancet 1:284, 1959.

78. Irwin, G.R., Jr., Hart, R.J., Martin, C.M., Pathogenesis and prevention of intravenous catheter infections. Yale J. Biol. Med. 46:85, 1973.

78a.James, P.M., Myers, R.T., Central venous pressure monitoring: Complications and a new technique. Am. Surg. 39:75, 1973.

78b.Jernigan, W.R., Gardner, W.C., Mahr, M.E., Use of the internal jugular vein for placement of central venous catheters. Surg. Gynecol. and Obstet. 130:520, 1970.

79. Johnson, C.L., Lazarchik, J., Lynn, H.B., Subclavian venipuncture: Preventable complications: Report of two cases. Mayo Clin. Proc. 45:712, 1970.

79a.Johnson, R.W., A complication of radical artery cannulation. Anesthesiology 40:598, 1974.

79b.Johnston, A.O.B., Clark, R.G., Malpositioning of cardiovascular catheters. Lancet 2:1395, 1972.

80. Kaltman, A.J., Indications for temporary pacemaker insertion in acute myocardial infarction. Am. Heart J. 81:837, 1971.

81. Kaplan, J.A., Miller, E.D., Insertion of the Swan-Ganz catheter. Anesthesiol. Rev., January, 1976, pp. 22.

82. Keeri-Szanto, M., The subclavian vein: a constant and convenient intravenous injection site. Arch. Surg. 72:179, 1956.

82a.Kellner, G.A., Smart, J.F., Percutaneous placement of catheters to monitor "central venous pressure." Anesthesiology 36:515, 1972.

83. Kerber, R.E., Electrocardiographic indications of atrial puncture during pericardiocentesis. N. Engl. J. Med. 282:1142, 1975.

84. Khalil, K.G., Thoracic duct injury: A complication of jugular vein catheterization. J.A.M.A. 221:908, 1972.

85. Killip, T., Kimball, J.T., Percutaneous techniques for introducing flexible electrodes for intracardiac pacing. Ann. N.Y. Acad. Sci. 167:597, 1969.

85a.Kimball, J.T., Killip, T., A simple method for transvenous intracardiac pacing. Am. Heart J. 70:35, 1965.

86. Kitterman, J.A., Phibbs, R.H., Tooley, W.H., Catheterization of umbilical vessels in newborn infants. Pediatr. Clin. North Am. 17:895, 1970.

87. Knopp, R., Dailey, R.H., Central venous cannulation and pressure monitoring. J.A.C.E.P. 6:358, 1977.

88. Krausz, M.M., Berlatzky, Y., Ayalon, A., et al., Percutaneous cannulation of the internal jugular vein in infants and children. Surg. Gynecol. Obstet. 148:591, 1979.

89. Kunz, H.W., A technique for obtaining blood specimens and giving transfusions in small infants. J. Pediatr. 42:80, 1953.

90. Land, R.E., The relationship of the left subclavian vein to the clavicle. J. Thorac. Cardiovasc. Surg. 63:564, 1972.

91. Larsen, H.W., Lindahl, F., Lesion of the internal mammarian artery caused by infraclavicular percutaneous catheterization of the subclavian vein. Acta Chir. Scand. 139:571, 1973.

92. Lee, Y.-H., Kerstein, M.D., Osteomyelitis and septic arthritis: A complication of subclavian venous catheterization. N. Engl. J. Med. 285:1179, 1971.

93. Lefrak, E.A., Noon, G. P., Management of arterial injury secondary to attempted subclavian vein catheterization. Ann. Thorac. Surg. 14:294, 1972.

94. Leonard, M.D., Sciatic nerve paralysis following anticoagulant therapy. J. Bone Joint Surg. 54B:152, 1972.

94a.Lowenstein, E., Little, J.W., Lo, H.H., Prevention of cerebral embolization from flushing radial artery cannulae. N. Engl. J. Med. 285:1414, 1971.

95. Luce, E.A., Futrell, J.W., Wilgis, E.F.S., et al., Compression neuropathy following brachial arterial puncture in anticoagulated patients. J. Trauma 16:717, 1976.

95a.Lumia, F.J., Rios, J.C., Temporary transvenous pacemaker therapy: An analysis of complications. Chest 64:604, 1973.

96. McConnell, R.Y., Experience with percutaneous internal jugular innominate vein catheterization. Calif. Med. 117:1, 1972.

97. McKay, R.J., Diagnosis and treatment: Risks of obtaining samples of venous blood in infants. Pediatrics 38:906, 1966.

98. Maki, D.G., Goldmnan, D.A., Rhame, F.S., Infection control in intravenous therapy. Ann. Intern. Med. 79:867, 1973.

99. Marlon, A.M., Cohn, L.H., Fogarty, T.J., et al., Retrieval of catheter fragments: Report of two cases. Calif. Med. 115:61, 1971.

100. Massumi, R.A., Ross, A.M., Atraumatic, nonsurgical technic for removal of broken catheters from cardiac cavities. N. Engl. J. Med. 277:195, 1967.

101. Matensen, J.D., Clinical sequelae from arterial needle puncture, cannulation, and incision. Circulation 35:1118, 1967.

102. Mattox, K.L., Fisher, R.G., Persistent hemothorax secondary to malposition of a subclavian venous catheter. J. Trauma 17:387, 1977.

103. Meister, S.G., Banka, V.S., Helfant, R.H., Transfemoral pacing with balloon-tipped catheters. J.A.M.A. 225:712, 1973.

104. Meister, S.G., DeVilla, M., Banka, V.S., et al., An improved method for temporary transvenous pacing without fluoroscopy (abstract). Circulation (Suppl. II) 45,46:II191, 1972.

105. Meister, S.G., Engel, T.R., Fisher, H.A., et al., Potential artifact in measurement of left ventricular filling pressure with flow-directed catheters. Cathet. Cardiovasc. Diagn. 2:175, 1976.

106. Merk, E.A., Rush, B.F., Emergency subclavian vein catheterization and intravenous hyperalimentation. Am. J. Surg. 129:266, 1975.

107. Michenfelder, J.D., Terry, H.R., Jr., Daw, E.F., et al., Air embolism during neurosurgery: A new method of treatment. Anesth. Analg. 45:390, 1966.

108. Mitchell, S.E., Clark, R.A., Complications of central venous catheterization. Am. J. Radiol. 133:467, 1979.

109. Mitty, W.F., Nealon, T.F., Complications of subclavian sticks. J.A.C.E.P. 4:24, 1975.

110. Mobin-Uddin, K., Smith, P.E., Lombardo, C., et al., Percutaneous intracardiac pacing through the subclavian vein. J. Thorac. Cardiovasc. Surg. 54:545, 1967.

111. Mogil, R.A., DeLaurentis, D.A., Rosemond, G.P., The infraclavicular venipuncture: Value in various clinical situations including central venous pressure monitoring. Arch. Surg. 95:320, 1967.

112. Mokrohisky, S.T., Levine, R.L., Blumhagen, J.D., et al., Low positioning of umbilical-artery catheters increases associated complications in newborn infants. N. Engl. J. Med. 299:561, 1978.

113. Moran, J.M., Atwood, R.P., Rowe, M.I., A clinical and bacteriologic study of infections associated with venous cutdowns. N.Engl. J. Med. 272:554, 1965.

113a.Morgan, W.W., Harkins, G.A., Percutaneous introduction of long-term indwelling venous catheters in infants. J. Pediatr. Surg. 7:538, 1972.

114. Mostert, J.W., Kenny, G.M., Murphy, G.P., Safe placement of central venous catheter into internal jugular veins. Arch. Surg. 101:431, 1970.

115. Nichols, W.A., Cutright, E.D., Intralingual injection site for emergency stimulant drugs. Oral Surg. 32:677, 1971.

116. Norden, C.W., Application of antibiotic ointment to the site of venous catheterization: A controlled trial. J. Infect. Dis. 120:611, 1969.

117. Northfield, T.C., Smith, T., Physiologic significance of central venous pressure in patients with hemorrhage. Surg. Gynecol. Obstet. 135:267, 1972.

118. Nowak, R.M., Tomlanovich, M.C., Venous cutdowns in the emergency department (letter). J.A.C.E.P. 8:245, 1979.

119. Oppenheimer, E.H., Esterly, J.R., Thrombosis in the newborn: Comparison between infants of diabetic and nondiabetic mothers. J. Pediatr. 67:549, 1965.

120. O'Reilly, M.V., The technique of subclavian vein cannulation. Can. Med. Assoc. Journal 108:63, 1973.

120a.Palm, T., Evaluation of peripheral arterial pressure in the thumb following radial artery cannulation. Br. J. Anaesth. 49:819, 1977.

121. Paskin, D.L., Hoffman, W.S., Tuddenham, W.J., A new complication of subclavian vein catheterization. Ann. Surg. 179:266, 1974.

122. Phillips, P.J., Pain, R.W., Brooks, G.E., The pain of venipuncture (letter). N. Engl. J. Med. 294:116, 1976.

123. Phillips, S.J., Okies, J.E., Inexpensive simple monitoring techniques. Surg. Gynecol. Obstet. 139:761, 1974.

124. Pomeroy, G.L.M., Loehr, M.M., Intralingual injection of lidocaine. J.A.C.E.P. 6:163, 1977.

125. Prince, S.R., Sullivan, R.L., Hackel, A., Percutaneous catheterization of the internal jugular vein in infants and children. Anesthesiology 44:170, 1976.

126. Qureshi, G.D., Lilly, E.L., Complications of CVP catheter insertion in cubital vein. J.A.M.A. 209:1906, 1969.

127. Randolph, J., Technique for insertion of plastic catheter into saphenous vein. Pediatrics 24:631, 1959.

128. Rosenberg, A.S., Grossman, J.I., Escher, D.J.W., et al., Bedside transvenous cardiac pacing. Am. Heart J. 77:697, 1969.

129. Schapira, M., Stern, W.Z., Hazards of subclavian vein cannulation for central venous pressure monitoring. J.A.M.A. 201:111, 1967.

130. Schnitzler, R.N., Caracta, A.R., Damato, A.N., "Floating" catheter for temporary transvenous ventricular pacing. Am. J. Cardiol. 31:351, 1973.

131. Simon, R.R., A new technique for subclavian puncture. J.A.C.E.P. 7:409, 1978.

132. Segall, M.M., Infraclavicular subclavian venous catheterization. Surg. Gynecol. Obstet. 148:925, 1979.

133. Shin, B., Ayella, R.J., McAslan, T.C., Pitfalls of Swan-Ganz catheterization. Crit. Care Med. 5:125, 1977.

134. Silva, Y.J., In vivo use of human umbilical vessels and the ductus venosus arantii. Surg. Gynecol. Obstet. 148:595, 1979.

135. Sink, J.D., Comer, P.B., James, P.M., Loveland, S.R., Evaluation of catheter placement in the treatment of venous air embolism. Ann. Surg. 183:58, 1976.

136. Sketch, M.H., Cale, M., Mohinddin, S.M., et al., Use of percutaneously inserted venous catheters in coronary care units. Chest 62:684, 1972.

137. Smith, B.E., Complications of subclavian vein catheterization. Arch. Surg. 90:228, 1965.

138. Smith, H., Freedman, L.R., Prolonged venous catheterization as a cause of sepsis. N. Engl. J. Med. 276:1229, 1967.

139. Smyth, N.P.D., Rogers, J.B., Transvenous removal of catheter emboli from the heart and great veins by endoscopic forceps. Ann. Thorac. Surg. 11:403, 1971.

140. Solomon, N., Escher, D.J.W., A rapid method for insertion of the pacemaker catheter electrode. Am. Heart J. 66:717, 1963.

140a.Stam, W.E., Colella, J.J., Anderson, R.C., et al., Indwelling arterial catheters as a source of nosocomial bacteremia. N. Engl. J. Med. 292:1099, 1975.

141. Stephenson, H.E., Treatment of ruptured abdominal aorta. Surg. Gynecol. Obstet. 144:855, 1977.

141a.Stillman, M.T., Richards, A.M., Perforation of the interventricular system by transvenous pacemaker catheter. Am. J. Cardiol. 24:269, 1969.

142. Swan, H.J.C., Guidelines for use of balloon-tipped catheter. Am. J. Cardiol. 34:119, 1974.

143. Swan, H.J.C., Balloon flotation catheters: Their use in hemodynamic monitoring in clinical practice. J.A.M.A. 233:865, 1975.

144. Symansky, M.R., Fox, H.A., Umbilical vessel catheterization: Indications, management and evaluation of the technique. J. Pediatr. 80:820, 1972.

145. Taylor, F.W., Rutherford, C.E., Accidental loss of plastic tube into venous system. Arch. Surg. 86:177, 1963.

146. Thomas, C.S., Carter, J.W., Lowder, S.C., Pericardial tamponade from central venous catheters. Arch. Surg. 98:217, 1969.

147. Thomas, T.V., Location of catheter tip and its impact on central venous pressure. Chest 61:668, 1972.

148. Thurer, R.J., Chylothorax: A complication of subclavian vein catheterization and parenteral hyperalimentation. J. Thorac. Cardiovasc. Surg. 71:465, 1976.

148a.Tintinalli, J.E., White, B.C., Transthoracic pacing during CPR. Ann. Emerg. Med. 10:113, 1981.

149. Tofield, J.J., A safer technique of percutaneous catheterization of the subclavian vein. Surg.

Gynecol. Obstet. 128:1069, 1969.

150. Torres, D.P., Massive hemothorax complicating subclavian venipuncture. J.A.C.E.P. 3:259, 1974.

150a.Voukydis, P.C., Cohen, S.I., Catheter-induced arrhythmias. Am. Heart J. 88:588, 1974.

151. Walters, M.B., Stanger, H.A.D., Rotem, C.E., Complications with percutaneous central venous catheters. J.A.M.A. 220:1455, 1972.

152. Ward, M.E., Lee, P.F.S., Pneumothorax and contralateral hydrothorax following subclavian vein catheterization. Br. J. Anaesth. 45:227, 1973.

153. Warden, G.D., Wilmore, D.W., Pruitt, B.A., Central venous thrombosis: A hazard of medical progress. J. Trauma 13:620, 1973.

153a.Webre, D.R., Aren, J.F., Use of cephalic and basilic veins for introduction of cardiovascular catheters. Anesthesiology 38:389, 1973.

154. Weinstein, R.A., Pressure monitoring devices: Overlooked source of nosocomial infection. J.A.M.A. 236:936, 1976.

155. Wigger, H.J., Bransilver, R.R., Blanc, W.A., Thromboses due to catheterization in infants and children. J. Pediatr. 76:1, 1970.

156. Wright, J.E., Cut-down technique for intravenous infusion in infants. Med. J. Aust. 37:1203, 1972.

156a.Wyatt, R., Glova, I., Coopa, E.J., Proximal skin necrosis after radial artery cannulation. Lancet 1:1135, 1974.

157. Yoffa, D., Supraclavicular subclavian venipuncture and catheterisation. Lancet 2:614, 1965.

158. Zelman, S., Notes on techniques of intramuscular injection. Am. J. Med. Sci. 241:563, 1961.

159. Zinner, S.H., Denny-Brown, B.C., Braun, P. et al., Risk of infection with intravenous indwelling catheters: Effect of application of antibiotic ointment. J. Infect. Dis. 120:616, 1969.

160. Zollinger, R.W. II, A useful intravenous access route. Surg. Gynecol. Obstet. 154:725, 1982.

Bibliography

1. Banks, D.C., Yates, D.B., Infection from intravenous catheters. Lancet 1:443, 1970.

2. Bernard, R.W., Subclavian vein catheters: A prospective study. Ann. Surg. 173:191, 1971.

3 Brereton, R.B., Incidence of complications from indwelling venous catheters. Del. Med. J. 41:1, 1969.

4. Greenblatt, D.J., Koch-Weser, J., Intramuscular injection of drugs. N. Engl. J. Med. 29:542, 1976.

5. Krauss, A.N., Albert, R.F., Kannan, M.M., Contamination of umbilical catheters in the newborn infant. J. Pediatr. 77:965, 1970.

6. Neal, W.A., Reynolds, J.W., Jarvis, C.W., et al., Umbilical artery catheterization: Demonstration of arterial thrombosis by aortography. Pediatrics 50:6, 1972.

7. Simon, R.R., A new technique for subclavian puncture. J.A.C.E.P. 7:409, 1978.

8. How to give an intramuscular injection. Anesth. Anal. 45:205, 1966.

Index